HANDBOOK

OF

INTER-RATER RELIABILITY

FOURTH EDITION

HANDBOOK OF INTER-RATER RELIABILITY

Fourth Edition

The Definitive Guide to Measuring the Extent of Agreement Among Raters

Kilem Li Gwet, Ph.D.

Advanced Analytics, LLC
P.O. Box 2696
Gaithersburg, MD 20886-2696
USA

Published by Advanced Analytics, LLC; in the United States of America.

Advanced Analytics, LLC
PO BOX 2696,
Gaithersburg, MD 20886-2696
e-mail : gwet@agreestat.com

This publication is designed to provide accurate and authoritative information in regard of the subject matter covered. However, it is sold with the understanding that the publisher assumes no responsibility for errors, inaccuracies or omissions. The publisher is not engaged in rendering any professional services. A competent professional person should be sought for expert assistance.

Publisher's Cataloguing in Publication Data:

Gwet, Kilem Li
Handbook of Inter-Rater Reliability
   The Definitive Guide to Measuring the Extent of Agreement Among Raters/ By Kilem Li Gwet - 4th ed.
      p. cm.
      Includes bibliographical references and index.
   1. Biostatistics
   2. Statistical Methods
   3. Statistics - Study - Learning. I. Title.
   ISBN 978-0-9708062-8-4

Preface to the Fourth Edition

The ratings assigned to the very same subjects may differ widely from one rater to another. Many researchers across various fields of research have acknowledged this issue for a long time. The extent of these discrepancies is unacceptable primarily because the analysis of ratings often ignores the presence of the rater-induced source of variation, and assumes most variation in the data to be due to a change in the subject's attribute being investigated. This variation between raters may jeopardize the integrity of scientific inquiries, and could potentially have a dramatic impact on subjects. In fact, a wrong drug or a wrong dosage of the correct drug may be administered to patients at a hospital due to a poor diagnosis, or an exam candidate may see her professional career or even her life plans take a negative turn due to inexplicably large discrepancies in the raters' scoring of her exam. It is the need to resolve these problems that led to the study of inter-rater reliability.

The focus of the previous edition (i.e. third edition) of this *Handbook of Inter-Rater Reliability* is on the presentation of various techniques for analyzing inter-rater reliability data. These techniques include chance-corrected measures, intraclass correlations, and a few others. However, inter-rater reliability studies must be optimally designed before rating data can be collected. Many researchers are often frustrated by the lack of well-documented procedures for calculating the optimal number of subjects and raters that will participate in the inter-rater reliability study. The fourth edition of the *Handbook of Inter-Rater Reliability* will fill this gap. In addition to further refining the presentation of various analysis techniques covered in previous editions, a number of chapters have been expanded considerably in order to address specific issues such as knowing how many subjects and raters to retain for the study, or finding the correct protocol for selecting these subjects and raters to ensure an adequate representation of their respective groups. In particular, the coverage of intra-rater reliability has been expanded and substantially improved.

Unlike the previous editions, this fourth edition discusses the concept of inter-rater reliability first, before presenting the techniques for computing it. The reader who has previously had limited or no exposure to the issues related to inter-rater reliability, will be able to learn about this concept, how it arises in practice, how it affects rating data, and what can be done about it. After a gentle introduction to the field of inter-rater reliability, I proceed in subsequent chapters with the presentation of simple statistical techniques for quantifying the extent of agreement among raters, and its precision from observed ratings. The reader will quickly notice that this book is detailed. Yes, I wanted it sufficiently detailed so that practitioners can gain considerably more insight into the different topics than would be possible in a book aimed simply at promoting concepts. I wanted a researcher to read this book and be able to implement the proposed solutions without having to figure out hidden steps or expressions not fully fleshed out.

This book is not exhaustive. It does not cover all topics of interest related to the field of inter-rater reliability. I selected topics, which are among the most commonly referenced by researchers in various fields of research. I have also come to the realization that in general, evaluating inter-rater reliability is only one specific task among many others during the conduct of an investigation. Consequently, the time one is willing to allocate to this task may not be sufficient to implement very elaborate techniques that require substantial experience in the use of statistical methods. Therefore, I have made considerable effort to confine myself to techniques that a large number of researchers will feel comfortable implementing. It is also partly because of this that I decided to exclude from the presentation all approaches based on the use of sophisticated theoretical statistical models (e.g. Rasch models, logistic regression models, ...) that generally require considerable time and statistical expertise to be successfully implemented.

I have accumulated considerable experience in the design and analysis of inter-rater reliability studies over the past 15 years, through teaching, writing and consulting. My goal has always been, and remains to gather in one place, detailed, well-organized, and readable materials on inter-rater reliability that are accessible to researchers and students in all fields of research. I expect readers with no background in statistics to be able to read this book. However, the need to provide a detailed account of the techniques has sometimes led me to present a mathematical formulation of certain concepts and approaches. In order to offer further assistance to readers who may not read some equations adequately, I present detailed examples, and provide downloadable Excel spreadsheets that show all the steps for calculating various agreement coefficients, along with their precision measures. Users of the R statistical package will find in appendix B several R functions implementing the techniques discussed in this book, and which can be downloaded for free. I expect the *Handbook of Inter-Rater Reliability* to be an essential reference on inter-rater reliability assessment to all researchers, students, and practitioners in all fields. If you have comments do not hesitate to contact the author.

Kilem Li Gwet, Ph.D.

Preface to the Third Edition

Here, I like to explain why I decided to write the third edition of this book. There are essentially 2 reasons for which I decided to write this third edition:

- The second edition covers various chance-corrected inter-rater reliability coefficients including Cohen's Kappa, Fleiss' Kappa, Brennan-Prediger coefficient, Gwet's AC_1 and many others. However, the treatment of these coefficients is limited to the situation where there is no missing ratings. That is, each rater is assumed to have scored all subjects that participated in the inter-rater reliability experiment. This situation rarely occurs in practice. In fact, most inter-rater reliability studies generate a sizeable number of missing ratings. For various reasons some raters may be unable to rate all subjects, or some reported ratings must be rejected due to coding errors. Therefore, it became necessary to revise the presentation of the various agreement coefficients in order to provide practitioners with clear guidelines regarding the handling of missing ratings during the analysis of inter-rater reliability data.

- Although the second edition offers an extensive account of chance-corrected agreement coefficients, it does not cover 2 important classes of measures of agreement. The first class includes all agreement coefficients in the family of Intraclass Correlation Coefficients (or ICC). The second class of agreement measures omitted in the second edition of this book belong to the family of association measures, whose objective is to quantify the extent of agreement among raters with respect to the ranking of subjects. In this second class of coefficients, one could mention for example the Kendall's coefficient of concordance, Kendall's tau, the Spearman's correlation and the likes. Given the importance of these coefficients for many researchers, there was a need to include them in a new edition.

In addition to expanding the coverage of methods, I have added more clarity into the presentation of many techniques already included in the second edition of this book. Those who read the second edition, will likely find the coverage of weighted agreement coefficients much more readable.

By writing this book, my primary goal was to allow researchers and students in all fields of research to access in one place, detailed, well-organized, and readable materials on inter-rater reliability. Although my background is in statistics, I wanted to ensure that the content of this book is accessible to readers with no background in statistics. Based the feedback I received about earlier editions of this book, this goal appears to have been achieved to a large extent. I expect the *Handbook of Inter-Rater Reliability* to be an essential reference on inter-rater reliability assessment to all researchers, students, and practitioners in all fields.

Kilem Li Gwet, Ph.D.

Table of Contents

ACKNOWLEDGMENTS

First and foremost, this book would never have been written without the full support of my wife Suzy, and our three girls Mata, Lelna, and Addia. They have all graciously put up with my insatiable computer habits and so many long workdays, and busy weekends over the past few years. Neither would this work have been completed without my mother inlaw Mathilde, who has always been there to remind me that it was time to have diner, forcing me at last to interrupt my research and writing activities to have a short but quality family time.

I started conducting research on inter-rater reliability in 2001 while on a consulting assignment with Booz Allen & Hamilton Inc., a major private contractor for the US Federal Government headquartered in Tysons Corner, Virginia. The purpose of my consulting assignment was to provide statistical support in a research study investigating the personality dynamics of information technology (IT) professionals and their relationship with IT teams' performance. One aspect of the project focused on evaluating the extent of agreement among interviewers using the Myers-Briggs Type Indicator Assessment, and the Fundamental Interpersonal Relations Orientation-Behavior tools. These are two survey instruments often used by psychologists to measure people's personality types. I certainly owe a debt of gratitude to the Defense Acquisition University (DAU) for sponsoring the research study, and to the Booz Allen & Hamilton's associates and principals who gave me the opportunity to be part of it.

Finally, I like to thank you the reader for buying this book. Please tell me what you think about it, either by e-mail or by writing a review at Amazon.com.

Thank you,

Kilem Li Gwet, Ph.D.

PART I

PRELIMINARIES

CHAPTER $\boxed{1}$

Introduction

OBJECTIVE

The primary objective of this chapter is to provide a broad view of the inter-rater reliability concept, and to highlight its importance in scientific inquiries. The difficulties associated with the quantification of inter-rater reliability, and some key factors affecting its magnitude are discussed as well. This chapter stresses out the importance of a clear statement of the study objectives, and a careful design of inter-rater reliability experiments. Different inter-rater reliability types are presented, and the practical context in which they can be used described. Also discussed in this chapter, are the types of reliability data the researcher may collect, and how they affect the way the notion of agreement is defined. I later insist on the need to analyze inter-rater reliability data according to the principles of statistical inference in order to ensure the findings can be projected beyond the often small samples of subjects and raters that participate in a reliability experiment. Figure 1.7.1 represents a flowchart that summarizes the process for identifying the correct type of agreement coefficient to use based on the type of ratings to be collected. The chapters where the recommended agreement coefficients are treated are also identified.

CONTENTS

"The man who grasps principles can successfully select his own methods.
The man who tries methods, ignoring principles, is sure to have trouble."
Ralph Waldo Emmerson (May 25, 1803 - April 27, 1882)

1.1   What is Inter-Rater Reliability ?

The concept of inter-rater reliability has such a wide range of applications across many fields of research that there is no one single definition that could possibly satisfy the specialists in any field. Nevertheless, introducing the general concept is straightforward. During the conduct of a scientific investigation, classifying subjects or objects into predefined classes or categories is a rather common activity. These categories are often values taken by a nominal or an ordinal characteristic. The reliability of this classification process can be established by asking two individuals referred to as raters, to independently perform this classification with the same set of objects. By accomplishing this task, these two individuals will have just participated in what is called an inter-rater reliability experiment expected to produce two categorizations of the same objects. The extent to which these two categorizations coincide represents what is often referred to as inter-rater reliability. If inter-rater reliability is high then both raters can be used interchangeably without the researcher having to worry about the categorization being affected by a significant rater factor. Interchangeability of raters is what justifies the importance of inter-rater reliability. If interchangeability is guaranteed, then the categories into which subjects are classified can be used with confidence without asking what rater produced them. The concept of inter-rater reliability will appeal to all those who are concerned about their data being affected to a large extent by the raters, and not by the subjects who are supposed to be the main focus of the investigation.

Our discussion of the notion of inter-rater reliability in the previous paragraph remains somehow superficial, and vague. Many terms are lousily defined. Although one can easily get a sense of what inter-rater is and how important it is, articulating a universal definition that is applicable in most situations is still problematic. For example the previous paragraph mentions two raters. But can we define inter-rater reliability without being specific about the number of raters ? If we cannot, then how many raters should be considered for this purpose ? What about the number of subjects being rated ? Consider for example faculty members rating the proficiency of nursing students on five aspects of patient care on the following four-point scale: (*i*) None, (*ii*) Basic, (*iii*) Intermediate, (*iv*) Advanced. Here the raters are humans (faculty members), and 4 categories representing an ordinal scale are used. Here, inter-rater (actually inter-faculty) reliability is the extent to which a nursing student is assigned a proficiency level, which is independent of the specific faculty member who performed the evaluation. The proficiency level should be an attribute of the nursing student and the particular test that is administered, and not an attribute of any particular faculty member. There is no reference to a particular student, nor to a particular faculty member. We do not worry about quantifying inter-rater reliability at the present. Instead, we want to explore the concept only.

So far our discussion has been limited to human raters and to categories as the measurements being produced by the inter-rater reliability experiment. This will not always be the case. Consider a situation where two medical devices designed by two manufacturers to measure the strength of the human shoulder in kilograms. The researcher wants to know whether both medical devices can be interchangeable. Before getting down to the analysis of shoulder strength data, you want to ensure that they are not contaminated by an important medical device factor. It is because what you are studying is the human shoulder, and not the medical device. What is peculiar about this experiment is that the raters are no longer humans, instead they are medical devices. Moreover, the measurements produced by the experiment are no longer categories. Instead, they are numerical values. This changes the notion of agreement entirely, and raises a whole host of new issues. Two medical devices from two manufacturers are unlikely to yield two identical values when used on the same subject. Therefore, we need to have a different way of looking at the closeness of the ratings. This is generally accomplished by looking at the variation in ratings that is due to raters only. A small variation is an indication of ratings that are very close, while a large variation suggests that the raters may have very different opinions. We are implicitly assuming here that isolating the component of the rating variation that is due to the raters alone is feasible.

There are situations where the rater can be seen as an abstract entity to some extent when defining inter-rater reliability, and other situations where the rater must be a concrete entity. For example when discussing about inter-rater reliability of medical devices, unless we clearly identify what medical devices we are referring to, our discussion will carry little interest. Our inter-rater reliability definition will clearly be limited to those devices, and any concrete statistical measure of reliability will directly refer to them. When we explore the inter-rater reliability among faculty members testing the proficiency of nursing students, then it is clearly in our interest not to exclude from consideration any faculty member who is a potential examiner now or in the future. Likewise, we would want to have our sight over all possible nursing students who may have to be evaluated at some point during their program. The general framework retained at this exploratory stage of the investigation will not just help define inter-rater reliability, it will also help to delineate the domain of validity of the concrete agreement measures that will be formulated in the form of inter-rater reliability coefficients.

In the inter-rater reliability literature, it is rather common to encounter other notions such as that of intra-rater reliability, or test-retest reliability. While inter-rater reliability is concerned about the reproducibility of measurements by different raters, intra-rater reliability on the other hand is concerned about self-reproducibility. It can be seen as a special case of inter-rater reliability. Instead of having several raters rate the same subject as in the case of inter-rater reliability, you would have the same rater rating the same subject on several occasions, also known as trials or replicates. In other words, intra-rater reliability can be seen as inter-trial or inter-replicate reliability. It does not raise any new challenges. Instead it requires an adaptation of existing ideas and approaches initially developed to assess inter-rater reliability. In addition to intra-rater reliability, the inter-rater reliability has several other branches that will be explored at a later time when the context is appropriate.

SOME APPLICATIONS OF INTER-RATER RELIABILITY

There is little doubt that it is in the medical field that inter-rater reliability has enjoyed an exceptionally high popularity. Perhaps this is due to medical errors having direct and possibly lethal consequences on human subjects. We all know stories of patients who have received the wrong medication or the right medication at a wrong dosage because the wrong illness was diagnosed by a medical personnel with insufficient training in the administration of a particular test. Therefore, improving the quality of medical tests was probably far more urgent than improving for example the quality of a video game. Patient care for example in the field of nursing is another highly sensitive area where inter-rater reliability has found a fertile ground. Chart abstractors in a neonatal intensive care unit for example play a pivotal role in the care given to newborn babies who present a potentially serious medical problem. Ensuring that the charts are abstracted in a consistent manner is essential for the reliability of diagnoses and other quality care indicators.

The field of psychometrics, which is concerned with the measurement of knowledge, abilities, attitudes, personality traits, and educational attainment, has also seen a widespread use of inter-rater reliability techniques. The use of inter-rater reliability is justified here by the constant need to validate various measurement instruments such as questionnaires, tests, and personality assessments. A popular personality test is the Myers-Briggs Type Indicator (MBTI) assessment, which is often used to categorize individuals according to their personality type (e.g. Introversion, Extraversion, Intuition, Sensing, Perception, ...). These classifications often help managers match job applicants to different job types, and build project teams. Being able to test the reliability of such a test is essential for their effective use. When used by different examiners, a reliable psychometric test is expected to produce the same categorization of the same human subjects. Eckes (2011) discusses eloquently the inter-rater reliability issues pertaining to the area of performance assessment.

Content analysis is another research field where inter-rater reliability has found numerous applications. One of the pioneering works on inter-rater reliability by Scott (1955) was published in this field. Experts in content analysis often use the terminology "inter-coder reliability." It is because raters in this field must evaluate the characteristics of a message or an artifact and assign to it a code that determines its membership in a particular category. In many applications, human coders use a codebook to guide the systematic examination of the message content. For example, health information specialists must often read general information regarding a patient's condition, the treatment received before assigning one of the numerous International Classification of Disease codes so that the medical treatment administered by doctors can be processed for payment. A poor intercoder reliability in this context would result in payment errors and possibly large financial losses. More information regarding the application of inter-reliability in content analysis can be found in Krippendorff (2012), or Zhao, Liu, and Deng (2013).

In the fields of linguistic analysis, computational linguistics, or text analytics, annotation is a big thing. Linguistic annotations can be used by subsequent applications such as a text-to-speech application with a speech synthesizer. There could be human annotators, or different annotation tools. Experts in this field are often concerned about different annotators or annotation techniques not being in agreement. This justifies the need to evaluate inter-rater reliability, generally referred to in this field of study as inter-annotator reliability. Carletta (1996) discusses some of the issues that are specific to the application of inter-rater reliability in computational linguistics. Even in the area of software testing or software process assessment, there have been some successful applications of inter-rater reliability. Software assessment is a complex activity where several process attributes are evaluated with respect to the capability levels that are reached. Inter-rater reliability, also known in this field as inter-assessor reliability is essential to ensure the integrity of the testing procedures. Jung (2003) summarizes the efforts that have been made in this area.

Numerous researchers have also used the concept of inter-rater reliability in the field of medical coding, involving the use of one or multiple systems of classification of diseases. The terminology used most often by practitioners in this field is intercoder reliability. Medical coding is a specialty in the medical field, which has specific challenges posed by inter-rater reliability assessment. The need to evaluate intercoder agreement generally occurs in one of the following two situations:

- Different coders evaluate the medical records of patients and assign one or multiple codes from a disease classification system. Unlike the typical inter-rater reliability experiment where a rater assigns each subject to one and only one category, here coders can assign a patient do multiple disease categories.

For example, Leone et al. (2006) investigated the extent to which neurologists agree when assigning ICD-9-CM[1] codes to patients who have suffered from stroke. The challenge here is to define the notion of agreement in this situation where one coder assigns 3 codes to a patient, while a second coder assigns a single code to the same patient.

Several approaches are possible depending on the study objective. One approach is to define agreement with respect to the primary diagnostic code only. They have to be identical for the coders to be in agreement. A second approach is to create groups of codes and to consider that two coders have agreed if they respective primary diagnosis codes (possibly different) fall into the same group of codes. Alternatively one may use both primary and secondary diagnosis codes provided group membership can be well defined.

- The concept of inter-rater reliability has also been successfully used in the field of medical coding to evaluate the reliability of mapping between two coding systems. Mapping between two coding systems is an essential activity for various reasons. For example behavioral health practitioners consider the Diagnostic and Statistical Manual (DSM) of Mental Disorders to be their nomenclature. However, the US federal government pays claims from the beneficiaries of public health plans using codes from the International Classification of Diseases, 9th revision, Clinical Modification (ICD-9-CM). Likewise, the Systematic Nomenclature of Medicine-Clinical Terms (SNOMED CT) was developed to be used in Electronic Health Records (EHR) for data entry and retrieval and is optimized for clinical decision support and data analysis.

In the context of inter-rater reliability, multiple coders may be asked to independently do the mapping between two systems so that the reliability of the mapping process can be evaluated. All raters take each code from one system, and map it to one or several codes from the second system. This data is generally analyzed as follows:

⇒ Suppose that a SNOMED code such as **238916002** is mapped to a single ICD-9-CM **60789** by coder 1, and to the three ICD-9-CM codes **60789**, **37454**, and **7041** by coder 2. The analysis of this data is made easier if the coders assign multiple codes by order of priority. One may consider one of the following two options for organizing this data:

OPTION 1

In option 1, all ICD-9-CM codes from each rater are displayed vertically following the priority order given to them. Each row of Table 1.1 is treated

[1]ICD-9-CM: International Classification of Diseases 9th Revision - Clinical Modification

as a separate subject that was coded independently from the others. The bullet point indicates that coder 1 did not code subjects 2 and 3.

Table 1.1: Option 1

Subject	SNOMED	Coder 1	Coder 2
1	238916002	60789	60789
2	238916002	•	37454
3	238916002	•	7041

This option more or less ignores subjects 2 and 3 in the calculation of agreement. It has nevertheless been used by some authors (c.f. Stein et al. - 2005).

OPTION 2

A better approach may be option 2 of Table 1.2, where the bullet points are replaced by the Coder 1's code with the lowest priority level. Now there is a "Weight" column that determines what weight (between 0 and 1) will be assigned to the disagreement. The use of weights in inter-rater reliability is discussed more thoroughly in the next few chapters.

Table 1.2: Option 2

Subject	SNOMED	Coder 1	Coder 2	Weight
1	238916002	60789	60789	1
2	238916002	60789	37454	0.75
3	238916002	60789	7041	0

⇒ Once an option for organizing rating data is retained, then one may use one of the many standard computation methods that will be discussed in the next few chapters.

THE STUDY OF INTER-RATER RELIABILITY

When defining the notion of inter-rater reliability, there will always be a degree of impreciseness in what we really mean by it. This issue is acknowledged by Eckes (2011, p. 24) when he says "... even if high interrater reliability has been achieved in a given assessment context exactly what such a finding stands for may be far from clear. One reason for this is that there is no commonly accepted definition of inter-rater reliability." Even the notion of agreement can sometimes be fuzzy. For example when categories represent an ordinal scale such as "none", "basic", "intermediate", "Advanced", and "Expert," it is not difficult to see to see that although "Advanced", and "Expert" represent a disagreement, these two categories are often justifiably seen as a "partial agreement", especially when compared to two categories such as "none" and "expert." Nevertheless, there is no doubt that the concept of inter-rater reliability is of great importance in all fields of research. Therefore, it is justified for us to turn to the question of which methods are best for studying it. Many ill-defined scientific concepts have been thoroughly investigated in the history of science, primarily because their existence and importance raise no doubt. For example the notion of probability has never been thoroughly defined as indicated by Kolmogorov (1999). However, very few statistical concepts have been applied more widely than this one.

1.2   Defining Experimental Parameters

Many articles about inter-rater reliability are characterized by a description of an experiment that produces ratings, and the method for analyzing those ratings. But these articles devote little space to discuss about the strength of the evidence presented, and its validity. The researcher who obtains a high inter-rater reliability coefficient of 0.95 may conclude that the extent of agreement among raters is very good and therefore the raters are interchangeable. But what raters exactly are interchangeable? Are we just referring to those two raters who participated in the reliability experiment? Can we extrapolate to other similar raters who may not have participated in the study? If the two participating raters agreed very well on the specific subjects that were rated, can we conclude that they still agree at the same level when rating other subjects? What subject population are we allowed to infer to? Generally many inter-rater reliability studies published in the literature do not address these critical questions. One of the reasons these issues are not addressed is that inter-rater reliability studies are not based on a precise definition of what should be quantified. Although starting with a general theoretical definition of inter-rater reliability may not connect directly with your specific application, we can still do a good job clarifying the scope of our investigation, and providing a detailed description of our ultimate goal. I will show in the next few paragraphs how this problem could be approached.

In a recent past, I was involved in the design of an inter-rater reliability study aimed at evaluating the extent to which triage nurses agree when assigning priority levels for care to pregnant women who present themselves in an obstetric unit with a health problem. If different triage nurses were to assign different priority levels to the same patients then one can see the potential dangers to which such disagreements may expose future mothers and their fetuses. Rather than rushing into the collection of priority data with a few triage nurses and a handful of mothers-to-be who happen to be available, it is essential to take the time to carefully articulate the ultimate goal of this study. Here are a few goals to consider:

- The concern here is to ensure that the extent of agreement among triage nurses is high in order to improve patient-centered care for the population of pregnant women.

- But what is exactly that population of pregnant women we are servicing by the way? Are they the women who visit a particular obstetric unit? Should other obstetric units be considered as well? Which ones?

- Who are the triage nurses targeted by this study? I am not referring to the triage nurses who may eventually participate in the study. Instead, I am referring to all triage nurses whose lack of proficiency in the triage process may have adverse effects on our predefined target population of pregnant women. They represent our target population of triage nurses. The possibly large number of nurses in this triage nursing population is irrelevant at this point, since we do not yet worry about those who will ultimately be recruited. Recruitment for the study will be addressed at a later time.

- In the ideal scenario where each triage nurse in the nursing population was to participate in the prioritization of all pregnant women in the target subject population, we want the extent of agreement among the nurses to be very high. But there is another important outstanding problem we need to address. If the triage patients must be classified into one of 5 possible priority categories, then we need to recognize that even after a maternal and fetal assessment are performed on the patient, two triage nurses may still be uncertain about the correct priority level the patient should be assigned to. This undesirable situation could lead them to assign a priority level that is not directly dictated by the patient's specific condition. An agreement among nurses that results from such an unpredictable situation is known in the inter-rater reliability literature as *Chance Agreement*. As badly as we may crave for high agreement among the nurses, this is not the type of agreements that we want. We want to prevent these types of agreement from giving us a false sense of security.

All the issues raised above could lead to the following definition of inter-rater reliability for this triage study:

> *Inter-rater reliability is defined as the propensity for any two triage nurses taken from the target triage nursing population, to assign the same priority level to any given pregnant woman chosen from the target women population, chance agreement having been removed from consideration.*

The above definition of inter-rater reliability does not provide a blueprint for calculating it. But that was not its intended purpose either. Instead, its purpose is to allow the management team to agree on a particular attribute of the nursing population that should be explored. Once this phase is finalized, the next step would be for the scientists to derive a formal mathematical expression to be associated with the attribute agreed upon, under the hypothetical situation where both target populations (raters and subjects) are available. This expression would then be the population parameter or coefficient (also known as inter-rater reliability coefficient) associated with the concept of inter-rater reliability. Now comes the experimental phase where a subset of raters and a subset of subjects are selected to derive an estimated inter-rater reliability coefficient, which is the concrete number ultimately produced by the inter-rater reliability experiment. An adequate presentation of the inter-rater reliability problematic cannot consist of detailed information, and computation procedures alone. It must also provide a proper and global view of the essential nature of the problem as a whole.

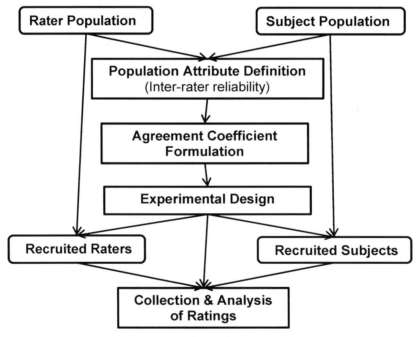

Figure 1.2.1: Phases of an Inter-Rater Reliability Study

Proving that the initial formulation of an inter-rater reliability coefficient as a population parameter is useful for studying the population attribute agreed upon can be a delicate task. What we can do in practice is to conduct an experiment and actually compute an estimated agreement coefficient. If the experiment is well designed, this estimated agreement coefficient will be a good approximation of the population inter-rater reliability coefficient. The interpretation of its value in conjunction with the subject-matter knowledge of the tasks the raters are accomplishing will help determine if the way inter-rater reliability is quantified is acceptable. We will further discuss some technical issues pertaining to the formulation of agreement coefficients in the next section.

An inter-rater reliability experiment must be carefully designed. This design involves determining how many raters and subjects should be recruited, and what protocol should be retained for selecting them. Since only a subset of the rater population is generally retained for the experiment, it is essential to have a formal link between the participating raters and their home universe to ensure that the agreement coefficient that will ultimately be calculated will have a connection to the target population of raters around which the population attribute agreed upon was articulated. The same thing can be said about the subjects that will be recruited to participate in the inter-rater reliability experiment. Although a complete discussion of these design issues will take place in subsequent chapters, we will further explore some of these issues in the next few sections.

Ratings collected from a reliability experiment are generally presented in the form of a data table where the first column represents the subjects, and the subsequent columns representing the raters and the different ratings they assigned to these subjects. Two types of analyzes can then be performed on such data:

- Some researchers simply want to summarize the extent of agreement among raters with a single number that quantifies the extent of agreement among raters (e.g. kappa, intraclass correlation, Spearman correlation, etc...). These agreement coefficients may be formulated in many different ways depending on the study objectives as will be seen later.

- Other researchers are primarily interested in studying the different factors that affect the magnitude of the ratings. This task is often accomplished by developing statistical models that describe several aspects pertaining to the rating process. These statistical models, which are often described in the form of logit or log-linear models are not covered in this book. Interested readers may want to read Agresti (1988), Tanner, and Young (1985), Eckes (2011), or Schuster and von Eye (2001) among others.

1.3   Formulation of Agreement Coefficients

I indicated in the previous section that after defining the population attribute considered to represent inter-rater reliability, the next step is to formulate the agreement coefficient that will quantify it. This formulation takes the form of an algebraic expression that shows how the ratings will be manipulated to produce a number representing the inter-rater reliability coefficient. Let us consider the maternal fetal triage study discussed in the previous, and assume that 75 triage nurses have been identified in the target nursing population (let us say in a more formal way that $R = 75$), and 1,000 patients in the patient population affected by the triage processes being investigated (that is $N = 1,000$). Although the inter-rater reliability experiment will likely not involve all 75 raters and all 1,000 potential patients, I still want to formulate the agreement coefficient under the ideal scenario where each of the 75 triage nurses prioritizes all 1,000 patients by assigning one of 5 priority levels to them.

Suppose for simplicity sake that you are only interested in the *"the propensity for any two triage nurses taken from the target triage nursing population, to assign the same priority level to any given pregnant woman chosen from the target women population."* Assuming we do not have to worry about the notion of chance agreement, this population attribute can be quantified by the relative number of pairs of triage nurses who assign a patient to the same priority level, averaged over all patients in the patient population. Let R_{ik} designate the number of nurses who assign patient i to priority level k. The total number of pairs of raters that can be formed out of R nurses in the population is $R(R-1)/2$. Likewise, the number of pairs of nurses that can be formed out of those R_{ik} who assigned patient i to priority k is $R_{ik}(R_{ik}-1)/2$. Now the relative number of pairs of nurses who assign the exact same priority level k to patient i is $P_{a|i,k} = R_{ik}(R_{ik} - 1)/R(R - 1)$. This means the relative number of pairs of nurses who assign any of the same priority level to patient i is obtained by summing the values $P_{a|i,k}$ for all 5 priority levels 1, 2, 3, 4, and 5. That is, $P_{a|i} = P_{a|i,1} + P_{a|i,2} + P_{a|i,3} + P_{a|i,4} + P_{a|i,5}$. Averaging all these values $P_{a|i}$ over all patients in the patient population will yield the agreement coefficient P_a we are looking for. All these operations can be codified mathematically as follows:

$$P_a = \frac{1}{N} \sum_{i=1}^{N} \sum_{k=1}^{5} \frac{R_{ik}(R_{ik} - 1)}{R(R - 1)}. \tag{1.3.1}$$

This quantity becomes the estimand that will later be approximated using actual ratings from the reliability experiment.

The formulation of the agreement coefficient I just discussed appears reasonable for a simple reason. The ratings that are collected from the experiment can only take five discrete values. Therefore the notion of agreement is straightforward and corresponds to an assignment of the same priority level by two raters. These ratings belong to the group of data known to be of nominal type. However, agreement co-efficients recommended for nominal scales will be inefficient for ordinal, interval or ratio scales. And vice-versa, agreement coefficients suitable for the analysis of ratio data may not be indicated for analyzing nominal data.

Consider for example a psychiatrist classifying his patients into one of five categories named "Depression", "Personal Disorder", "Schizophrenia", "Neurosis", and "Other.[2]" This five-item scale is *Nominal* since no meaningful ordering of items is possible (i.e. no category can be considered closer to one category than to another one). On the other hand, patients classified as "Certain," "Probable," "Possible," or "Doubtful" after being tested for Multiple Sclerosis, are said to be rated on an *Ordinal Scale*. The "Certain" category is closer to the "Probable" category than it is to the "Doubtful" category. Consequently, disagreements on an ordinal scale should be treated differently from disagreements on a nominal scale. This is a situation where the type of rating data (Nominal or ordinal) will have a direct impact on the way the data is being analyzed. Some inter-rater reliability studies assign continuous scores such as the blood pressure level to subjects. The data scale in this example is a continuum. As result, it is unreasonable to require agreement between two raters to represent an assignment of the exact same score to a subject. Agreement in this context is often measured by the within-subject variation of scores. With a different notion of agreement comes different ways of formulating agreement coefficients.

NOMINAL RATINGS

With a nominal scale, two raters agree when their respective ratings assigned to a subject are identical, and are in disagreement otherwise. In this context, agreement and disagreement are two distinct and opposite notions, and the relative number of times agreement occurs would normally be sufficient to determine the extent of agreement among raters. Unfortunately the limited number of values that raters can assign to subjects increases the possibility of an agreement happening by pure chance. Intuitively, the smaller the number of categories the higher the likelihood of chance agreement. Consequently, our initial intuition that the relative number of agreement occurrences can be used as an inter-rater reliability measure is unsatisfactory and must be adjusted for chance agreement. A key motivation behind the development of the well-know Kappa coefficient by Cohen (1960) was to propose an agreement coefficient that will be corrected for chance agreement.

The notion of agreement sometimes appears in the form of internal consistency

---

[2]Although the same patient may present multiple symptoms, we assume that the rating will be determined by the most visible symptom.

in scale development. When a set of questions are asked to a group of participating subjects in order to measure a specific construct, the scale developer expects all of the questions to show (internal) consistency towards the measurement of a unique latent construct. High internal consistency is an indication of a high degree of agreement among the questions (called items in the jargon of item response theory) with respect to the construct associated with the subjects. One of the best known measures of internal consistency is Cronbach's alpha coefficient (Cronbach, 1951) discussed in Part IV of the book.

ORDINAL RATINGS

When the measurement is ordinal, agreement and disagreement are no longer two distinct notions. Two raters A and B who rate the same patient as "Certain Multiple Sclerosis" and "Probable Multiple Sclerosis" are not quite in total agreement for sure. But are they in disagreement? Maybe to some extent only. That is, with ordinal scales, a disagreement is sometimes seen as a different degree of agreement, a *Partial Agreement*. An ordinal scale being nominal and ordered, the chance-agreement problem discussed previously remains present and becomes more complex with a changing notion of disagreement. This problem has been addressed in the literature by assigning weights to different degrees of disagreement as shown by Cohen (1968) among others.

With ordinal ratings, there is another kind of agreement that may be of interest to some researchers. It is the agreement among raters with respect to the ranking of subjects. Since the subjects participating in the reliability experiment can be ranked with respect to the scores assigned by one rater, a researcher may want to know whether all raters agree on which subject is the best, which one is the second best, and so on. For government examiners who score proposals submitted by potential contractors, the actual score may not matter as much as the ranking of the proposals. In this case, the most appropriate agreement coefficients would belong to the family of measures of concordance, or association as will be seen later in this book.

INTERVAL AND RATIO RATINGS

The distinction between the notions of interval and ratio data is not as important in the field of inter-rater reliability assessment, as it would in other fields. Nevertheless knowing that distinction will help researchers make a better choice of agreement coefficients. An example of interval data, which is not of ratio type, is the temperature expressed either in degree Celsius or in degree Fahrenheit. The difference between 35^0F and 70^0F is 35^0F, which represents a drastic change in the intensity of heat we feel. However, only a comparison between 2 temperature values can give meaning to each of them. An isolated value such as 35^0F does not represent a concrete measure in the absence of a natural origin, making it meaningless to apply certain arithmetic operations such as the multiplication or the division[3]. Ratio data on the other hand, such as the weight, the height, or the body mass index possess all the properties of the nominal, ordinal, and interval data, in addition to allowing for the use of all arithmetic operations, including the multiplication and the division.

Why should we care about rating data being of interval or ratio type? It is because interval/ratio-type ratings would require special methods for evaluating the extent of agreement among raters. The very notion of agreement must be revised. Given the large number of different values a score may take, the likelihood of two raters assigning the exact same score to a subject is slim. Consequently, the extent of agreement among raters is best evaluated by comparing the variation in ratings caused by the raters to the variation in ratings caused by random errors.

1.4 Different Reliability Types

The inter-rater reliability literature is full of various notions of reliability. Different terms are used to designate similar notions (e.g. intra-rater reliability, and test-retest reliability), while the word inter-rater reliability has been used with different meanings in different contexts. There is also an important distinction to be made between validity and reliability. While reliability is necessary (although insufficient) to ensure validity, validity is unnecessary for a system to be reliable. This section reviews some uncommon reliability types often encountered in the literature, and will discuss the relationship between reliability and validity.

1.4.1 *Undefined Raters and Subjects*

There are studies where identifying what entities represent subjects and raters can be unclear. As an example consider a reliability study discussed by Light (1971) where 150 mother-father pairs are asked a single 3-item multiple choice question. The ratings obtained from this experiment are reported in Table 1.3. The problem is to evaluate the extent to which mothers and fathers agree on a single issue, which could be related to children education for example. Instead of having two raters (one mother and one father) rate 150 subjects as is often the case, this special expe-

---

[3]For example, if you write 70^0F $= 2 \times 35^0$F then you will be giving the false impression that at 70^0F the heat intensity is twice higher than at 35^0F. The only thing we really know for sure is that the intensity of the heat at 70^0F is substantially higher than at 35^0F. By how much? Twice? Three times? We cannot really say it in any meaningful way.

riment involves 150 raters rating a single subject[4]. This could nevertheless be seen as a classical inter-rater reliability as long as 75 raters of one type (e.g. fathers) are paired with 75 raters of a different type (e.g. mothers). However, it is unwise to treat these raters as raters. Instead, you should see inter-rater reliability in this context as being calculated not between two human raters, but rather between two types of raters: "Mothers," and "Fathers." The different mother-father pairs can be seen as distinct "subjects." "Mothers," and "Fathers" are virtual raters, whose ratings come from specific mother-father pairs.

Table 1.3: Distribution of Mother-Father Pairs by Response Category

Fathers	Mothers			Total
	1	2	3	
1	40	5	5	50
2	8	42	0	50
3	2	3	45	50
Total	50	50	50	150

The main advantage of this design lies in the possibility it offers to extrapolate the calculated extent of agreement to a population of mothers and fathers larger than the 150 study participants.

1.4.2 *Conditional Reliability*

When the extent of agreement among raters on a nominal or ordinal scale is unexpectedly low, it is common for researchers to want to identify the specific category or categories on which raters have difficulties agreeing. This effort aims at finding some of the root causes of the weak rater agreement. The method used consists of calculating the extent of agreement among raters based on the pool of subjects known to have been classified by a given rater into the category to investigate. The resulting agreement coefficient is constrained by the requirement (or condition) to use only subjects whose membership in one category was determined by a given rater, and is known as the conditional agreement coefficient.

The reference rater whose ratings are used to select the subjects for conditional analysis, could be chosen in a number of ways. In a two-rater reliability experiment for example, the reference rater will necessarily be one of the two participants. In

---

[4]Rating a subject in this context amounts to one mother-father pair providing a personal opinion on a social issue.

a multiple-rater reliability experiment however, the reference rater may be chosen arbitrarily, or may represent the most experienced of all raters whose ratings may be considered as the gold standard. Fleiss (1971), or Light (1971) among others studied such conditional analyzes.

1.4.3   *Reliability as Internal Consistency*

In the social sciences, survey questionnaires often contain groups of questions aimed at collecting the same information from different perspectives. If a specific set of questions provides highly correlated information from different respondents in a consistent manner, it is considered to be reliable. This reliability is known as *Internal Consistency Reliability*. There are numerous situations in practice that lead to special forms of the internal consistency reliability. Internal consistency does not deal with raters creating scores. Instead, it deals with item questions used to create summary scores (also known as scales) based on information collected from the subjects. This topic is discussed in part IV of this book.

The discussion on internal consistency evaluation in this book will focus on Cronbach's alpha proposed by Cronbach (1951). Additional information on this topic could be found in other textbooks on social research methods such as those of Carmines and Zeller (1979), or Traub (1994).

1.4.4   *Reliability versus validity*

Reliability coefficients quantify the extent to which measurements are reproducible. However, the existence of a " true" score associated with each subject or object raises the question as to whether the scores that the raters agreed upon match the "true" scores. Do raters who achieve high inter-rater reliability also agree on the correct category, when it exists ? Or do they simply agree on any category ? These are some important questions a researcher may want to consider in order to have an adequate interpretation of the magnitude of agreement coefficients.

If two raters agree frequently, then the scores they assign to subjects are considered reliable. If both raters agree on the subject's "true" score, then these scores are considered valid. Valid scores are scores that are both reliable and match the reference score, also known as the "Gold Standard." Classical inter-rater reliability coefficients will generally not measure the validity of scores. Validity is measured with special validity coefficients to be discussed in chapter 11.

As seen earlier in this chapter, the "true" score does not always exist. The scoring of the quality of customer service in a department store for example reflects the rater's personal taste or opinion. No score in this case can a priori be considered standard or true, although if customer service consistently receives low ratings, it could reasonably be considered to be of poor quality. This may still provide valuable information to managers, primarily because it shows that the raters (i.e. the store customers) agree on something that has the potential to affect the business profitability.

1.5 Statistical Inference

The analysis of ratings often leads researchers to draw conclusions that go beyond the specific raters and subjects that participated in the experiment. This process of deducing from hard facts is known as inference. However, I recommend this inference to be statistical. Before enumerating some of the benefits of statistical inference, I must stress out that what distinguishes statistical inference from any other type of inference is its probabilistic nature. The foundation of statistical inference as it applies in this context of inter-rater reliability, and as presented in this book is the law of probability that governs the selection of raters from the rater population and the selection of subjects from the subject population. I expect to be able to pick any rater from the rater population (or one subject from the subject population) and tell precisely the likelihood that it will be recruited to participate in the experiment. These laws of probabilities tie the set of recruited raters and subjects to their respective populations. These links will make it possible to evaluate the chance for our calculated agreement coefficient to have the desired proximity with its population-based estimand. Here is where you find one of the main benefits of statistical inference.

In the past few sections, I indicated that before an inter-rater reliability study is formally designed the target rater and subject populations must be carefully defined first. Then inter-rater reliability is defined as an attribute of the rater population, which in turn should be codified mathematically with respect to both the rater and subject populations. This expression represents the population parameter or the estimand or the inter-rater reliability parameter to be estimated using actual ratings from the reliability experiment. Note that the expression showing how the ratings produced by the experiment are manipulated is called the inter-rater reliability estimator. In sequence we have three things to worry about, the attribute, the estimand, and the estimator. Most published papers on inter-rater reliability tend to limit the discussions to the estimator that produces the numbers. For the discussion to be complete, it must tie the estimator to the estimand and to the attribute.

Note that the inter-reliability coefficient generated by the estimator changes each time the raters or subjects who participate in the study change. It is directly affected by the experimental design. The estimand on the other hand solely depends upon both the rater and the subject populations, and are not affected in any way by the experiment. It may change only if you decide to modify the pool of raters and subjects that are targeted by the study. The attribute is the most stable element of all. It can only be affected if the study objective changes. The discrepancy between the estimator and the estimand is what is known as the statistical error. This one can be and should be estimated. It shows how well the experiment was designed. Many different groups of raters and subjects can be formed out of the rater and subject populations. Each of these rater-subject combinations will generate different values for the agreement coefficient. How far you expect any given coefficient to stray away from their average value is measured by the agreement coefficient's standard deviation

Chapter 5 is entirely devoted to the treatment of this important topic. Although I have decided to use the laws of probability governing the selection of raters and subjects as the foundation of statistical inference, this is not to claim that it is the only possible foundation that is available. Researchers who based these analyzes on theoretical statistical models may decide to use the hypothetical laws of probability that come with these models as their foundation. This alternative approach for inference is not considered in this book.

1.6   Book's Structure

This book presents various methods for calculating the extent of agreement among raters for different types of ratings. Although some of the methods were initially developed for nominal ratings only, they have been extended in this book to handle ordinal, interval, and ratio scales as well. To ensure an adequate level of depth in the treatment of this topic, I decided to discuss the precision aspects of the agreement coefficients being calculated, and to expand the methods so that datasets containing missing ratings can be analyzed as well. I always start the presentation of new methods with a simple scenario involving two raters only before extending it to the more general context of multiple raters, and nominal, ordinal, interval, or ratio ratings. The book is divided into five parts:

- Part I has a single chapter, which is the current one.
- Part II is made up of five chapters. These are chapters 2, 3, 4, 5, and 6. They deal with many different types, and aspects of the chance-corrected agreement coefficients (CAC). Agreement coefficients are discussed in these chapters for ratings that are of nominal, ordinal and interval types. Also discussed in part II chapters are the benchmarking methods for qualifying the magnitude of the agreement coefficients as well as the techniques for evaluating associated statistical errors.
- Part III covers the Intraclass Correlation Coefficients (ICC), which are recommended for use with quantitative measurements. This part of the book is made

up of the four chapters 7 to 10.

- Part IV is essentially about miscellaneous topics, which include the study of agreement coefficients conditionally upon specific categories, as well as a discussion of various measures of association or measures of agreement based on ranks. The two chapters 11 and 12 are included in this part of the book.

- Part V of the book includes appendices A and B. Appendix A contains a number of datasets that the reader may use for practice, while appendix B discusses a number of software options that may be considered for analyzing inter-rater reliability data.

Part II of this book starts in chapter 2 with a detailed critical review of several agreement coefficients as proposed in the literature for the analysis of nominal ratings. This review includes Cohen's Kappa coefficient, its generalized versions to multiple raters, Gwet AC_1, Krippendorff's alpha, or Brennan-Prediger coefficients among others. In chapter 3, I show that with the use of proper weights, the agreement coefficients discussed in chapter 2 can be adapted to produce a more efficient analysis of ordinal and interval ratings. In chapter 4, I use the AC_1 coefficient proposed by Gwet (2008a), and Aickin's alpha coefficient of Aickin (1990) as examples to show how agreement coefficients can be constructed from scratch, and why these two particular coefficients are expected to yield valid measures of the extent of agreement among raters. The theory underlying these two coefficients is also discussed in details. In chapter 5, I introduce the basic principles of statistical inference in the context of inter-rater reliability assessment. I stress the importance of defining the population of raters and the population of subjects that are targeted by the inter-rater reliability study. I did not use the model-based approach to statistical inference of Kraemer et al. (2002) and others. Instead, I decided to introduce for the first time the design-based approach to statistical inference in the field of inter-rater reliability assessment. The design-based approach to statistical inference is widely used in sample surveys and relies on the random selection of the sample of subjects from a well-defined finite population, as well as from the random selection of raters from a well-defined population of raters. Chapter 6 addresses the important problem of benchmarking the inter-rater reliability coefficient. The problem consists of determining different thresholds (or benchmarks) that could be used to interpret inter-rater reliability as poor, good, or excellent. We review different benchmarks that have been proposed in the literature before proposing a new benchmarking model specific to each inter-rater reliability coefficient.

Part III of this book starts with chapter 7, which provides a general introduction to the problem of analyzing continuous or quantitative ratings. In chapter 8, I discuss the intraclass correlation in one-factor studies. In these studies, the rater's quantitative score is investigated as a function of the rater effect alone, or as a function of the subject effect alone. These are typically studies where each subject may be rated by a different group of raters, or where each rater may rate a different group of subjects. Chapter 9 covers the intraclass correlation in two-factor studies based on a random factorial design. In this chapter, the rater's quantitative score is investigated as a function of both the rater and the subject effect. The group of subjects is assumed to be representative of the larger population of subjects it was randomly selected from. Likewise, the group of raters is assumed to be representative of the larger group it was selected from. Chapter 10 is the last chapter of part III of the book, and deals with the intraclass correlation in two-factor studies based on a the mixed factorial design. That is, while the group of subjects is assumed to be representative of a larger group of subjects, the participating raters on the other hand are the only raters of interest.

Part IV of this book focuses on miscellaneous topics, and starts with chapter 11 on the conditional analysis of inter-rater reliability. Validity coefficients are discussed in this chapter, as well as agreement coefficients conditionally upon specific categories. The conditioning is done on the "true" category when one exists, or on the category chosen by a given rater otherwise. This chapter explores additional methods for enhancing the analysis of inter-rater reliability data beyond a single statistic. Chapter 12 is devoted to the study of various measures of association or concordance, in addition to discussing Cronbach's alpha, a popular statistic in the field of item analysis.

1.7 Choosing the Right Method

How your ratings should be analyzed depends heavily on the type of data they represent, and on the ultimate objectives of your analysis. I previously indicated that your ratings may be of nominal, ordinal, interval, or ratio types. Figure 1.7.1 is a flowchart that shows what types of agreement coefficients should be used and the chapters where they are discussed, depending on the rating data type. Note that this chart describes my recommendations, which should not preclude you from treating ordinal ratings for example as if they were nominal, ignoring their ordinal nature if deemed more appropriate.

Figure 1.7.1 does not identify a specific agreement coefficient that must be used. Instead, it directs you to the chapters that discuss the topics that must be of interest to you. These chapters provide more details that will further help you decide ultimately what coefficients are right for your analysis. You will also notice that this chart does not include the special topics that are addressed in part IV of this book. You may review the content of these chapters if your analysis needs are out of the ordinary.

Figure 1.7.1 indicates that if you are dealing with ratio or interval ratings, then you can use one of the chance-corrected agreement coefficients of chapters 2 or 3 only if these ratings are predetermined before the experiment is conducted. Otherwise, you will need the intraclass correlation coefficients of chapters 7 to 10. The ratings are predetermined if before the experiment the researcher knows that each subject can for example only be assigned one of the values 1.35, 3.7, 4.12, and 6.78. However, if the rating is the subject's height, or weight whose values can be determined only after the measurement had been taken, then the intraclass correlation is what I recommend.

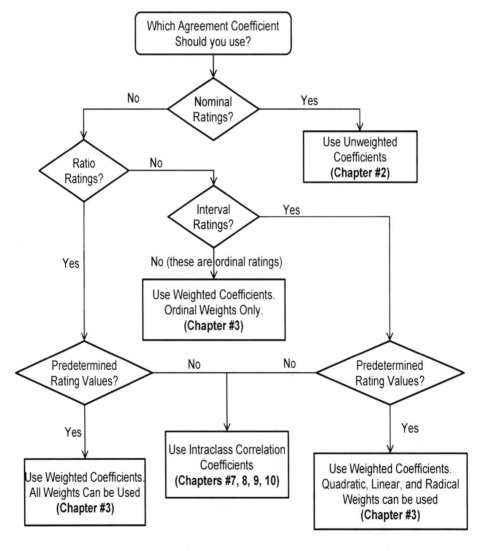

Figure 1.7.1: Choosing an Agreement Coefficient

PART II

CHANCE-CORRECTED AGREEMENT COEFFICIENTS

CHAPTER 2

Agreement Coefficients for Nominal Ratings: A Review

OBJECTIVE

This chapter presents a critical review of several agreement coefficients proposed in the literature in the past few decades for analyzing nominal ratings. Among other coefficients, I discuss the Kappa coefficient of Cohen (1960), its meaning, and its limitations. The different components of Kappa are teased apart and their influence on the agreement coefficient discussed. I explore the case of two raters and two response categories first before expanding to the more general situation of multiple raters and multiple-item response scales. This chapter also treats the important problem of missing ratings often overlooked in the literature. Figure 2.8.1 is a flowchart that shows the different agreement coefficients reviewed, the conditions under which they can be used, and their equation numbers that provide a convenient way to locate them in this chapter.

CONTENTS

"When you can measure what you are speaking about, and express it in numbers, you know something about it. But when you cannot – your knowledge is of meager and unsatisfactory kind. —" .
                                                              - Lord Kelvin (1824-1907) -

2.1   The Problem

The objective of this chapter is to present a number of agreement coefficients that have been proposed in the literature for quantifying the extent of agreement among raters when the ratings are data of the nominal type. Such ratings are independent categories, which cannot be ranked neither by order of importance, severity nor any other attribute. Table 2.1 for example shows the distribution of 223 psychiatric patients by diagnosis category and method used to obtain the diagnosis. The first method named "Clinical Diagnosis" (also known as "Facility Diagnosis") is used in a service facility (e.g. public hospital, or a community unit), and does not rely on a rigorous application of research criteria. The second method known as "Research Diagnosis" is based on a strict application of research criteria. Fenning, Craig, Tanenberg-Karant, and Bromet (1994) conducted this study to investigate the extent of agreement between clinical and Research Diagnoses, using the following 4 diagnostic categories:

- Schizophrenia
- Depression
- Bipolar Disorder
- Other

This inter-rater reliability experiment involves two raters, and four possible categories into which the patients may be classified. The two raters are the diagnosis methods "Clinical Diagnosis" and "Research Diagnosis." The rating scale is considered nominal because the four categories cannot be ranked, although it is more accurate to state that this study does not consider the ranking of these categories to be of any interest. The basic problem is to quantify the extent to which the two methods agree about the diagnoses they produce.

The most fundamental and intuitive approach to this problem is to consider the percent agreement as an agreement coefficient. The percent agreement is calculated by summing all four diagonal numbers of Table 2.1 and dividing the sum by the total number of patients. That is,

Percent Agreement $= (40 + 25 + 21 + 45)/223 = 131/223 = 58.7\%$.

Several authors have attempted to identify who first proposed this coefficient. There is still a confusion regarding this issue. While some authors refer to the percent agreement as the Osgood's coefficient, others refer to it as the Holsti's coefficient due to Osgood(1959) and Holsti (1969) recommending its use at a given point in time. There is ample evidence that the percent agreement has been used numerous times well before these works were released. Since the percent agreement is a crude application of the notion of empirical probability that did not require much investigation, my recommendation would be to put this debate to rest so we can move on to other things.

Researchers observed early in the history of inter-rater reliability estimation that two raters may agree for cause following a clear deterministic rating procedure, or they may agree by pure chance. The problem of chance agreement is best seen in a two-category inter-rater reliability experiment, where two raters must assign subjects to a positive and a negative categories. If two raters are unclear about the categorization of a subject and independently decide to make a subjective choice, they still have a chance to agree that is considerably high given the limited number of options they have to chose from. Because this type of agreement is unpredictable, and difficult to justify, it is clearly not the way any researcher will want the raters to agree. Therefore, agreement by chance is undesirable since it cannot be seen as evidence that the raters master the rating process. Unfortunately the percent agreement accounts for both types of agreement, and can be expected to overstate the "true" extent of agreement among raters. This is the problem that led several authors to propose what is known today as chance-corrected agreement coefficients. The important notion of chance agreement is further discussed in section 2.2.

Psychiatric diagnoses for example, are difficult to make due to the fuzzy boundaries that define various psychiatric disorders. A high degree of consistency between different methods permits each method to validate the other, and eventually be used with confidence and interchangeably on a routine basis. We saw in an example earlier that the clinical and research methods yield the same diagnosis on approximately 58.7% of patients. One can assume that some of these agreements did occur by pure chance. An agreement by chance is not a false agreement. It represents a form of gift or bonus that inflates the relative number of subjects in agreement without resulting from the diagnostic methods' inherent properties. Therefore a patient associated with an agreement by chance does not carry useful information regarding the degree of consistency that can be expected from the methods' intrinsic properties. Consequently, the figure 58.7% overestimates the extent of agreement between the two methods.

If we are able to identify all patients that are susceptible to chance agreement, then we could remove them from our pool of study participants before evaluating the percent agreement. But the sole existence of these special patients does not make them identifiable. A patient is associated with an agreement by chance if the processes that led to a particular diagnosis are not an integral part of the methods.

However, Table 2.1, which constitutes the basis for our analysis, contains no information regarding the processes behind the diagnoses. Moreover, some of these processes may even be cognitive and difficult to capture with precision. Still, an inter-rater reliability coefficient will yield a useful measure of the extent to which two methods are concurrent, only if it is corrected for chance agreement. How one defines chance agreement will determine the form a particular inter-rater reliability coefficient will take.

The oldest chance-corrected agreement coefficient mentioned in the literature is likely from Benini (1901). Other early efforts to solve the chance agreement issue include authors such as Guttman (1945), Bennett et *al.* (1954), Holley and Guilford (1964), Maxwell (1977), Janson and Vegelius (1979), and Brennan-Prediger (1981) who independently developed the same coefficient giving it different names. This simple coefficient, often referred to in the literature as the Brennan-Prediger coefficient is given by the ratio $(p_a - 1/q)/(1 - 1/q)$, where p_a is the percent agreement and q the number of nominal categories in the rating scale.

Brennan and Prediger (1981) recommended their coefficient in the case of two raters and an arbitrary number q of categories, while most authors before recommended it in the simpler case of two raters and two categories only. It can further be extended to the more general case of three raters or more as will be seen in subsequent sections. Holley and Guilford (1964) were the first to formally study this coefficient as a way to compute inter-rater reliability, even though others mentioned it before in various contexts. They named this coefficient the G-Index. These agreement coefficients and many others will be discussed in greater details in subsequent sections.

Some authors have criticized this coefficient under the ground that a practitioner may artificially increase the number of categories. The benefit of this operation would be a smaller chance-agreement probability (i.e. $1/q$), which in turn would increase the magnitude of the agreement coefficient. I believe that this criticism is unfounded. A practitioner who adds dummy categories for the sole purpose of jacking up the agreement coefficient engages in malpractice to obtain an undeserving reward. This is a behavioral problem. Time spent looking for a statistical fix to a problem that stems from a rigged experimental design is not time well spent.

While several inter-rater reliability coefficients have been proposed in the literature since the late forties and early fifties, the Kappa statistic proposed by Cohen (1960) became overtime the most widely-used agreement index of its genre. Despite its popularity, Kappa has many well-documented weaknesses that researchers have been slow to take into consideration when selecting an agreement coefficient. In the next few sections, I will discuss various properties of this coefficient, and will highlight some of its shortcomings.

Table 2.1: Distribution of 223 Psychiatric Patients by Type of Psychiatric Disorder, and Diagnosis Method

Clinical Diagnosis	Research Diagnosis				Total
	Schizo	Bipolar	Depress	Other	
Schizo	40	6	4	15	65
Bipolar	4	25	1	5	35
Depress	4	2	21	9	36
Other	17	13	12	45	87
Total	65	46	38	74	223

2.2   Agreement for two Raters and two Categories

A simple inter-rater reliability study consists of evaluating the extent of agreement between two raters who have each classified for example the same 100 individuals into one of two non-overlapping response categories. To be concrete, I will refer to the two raters as A and B and to the two categories as 1 and 2. Ratings obtained from such a study are often organized in a contingency table such as Table 2.2, which contains fictitious data. This table will be used later in this chapter for illustration purposes. Table 2.3 on the other hand, contains similar agreement data in their abstract form. I will appeal to the abstract agreement table throughout this chapter to describe the computational methods in their general form.

Table 2.2 shows that raters A and B both classified 35 of the 100 subjects into category 1, and 40 of the 100 subjects into category 2. Therefore, both raters agreed about the classification of 75 subjects for a percent agreement of 75%. However, they disagreed about the classification of 25 subjects, classifying 5 into categories 2 and 1, and 20 into categories 1 and 2 respectively. Likewise, using the abstract Table 2.3, I would say that raters A and B agreed on the classification of $n_{11} + n_{22}$ subjects out of a total of n subjects for a percent agreement $(n_{11} + n_{22})/n$. If p_a denotes the percent agreement then its value based on Table 2.2 data is given by:

$$p_a = (35 + 40)/100 = 0.75,$$

and its formula given by:

$$p_a = (n_{11} + n_{22})/n. \tag{2.2.1}$$

Table 2.2: Distribution of 100 Subjects by Rater and Category

Rater A	Rater B		Total
	1	2	
1	35	20	55
2	5	40	45
Total	40	60	100

Table 2.3: Distribution of n Subjects by Rater and Category

Rater A	Rater B		Total
	1	2	
1	n_{11}	n_{12}	n_{1+}
2	n_{21}	n_{22}	n_{2+}
Total	n_{+1}	n_{+2}	n

It would seem natural to consider 0.75 as a reasonably high extent of agreement between raters A and B. In reality, this number may overstate what one expects the inter-rater reliability between A and B to be, due to possible chance agreement as discussed in section 2.1. In this section, I will show how Cohen (1960) adjusted p_a for chance agreement to obtain the Kappa coefficient.

CHANCE-AGREEMENT CORRECTION

The idea of adjusting the percent agreement p_a for chance agreement is often controversial, and the definition of what constitutes chance agreement is part of the problem. Rater A for example, ignoring a particular subject's specific characteristics may decide to categorize it randomly[1]. With the number of response categories as small as 2, rater A could still categorize that subject into the exact same group as rater B, creating a lucky agreement that reflects neither the intrinsic properties of the classification system, not rater A's proficiency to use it.

2.2.1   *Cohen's Kappa Definition*

What researchers need, is an approach for measuring agreement beyond chance. To address this problem, Cohen (1960) estimated the expected percent chance agreement (denoted by p_e), and used it to adjust the percent agreement p_a to obtain the Kappa coefficient shown in equation 2.2.3. The percent chance agreement p_e is calculated by summing what Cohen considers to be the two probabilities for the two response categories 1 and 2. Note that the probabilities that raters A and B classify a subject into category 1 are respectively 0.55 and 0.40. These numbers correspond to the raw and column marginal percentages. According to Cohen the two raters are expected to reach agreement on category 1 with probability $0.55 \times 0.40 =$

---

[1]I consider a subject categorization to be random if it is not based on any known and predetermined process

0.22. Likewise they are expected to reach agreement on category 2 with probability $0.45 \times 0.60 = 0.27$. Consequently, Cohen's percent chance agreement is given by:

$$p_e = \frac{55}{100} \times \frac{40}{100} + \frac{45}{100} \times \frac{60}{100} = \frac{49}{100} = 0.49.$$

The formula for calculating the percent chance agreement is given by:

$$p_e = p_{1+}p_{+1} + p_{2+}p_{+2} = \frac{n_{1+}}{n} \times \frac{n_{+1}}{n} + \frac{n_{2+}}{n} \times \frac{n_{+2}}{n},$$
$$= p_{1+}p_{+1} + (1 - p_{1+})(1 - p_{+1}), \tag{2.2.2}$$

where $n_{1+} = n_{11} + n_{12}$, and $n_{+1} = n_{11} + n_{21}$ are the marginal counts, and p_{1+} and p_{+1} the associated marginal probabilities. Cohen (1960) defined the Kappa coefficient as follows:

$$\widehat{\kappa}_C = \frac{p_a - p_e}{1 - p_e}. \tag{2.2.3}$$

Although Cohen's original notation for the Kappa was κ (the Greek character "kappa"), I am using a different notation $\widehat{\kappa}_C$ (read "kappa hat-C"). In this new notation, the subscript C is a specific label that identifies Cohen's version of Kappa among other versions to be studied later, κ_C (without the hat) represents the true and error-free value of Kappa also known as the estimand, and the hat ($\widehat{}$) indicates an approximation of the estimand based on observed ratings. The notion of "true" value or estimand reminds us that calculated numbers are always one concrete representation of an abstract (and elusive) reality (some authors will refer to it as a construct) that constitutes our primary interest. These subtleties appeal to more sophisticated statistical concepts in the field of statistical inference, to be discussed in chapter 5.

To understand the meaning of the proposed notation $\widehat{\kappa}_C$, which is further discussed in chapter 5, the reader should remember that the Kappa value is calculated using one specific sample[2] of subjects. Consequently, a different sample of subjects selected by another researcher is expected to lead to a different value of Kappa. One may then wonder whether there exists a "true", fixed, and unique value for Kappa. The answer is yes, there is a unique "true" Kappa specific to a predefined universe or population of subjects. The subject population of interest is made up of subjects that participated in the reliability study, as well as all those subjects that could

---

[2] A sample of subjects in this context does not represent a single unit as is often the case in some medical fields(e.g. a blood sample). Instead, it represents the entire pool of subjects that participated in the reliability study.

potentially be rated in the future and to whom the researcher wants to extend the findings of the inter-rater reliability experiment. Defining this subject population at the beginning of any reliability study is an important task often overlooked by researchers, but which is essential for calculating the precision of our statistics.

Kappa's denominator represents the percent of subjects for which one would not expect any agreement by chance, while its numerator according to Cohen (1960) represents " ... *the percent of units in which beyond-chance agreement occurred ...*" Cohen (1960) sees Kappa as a measure of "... *the proportion of agreement after chance agreement is removed from consideration ...*" I will show in chapter 4 that this fundamental goal set by Cohen for Kappa can be achieved with alternative and more efficient methods.

It follows from Table 2.2 data, and from the values of p_a and p_e obtained earlier in this section that the inter-rater reliability between raters A and B as measured by Kappa is given by:

$$\widehat{\kappa}_{\mathrm{C}} = \frac{0.75 - 0.49}{1 - 0.49} \cong 0.51.$$

That is, the Kappa-based extent of agreement between raters A and B is approximately equal to 0.51. This represents a "Moderate" agreement level between two raters according to the Landis-Koch benchmark scale (see Landis and Koch, 1977). Although widely-used by researchers, this benchmark scale is not without flaws and is further discussed in chapter 6.

2.2.2   *What is Chance Agreement ?*

While the idea of correcting agreement coefficients for chance agreement is justified, the very notion of chance agreement introduced in the previous section is loosely defined. When we claim that two raters A and B have agreed by chance, what do we really mean ? Does p_e (Cohen's percent chance agreement) measure what it is supposed to measure ? These are two important questions that need to be addressed.

- By claiming that raters A and B have agreed by chance about the classification of a subject, do we mean that one of the two raters not knowing in which category the subject belongs, took a chance by randomly classifying it (perhaps with an equal probability of 0.5 (i.e. the 50:50 rule)) into one of the two possible categories ? This view ties the notion of chance agreement to that of random rating.

- Rather than using the 50:50 rule when randomly categorizing a subject, one may consider the marginal classification probabilities p_{1+} and p_{+1} as being the raters' propensity for classifying a subject into category 1. Even if the rating is random, raters A and B would choose category 1 with probabilities p_{1+} and p_{+1} respectively. They will then agree by chance if one of them performs a random classification according to the observed marginal probabilities. The classification can be seen as having been carried out either independently of the subject's specific characteristics, or following an unknown judgmental process with no apparent logic connecting the subject to the rating.

In both situations described above one of the raters must perform a random classification for concurrence to be considered chance agreement. Based on the second scenario, Cohen (1960) evaluated the chance-agreement probability as shown in equation 2.2.2. This equation could be problematic for the following reason:

> *The expression $p_{1+}p_{+1} + (1 - p_{1+})(1 - p_{+1})$ represents a probability of agreement between raters A and B only if the ratings are known to be independent[3]. In case of independence, the percent agreement p_a and the percent chance agreement p_e will be very close. If the ratings are not independent then the expression $p_{1+}p_{+1} + (1 - p_{1+})(1 - p_{+1})$ does not have any particular meaning and does not represent a measure of agreement. Using it in the Kappa equation may yield unpredictable results.*

Krippendorff (2011) argues that Cohen's percent chance agreement is based on the concept of statistical independence, which in his opinion *"... is only marginally related to how units are coded and data are made and does not yield valid coefficients for assessing the reliability of coding processes ..."*. One of the few instances in statistical science where both expressions p_a ("observed proportion" of agreement) and p_e ("expected proportion" of agreement due to chance) are part of the same equation, occurs when testing the statistical hypothesis of independence between two events with the Chi-Square test. In this case, the two expressions are used to define the test statistic, which does not represent any particular metric. Instead, the role of the test statistic is to determine whether the difference between observed and expected values under the hypothesis of independence, is sufficiently large to exclude the possibility that it may have been caused by the sampling variation alone. I will further discuss the limitations of Kappa in section 2.5.

---

[3]Note that two ratings from two raters A and B are independent if the knowledge of one rating makes the other neither more probable nor less probable. This may be the case for a small percent of subjects only. If two raters have high agreement, then for the majority of subjects, the knowledge of one rating provides a strong indication of what the other rating is (they are likely to be the same).

2.2.3   *Dealing with Missing Data*

Until now, I have only considered reliability experiments based on a fully-crossed design where each rater must classify all subjects. In practice however, raters may only have the opportunity to classify a portion of the participating subjects. Therefore one rating will be missing for those subjects not rated by both raters. Although the percent agreement will be based on the set of subjects rated by both raters, the percent chance agreement on the other hand could use all subjects classified by either rater. Using all subjects will make the marginal probabilities p_{1+} and p_{+1} more accurate.

When dealing with missing ratings, it is convenient to organize the rating data in a contingency table as shown in Table 2.4. Each rater classifies subjects into categories 1 and 2, and all subjects not rated by both raters are classified into a dummy category called X. For example, n_{1X} represents the number of subjects that rater A classified into category 1 and that rater B did not rate at all. Note from Table 2.4 that cell (X, X) always contains 0 (i.e. $n_{XX} = 0$). This indicates that subjects not rated by either rater are excluded from the analysis altogether.

Table 2.4: Distribution of n Subjects by Rater and Response Category with Missing Ratings

Rater A	Rater B			Total
	1	2	X	
1	n_{11}	n_{12}	n_{1X}	n_{1+}
2	n_{21}	n_{22}	n_{2X}	n_{2+}
X	n_{X1}	n_{X2}	0	n_{X+}
Total	n_{+1}	n_{+2}	n_{+X}	n

Considering missing ratings, the percent agreement p_a is defined as follows :

$$p_a = \frac{n_{11} + n_{22}}{n - (n_{+X} + n_{X+})}. \tag{2.2.4}$$

This equation indicates that the baseline for evaluating the percent agreement p_a must be restricted to subjects that both raters A and B have rated. Otherwise, the percent agreement will be underestimated since X will be treated as a regular category on which an agreement cannot be reached by design.

Cohen's percent chance agreement on the other hand will still be given by equation 2.2.2, with the difference that this time $n_{1+} = (n_{11} + n_{12}) + n_{1X}$, and $n_{+1} =$

$(n_{11} + n_{21}) + n_{X1}$ represent the total count of subjects that raters A and B classified into category 1. These counts include subjects rated by a single rater.

Example 2.1 _____

Let us consider a simple and fictitious inter-rater reliability study where two raters named A and B classified 100 subjects into one of two categories labeled as 1 and 2. As shown in Tables 2.5, rater B rated 8 subjects that rater A did not have the opportunity to rate. Similarly, rater A rated 5 raters that B did not rate.

Table 2.5: Distribution of 100 subjects by rater
and response category with missing ratings

Rater A	Rater B			Total
	1	2	X	
1	30	18	2	50
2	5	34	3	42
X	5	3	0	8
Total	40	55	5	100

The percent agreement p_a, and Kappa's percent chance agreement p_e are calculated as follows:

$$p_a = \frac{n_{11} + n_{22}}{n - (n_{X+} + n_{+X})} = \frac{30 + 34}{100 - (5 + 8)} = \frac{64}{87} \approx 0.74.$$

$$p_e = p_{1+}p_{+1} + p_{2+}p_{+2} = \frac{50}{100} \times \frac{40}{100} + \frac{42}{100} \times \frac{55}{100} = 0.431.$$

It follows from equation 2.2.3 that Kappa is given by:

$$\widehat{\kappa}_C = \frac{0.74 - 0.431}{1 - 0.431} = \frac{0.309}{0.569} \approx 0.54.$$

Using all 100 subjects of example 2.1 to compute the percent agreement p_a would reduce it to 0.64 (=64/100) from 0.74. This would be the consequence of considering X as a regular category, and the rating of 13 subjects by only one rater as a disagreement. Ignoring the X category (i.e. missing ratings) will yield a marginal probability[4] p_{+1} of approximately 0.38 ($\approx (30 + 5)/(50 + 42)$) as opposed to 0.40 (i.e. 40/100) obtained when all 100 subjects are used in the calculation. However, the marginal probability based on 100 subjects is more precise (i.e. has a smaller standard error) than when it is based on fewer subjects.

Although this section focuses on simple reliability experiments where two raters classify subjects into two distinct categories, many experiments in practice use more categories. This generalization is discussed in section 2.3.

_____
[4]Note that p_{+1} represents the probability that rater B classifies a subject into category 1

2.2.4   *Scott's Pi Coefficient*

About 5 years before Cohen's Kappa was published, Scott (1955) recommended the use of an agreement coefficient named Pi (Scott used the Greek character π to designate his coefficient). Scott's coefficient too is based on the same percent agreement of equation 2.2.1 (or equation 2.2.4 if some ratings are missing), and on a new percent chance agreement that is calculated with Table 2.2 data as follows:

$$p_e^2 = \left(\frac{(55/100) + (40/100)}{2}\right)^2 + \left(\frac{(45/100) + (60/100)}{2}\right)^2,$$
$$= (0.95/2)^2 + (1.05/2)^2 = 0.5013 \cdot$$

The abstract equation based on Table 2.3 is given by $p_e = \widehat{\pi}_1^2 + (1 - \widehat{\pi}_1)^2$, where $\widehat{\pi}_1 = (p_{1+} + p_{+1})/2$ and is defined by Scott (1955) as the frequency with which category 1 is used by coders[5]. This formulation of the percent chance agreement was later criticized by Cohen (1960) as one that assumes a unique propensity for classification into a particular category for all coders. Scott did not explicitly make such an assumption. Instead he was interested in the frequency of use of each category by either rater.

Scott's agreement coefficient is formally defined as follows:

$$\widehat{\kappa}_S = \frac{p_a - p_e}{1 - p_e}, \text{ where } p_e = \widehat{\pi}_1^2 + (1 - \widehat{\pi}_1)^2. \tag{2.2.5}$$

Using Table 2.2 data, this agreement coefficient is obtained as, $\widehat{\kappa}_S = (0.75 - 0.5013)/(1 - 0.5013) = 0.4988$. Scott's Pi coefficient has limitations that have been abundantly documented in the literature, and are known to be similar to those of Cohen's kappa. These limitations are discussed in section 2.5 with a particular focus on the Kappa coefficient. The main problem with Scott's Pi coefficient revolves around the calculation of the percent chance agreement p_e, which appears to be disconnected from experimental facts. Does p_e describe a phenomenon that occurred during the rating process, and which must be subtracted from the percent agreement p_a? It is well conceivable that some agreements did happen by pure chance, but certainly not all of them. This is one of the issues that led some authors to raise doubts about the quality of Scott's coefficient.

---

[5]The frequency is denoted as $\widehat{\pi}_1$ (read "Pi Hat One"), which is the Greek character π with a hat. The hat indicates that this quantity is an estimation from a sample and is subject to sampling errors. π_1 would be the "true" and unknown frequency.

2.2.5   *Krippendorff's Alpha Coefficient*

Krippendorff (1970, 2012) proposed an agreement coefficient names α (read "alpha"), which is often used by researchers in the field of communication. The procedure for computing Krippendorff's alpha is often described in terms of coincidence tables and difference functions (see Krippendorff, 2007). I will stay away from these two concepts, and replace them with the more common notations and concepts along the lines of Cohen (1960, 1968).

It is essential to realize that Krippendorff's alpha is solely based on subjects that are rated by two raters or more. All subjects rated by a single rater must be eliminated upfront before the calculations begin. For simple data such as described in Tables 2.2 and 2.3, this coefficient is fairly simple to describe. Let $\varepsilon_n = 1/(2n)$, where n is the number of subjects rated by both raters. Krippendorff's coefficient is calculated as follows:

$$\alpha_{\mathrm{K}} = (p'_a - p_e)/(1 - p_e), \ \text{where} \ \begin{cases} p_e & = \widehat{\pi}_1^2 + (1 - \widehat{\pi}_1)^2, \\ p'_a & = (1 - \varepsilon_n)p_a + \varepsilon_n, \end{cases} \tag{2.2.6}$$

with p_a being the percent agreement of equation 2.2.1. Note that the expression defining ε_n will be different when 3 raters or more are involved. Moreover, one may get the false impression that the percent chance agreement associated with Krippendorff's alpha is identical to that of Scott's Pi coefficient. This is true only if your dataset does not contain missing ratings. With missing ratings, the two quantities will be different. Krippendorff's percent chance agreement uses only subjects that are rated by both raters, while Scott's percent chance agreement uses all subjects including those rated by a single rater.

Equation 2.2.6 shows that Krippendorff's alpha and Scott's Pi are almost identical, with the only exception being the percent agreement. Krippendorff's version of the percent agreement is a weighted average of the observed percent agreement and its maximum value of 1, which always makes it higher than the observed percent agreement. If the number of subjects is limited to two, then Krippendorff's percent agreement will be $p'_a = 0.75 \times p_a + 0.25$. It is because of this weighting scheme that Krippendorff alpha is often said to apply a small-sample correction. This essentially means that when the number of subjects is small then the percent agreement is adjusted upwards, and the magnitude of the adjustment decreases as the number of subjects increases. This adjustment becomes almost insignificant as soon as the number of subjects reaches a modest size as 10. How critical is this adjustment is unclear. The need for such an adjustment and its potential benefits have not been documented. If the number of subjects is small then why do we even need to correct the percent agreement? If we do need such a correction then should the adjustment be done upwards or downwards? All these are unanswered questions?

2.2.6   Gwet's AC_1 Coefficient

Gwet (2008a) recommended an agreement coefficient named AC_1, which was developed to overcome many of the limitations associated with Cohen's Kappa. The limitations of Kappa are extensively discussed in section 2.5, and a more detailed discussion of Gwet's AC_1 can be found in chapter 4. What I like to do here is to provide a very brief review of AC_1 for simple inter-rater reliability experiments where the number of raters, and the number of categories are both limited to two.

Gwet's AC_1 is based on the same percent agreement p_a of equation 2.2.1 (or equation 2.2.4 if some ratings are missing), and on a new percent chance agreement calculated with Table 2.2 data as $p_e = 2 \times 0.475 \times (1 - 0.475) = 0.49875$, where 0.475 is the probability that a subject is classified into category 1 by a random rater.

Gwet's AC_1 coefficient, denoted here by $\widehat{\kappa}_G$ is formally defined as,

$$\widehat{\kappa}_G = \frac{p_a - p_e}{1 - p_e}, \text{ where } p_e = 2\widehat{\pi}_1(1 - \widehat{\pi}_1).$$

(2.2.7)

Using Table 2.2 data, this agreement coefficient is obtained as, $\widehat{\kappa}_G = (0.75 - 0.49875)/(1 - 0.49875) = 0.5012$. The percent chance agreement of equation 2.2.7 is actually calculated as $[\widehat{\pi}_1(1 - \widehat{\pi}_1) + \widehat{\pi}_2(1 - \widehat{\pi}_2)]/(2 - 1)$, and takes into consideration the fact that $\widehat{\pi}_1(1 - \widehat{\pi}_1) = \widehat{\pi}_2(1 - \widehat{\pi}_2)$. The number 2 in the denominator represents the number of categories. Readers interested in learning more about this coefficient, its merits and motivations are invited to read chapter 4.

2.2.7   G-Index

The G-index is the simplest chance-corrected agreement coefficient initially introduced by Holley and Guilford (1964), and later generalized to three categories or more by Brennan and Prediger (1981). It is based on the same percent agreement of equations 2.2.1 and 2.2.4. However, the percent chance agreement is simply 1/2, where 2 represents the number of categories used in the experiment.

The Holley-Guilford G-index denoted here by $\widehat{\kappa}_2$ is formally defined as,

$$\widehat{\kappa}_2 = \frac{p_a - 0.5}{1 - 0.5}.$$

(2.2.8)

Based on Table 2.2 data, this agreement coefficient is calculated as $\widehat{\kappa}_2 = (0.75 - 0.5)/(1 - 0.5) = 0.5$. The magnitude of the Holley-Guilford coefficient is generally reasonable compared to that of the percent agreement.

2.3 Agreement for two Raters and a Multiple-Level Scale

The Kappa coefficient introduced in section 2.2 within the basic framework of two raters and two response categories is extended in this section to the more general situation of two raters and an arbitrary number q (greater than 2) of nominal response categories. Such an extension does not present any new conceptual difficulties except when the categories are ordinal instead of nominal. For an ordinal multiple-level scale such as "No", "Possible", "Probable", and "Definite", two adjacent categories (e.g. "Probable" and "Definite") although different, still represent a higher degree of agreement[6] than two non-adjacent categories (e.g. "No" and "Definite"). Therefore using the Kappa coefficient of section 2.2 with ordinal scales will underestimate the "real" extent to which raters agree. For such scales, the most effective methods will take into consideration the hierarchical nature of ordinal categories. The problem of ordinal measurement scales is addressed briefly in section 2.6 and in greater details in chapter 3. We confine ourselves in this section to the case where the subjects are scored on a pure nominal measurement scale, where the notion of partial agreement does not apply.

Table 2.6 initially from Sim and Wright (2005) contains reliability data on two clinicians (1 & 2) who examined 102 individuals suffering from spinal pain and classified them according to their syndrome type (e.g. "Derangement", "Dysfunction", or "Postural"). For example, the same 11 individuals that clinician 1 diagnosed with a dysfunctional syndrome were diagnosed with a Postural syndrome by clinician 2. The measurement scale used in Table 2.6 is nominal as the three response categories $(q = 3)$ cannot a priori be ranked in any meaningful way. The extent of agreement between clinicians 1 and 2 can be evaluated using the Kappa coefficient of Cohen (1960).

In general, reliability data involving two raters and q categories will be organized as shown in Table 2.7. This table assumes that each rater had categorized all subjects (i.e. there is no missing rating), and is said to be balanced. Unbalanced tables are discussed later in this section.

---

[6]This special type of agreement on different categories has been referred to as "Partial Agreement" in the literature.

Table 2.6:

Ratings of Spinal Pain by Clinician and Syndrome Type

Clinician 1	Clinician 2			
	Derangement Syndrome	Dysfunctional Syndrome	Postural Syndrome	Total
Derangement Syndrome	22	10	2	34
Dysfunctional Syndrome	6	27	11	44
Postural Syndrome	2	5	17	24
Total	30	42	30	102

The diagonal elements $\{n_{11}, \cdots, n_{qq}\}$ represent counts of subjects classified into the same category by both raters, while the "Total" column and "Total" row respectively represent raters A and B marginal counts. In practice, percentages will sometimes be used in place of counts. For example $p_{kl} = n_{kl}/n$ represents the percentage of subjects classified into category k by rater A and into category l by rater B, while p_{k+} is the percentage of subjects that rater A classified in category k, and p_{+k} the percentage of subjects that rater B classified in category k. Here are some of the agreement coefficients defined with respect to the abstract numbers of table 2.7:

- **Kappa Coefficient**

  The Kappa statistic associated with Table 2.7 data is given by:

$$\widehat{\kappa}_{\mathrm{C}} = \frac{p_a - p_e}{1 - p_e} \text{ where } p_a = \sum_{k=1}^{q} p_{kk}, \text{ and } p_e = \sum_{k=1}^{q} p_{k+} p_{+k}. \qquad (2.3.1)$$

- **Scott's Pi Coefficient**

  Before Cohen's Kappa, Scott (1955) suggested the π statistic (read Pi statistic) given by:

$$\widehat{\kappa}_{\mathrm{S}} = \frac{p_a - p_e}{1 - p_e} \text{ where } p_e = \sum_{k=1}^{q} \hat{\pi}_k^2 \text{ with } \hat{\pi}_k = (p_{k+} + p_{+k})/2. \qquad (2.3.2)$$

Along the lines of Fleiss (1971), I define $\hat{\pi}_k$ as the probability that a rater selected randomly, classifies a randomly selected subject into category k. The hat symbol at the top of the π_k character indicates that $\hat{\pi}_k$ is a sample-based estimated value of the "true" (and unknown) probability π_k, and is likely to change from one group of participating subjects to another. Readers more interested in these notions of "estimated values" and "true" (unknown) parameters will find a more detailed discussion in chapter 5.

- **Gwet's AC$_1$ coefficient**

The AC$_1$ coefficient associated with Table 2.7 data is given by:

$$
\hat{\kappa}_{\mathrm{G}} = \frac{p_a - p_e}{1 - p_e}, \text{ where } \begin{cases} p_e = \dfrac{1}{q-1} \displaystyle\sum_{k=1}^{q} \hat{\pi}_k (1 - \hat{\pi}), \\ \hat{\pi}_k = (p_{k+} + p_{+k})/2. \end{cases} \tag{2.3.3}
$$

The percent agreement associated with the AC$_1$ coefficient is the same defined in equation 2.3.1, and q represents the number of categories.

- **Brennan-Prediger**

The agreement coefficient of Brennan and Prediger (1981) associated with Table 2.7 data is given by,

$$
\hat{\kappa}_q = \frac{p_a - p_e}{1 - p_e} \text{ where } p_e = 1/q. \tag{2.3.4}
$$

- **Krippendorff's Alpha**

The Krippendorff's alpha coefficient associated with Table 2.7 data is given by,

$$
\hat{\alpha}_{\mathrm{K}} = \frac{p'_a - p_e}{1 - p_e} \text{ where } \begin{cases} p'_a = (1 - \varepsilon_n)p_a + \varepsilon_n, \\ p_a = \displaystyle\sum_{k=1}^{n} p_{kk}, \text{ and } p_e = \displaystyle\sum_{k=1}^{q} \hat{\pi}_k^2. \end{cases} \tag{2.3.5}
$$

Note that $\varepsilon_n = 1/(2n)$, p_a is the percent agreement of equation 2.3.1, and $\hat{\pi}_k = (p_{k+} + p_{+k})/2$. When there are missing ratings, the probabilities $\hat{\pi}_k$ associated with Krippendorff's alpha will be calculated using only subjects that are rated by two raters or more. This is a potentially big difference between the ways Krippendorff's alpha and other agreement coefficients are calculated.

Table 2.7: Distribution of n subjects by rater and response category.

Rater A	Rater B				Total
	1	2	$\cdots$	q	
1	n_{11}	n_{12}	$\cdots$	n_{1q}	n_{1+}
2	n_{21}	n_{22}	$\cdots$	n_{2q}	n_{2+}
$\vdots$			$\cdots$		$\vdots$
q	n_{q1}	n_{q2}	$\cdots$	n_{qq}	n_{q+}
Total	n_{+1}	n_{+2}	$\cdots$	n_{+q}	n

Example 2.2

For illustration purposes, let us evaluate the extent of agreement between clinicians 1 and 2 based on Table 2.6 data, which are reported in Table 2.8 in terms of percentages to facilitate the use of equations 2.3.1 through 2.5.

Table 2.8:
Percentages of Patients with Back Pain, by Pain Type and Clinician

Clinician 1	Clinician 2			Total
	Derangement Syndrome	Dysfunctional Syndrome	Postural Syndrome	
Derangement Syndrome	0.2157	0.0935	0.0196	0.3333
Dysfunctional Syndrome	0.0588	0.2647	0.1078	0.4314
Postural Syndrome	0.0196	0.0490	0.1666	0.2353
Total	0.2941	0.4118	0.2941	1.0000

The reader must be aware that rounding errors in the calculations to follow may cause some minor discrepancies between the agreement coefficients calculated here, and estimates obtained from other software packages. This is inevitable here since I am attempting to show many computational steps, which require that I use approximate intermediate results causing a loss of precision. The percent agreement p_a of equation (2.3.1) is calculated as $p_a = 0.2157 + 0.2647 + 0.1666 = 0.647$.

- Cohen's Kappa Coefficient.
  Kappa's percent chance agreement (c.f. equation 2.3.1) is given by $p_e = 0.3333 \times 0.2941 + 0.4314 \times 0.4118 + 0.2353 \times 0.2941 = 0.3449$. Consequently, the Kappa coefficient is $\hat{\kappa}_c = (0.647 - 0.3449)/(1 - 0.3449) = 0.3021/0.6551 = 0.4612$.

- Scott's Pi Coefficient.
  To compute Scott's chance-agreement probability p_e (equation 2.6), we need the marginal probabilities $\hat{\pi}_1$, $\hat{\pi}_2$, and $\hat{\pi}_3$. These are obtained as follows: $\hat{\pi}_1 =$

$(0.3333+0.2941)/2 = 0.6274/2 = 0.3137$, $\hat{\pi}_2 = (0.4314+0.4118)/2 = 0.8432/2 = 0.4216$, and $\hat{\pi}_3 = (0.2353 + 0.2941)/2 = 0.5294/2 = 0.2647$. Consequently, $p_e = 0.3137^2 + 0.4216^2 + 0.2647^2 = 0.3462$, and $\widehat{\kappa}_{\rm s} = (0.647 - 0.3462)/(1 - 0.3462) = 0.3008/0.6538 = 0.4600$.

- Gwet's AC_1 Coefficient.
  Using the marginal probabilities $\hat{\pi}_1$, $\hat{\pi}_2$, and $\hat{\pi}_3$, one can compute the AC_1's percent chance agreement as $p_e = \big[0.3137 \times (1-0.3137)+0.4216 \times (1-0.4216)+ 0.2647 \times (1 - 0.2647)\big]/(3 - 1) = 0.3269$. This leads to an AC_1 value of $\widehat{\kappa}_{\rm G} = (0.647 - 0.3269)/(1 - 0.3269) = 0.3201/0.6731 = 0.4756$.

- Brennan-Prediger Coefficient.
  Since the number of categories is $q = 3$, Brennan-Prediger's percent chance agreement is $p_e = 1/3 \simeq 0.3333$, and the agreement coefficient can be obtained as $\widehat{\kappa}_3 = (0.647 - 0.3333)/(1 - 0.3333) = 0.3137/0.6667 = 0.4706$.

- Krippendorff's Alpha Coefficient.
  Since $\varepsilon_n = 1/(2n) = 1/(2 \times 102) = 0.004902$, the percent agreement associated with Krippendorff's alpha is calculated as (c.f. equation 2.3.5) $p'_a = (1 - 0.004902) \times 0.647 + 0.004902 = 0.6487304$. Consequently, Krippendorff's alpha coefficient is $\widehat{\alpha}_{\rm K} = (0.6487304 - 0.3462)/(1 - 0.3462) = 0.4627$.

Dealing with Missing Ratings

The approach I previously used to dealt with missing ratings in the context of two categories, will be used again here to adapt the agreement coefficients to a q-level measurement scale. When one rater does not rate some subjects the ratings may be organized as shown in Table 2.9 where the "X" column contains the number of subjects that only rater A has classified (and not rater B). That is, rater B did not classify a total of n_{+X} subjects. Similarly, the "X" row contains the number of subjects that only rater B has classified. Therefore, rater A did not classify n_{X+} subjects.

The agreement coefficients defined by equations 2.3.1 through 2.3.5 will still have the same general form in the presence of missing ratings. However, the various probabilities that go into these equations must be calculated differently. To calculate the percent agreement p_a between raters A and B for example, all $n_{+X} + n_{X+}$ missing ratings should be removed from consideration since they offer no possibility for both raters to agree. This is accomplished by defining p_a as follows:

$$p_a = \sum_{k=1}^{q} p_{kk}^{\star}, \ \ where \ p_{kk}^{\star} = \frac{p_{kk}}{1 - (p_{+X} + p_{X+})}, \qquad (2.3.6)$$

$p_{+X} = n_{+X}/n$, $p_{X+} = n_{X+}/n$, and $p_{kk}^{\star}$ represents the relative number of subjects scored by both raters, and that were classified into the same category k.

Calculating the percent chance agreement generally involves evaluating the marginal probabilities p_{k+} and p_{+k}, which are defined as follows:

$$p_{k+} = p_{kX} + \sum_{l=1}^{q} p_{kl}, \ and \ p_{+k} = p_{Xk} + \sum_{l=1}^{q} p_{lk}. \qquad (2.3.7)$$

Table 2.9: Distribution of n subjects by rater and response category.

Rater A	Rater B					Total
	1	2	$\cdots$	q	X	
1	n_{11}	n_{12}	$\cdots$	n_{1q}	n_{1X}	n_{1+}
2	n_{21}	n_{22}	$\cdots$	n_{2q}	n_{2X}	n_{2+}
$\vdots$			$\cdots$		$\vdots$	
q	n_{q1}	n_{q2}	$\cdots$	n_{qq}	n_{qX}	n_{q+}
X	n_{X1}	n_{X2}	$\cdots$	n_{Xq}	0	n_{X+}
Total	n_{+1}	n_{+2}	$\cdots$	n_{+q}	n_{+X}	n

Example 2.3

To illustrate the handling of missing values, let us consider the spinal pain reliability experiment that produced Table 2.6 data, and supplement it with 18 subjects scored by a single clinician and distributed as shown in Table 2.10. Counts are shown on the left side of the table and corresponding percentages on the right side.

Table 2.10: Counts of Patients with Back Pain, by Pain Type and Clinician.

Clinician 1	Clinician 2				Total
	DER	DYS	POS	X	
DER	22	10	2	3	37
DYS	6	27	11	2	46
POS	2	5	17	3	27
X	3	1	6	0	10
Total	33	43	36	8	120

The next few steps summarize how the different agreement coefficients should be computed in the presence of missing ratings. For further details the reader is invited to download the Excel spreadsheet www.agreestat.com/book4/chapter2examples.xlsx, and to look at the worksheet entitled "Example 2.3."

The percent agreement (equation 2.3.6) is given by: $p_a = (0.1833+0.2250+0.1417)/(1-(0.0667+0.0833)) = 0.6471$.

- Cohen's Kappa
  Kappa's percent chance agreement is obtained as follows: $p_e = 0.275 \times 0.308 + 0.358 \times 0.383 + 0.300 \times 0.225 + 0.067 \times 0.083 = 0.295$. This leads to a Kappa coefficient of,

  $$\widehat{\kappa}_\mathrm{C} = (0.6471 - 0.295)/(1 - 0.295) = 0.4992.$$

- Scott's Pi Coefficient
  Computing the Pi chance-agreement probability (equation 2.3.2) requires the 3 marginal probabilities $\hat{\pi}_1$, $\hat{\pi}_2$, and $\hat{\pi}_3$ to be calculated. These probabilities are respectively given by 0.3155, 0.4011, and 0.2834 (obtained by pairwise averaging Total2 and Total5 marginals of Table 2.11 - see equation 2.3.2). Squaring these numbers and summing the squared probabilities leads to the Pi percent chance agreement $p_e = 0.0995 + 0.1608 + 0.0803 = 0.3407$. Consequently, Scott's Pi coefficient is calculated as,

  $$\widehat{\kappa}_\mathrm{S} = (0.6471 - 0.3407)/(1 - 0.3407) = 0.4647.$$

- Gwet's AC$_1$ Coefficient
  Using the same 3 marginal probabilities $\hat{\pi}_1$, $\hat{\pi}_2$, and $\hat{\pi}_3$ calculated for Scott's coefficient, Gwet's percent chance agreement is obtained as $p_e = [0.3155 \times (1 - 0.3155) + 0.4011 \times (1 - 0.4011) + 0.2834 \times (1 - 0.2834)]/(3 - 1) = 0.3296$. Therefore, Gwet's AC$_1$ coefficient is calculated as,

  $$\widehat{\kappa}_\mathrm{G} = (0.6471 - 0.3296)/(1 - 0.3296) = 0.4735.$$

- Brennan-Prediger Coefficient
  The Brennan-Prediger coefficient is calculated as,

  $$\widehat{\kappa}_3 = (0.6471 - 1/3)/(1 - 1/3) = 0.4706.$$

- Krippendorff's Alpha Coefficient
  To compute Krippendorff's percent chance agreement, one needs to recalculate the 3 marginal probabilities $\hat{\pi}_1$, $\hat{\pi}_2$, and $\hat{\pi}_3$ using solely the subjects that were rated by both clinicians. These probabilities are calculated using the Total3 and Total6 marginals of Table 2.11 and equation 2.3.5, and are given by $\hat{\pi}_1 = 0.3137$, $\hat{\pi}_2 = 0.4216$, and $\hat{\pi}_3 = 0.2647$. Krippendorff's percent chance agreement is $p_e = 0.3137^2 + 0.4216^2 + 0.2647^2 = 0.3462$, and the percent agreement is $p_a = (1 - 0.00490) \times 0.64706 + 0.00490 = 0.6488$. Therefore, Krippendorff's alpha is,

  $$\widehat{\alpha}_\mathrm{K} = (0.6488 - 0.3462)/(1 - 0.3462) = 0.4628.$$

Many inter-rater reliability studies have implemented the techniques I discussed until now to quantify the extent of agreement between two raters only. Occasionally researchers want to evaluate the extent of agreement among a group of three raters or more. Two-rater techniques cannot deal with this situation, and must be extended to larger groups of raters. These extensions are the subject of section 2.4.

Table 2.11: Percentages of Patients with Back Pain, by Pain Type and Clinician.

Clinician 1	Clinician 2 (%)				Total1[a]	Total2[b]	Total3[c]
	DER	DYS	POS	X			
DER	0.183	0.083	0.017	0.025	0.308	0.33636	0.33333
DYS	0.050	0.225	0.092	0.017	0.383	0.41818	0.43137
POS	0.017	0.042	0.142	0.025	0.225	0.24545	0.23529
X	0.025	0.008	0.050	0.0	0.083	-	-
Total4[d]	0.275	0.358	0.300	0.067	1.0	1.0	1.0
Total5[e]	0.295	0.384	0.321	-	1.0		
Total6[f]	0.324	0.422	0.353	-	1.0		

[a]Clinician 1's marginals based on all subjects
[b]Clinician 1's marginals based on all subjects rated by clinician 1
[c]Clinician 1's marginals based on subjects rated by both raters
[d]Clinician 2's marginals based on all subjects
[e]Clinician 2's marginals based on all subjects rated by clinician 2
[f]Clinician 2's marginals based on subjects rated by both raters

2.4 Agreement for Multiple Raters on a Multiple-Level Scale

Let us consider a government agency that employs 7 contracting officers to make contract award decisions. To be fair to all contractors, this agency wants to ensure that all 7 assessors would assign comparable scores to similar bid submissions. This will make award decision-making processes independent of particular individuals and will be reassuring to the bidders. Using the two-rater techniques of the previous section would require the computation of a separate agreement coefficient for each of the 21 possible pairs of assessors one can form out of a group of 7 assessors. These 21 agreement coefficients will take different values, making it impossible to issue a general statement regarding the overall extent of agreement among the 7 assessors. Therefore, there is a need to have a single and global multiple-rater inter-rater reliability coefficient.

2.4.1 *Defining Agreement Among 3 Raters or More*

Seemingly obvious when applied to two raters, the notion of rater agreement does not generalize to the case of three raters or more in a natural way. For the sake of simplicity let us consider a situation where a researcher must quantify the extent of agreement among three raters named A, B, and C. When can you claim that there is agreement among the three raters about the classification of a subject? Is it when all three raters classify the subject into the exact same category? If only two of the three raters agree, should one treats this as a disagreement the same way you would treat the extreme situation where all three raters classify the subject into three different categories? Should it be treated as partial agreement? These are some of the fundamental questions that should be addressed.

The rating of a subject by two raters involves a single pair of raters, who will or will not agree. An intuitive approach for generalizing this notion to the case of three raters for example, is to consider all three pairs of raters[7] that can be formed out of a group of three raters. Only 0, 1, or all three pairs can be in agreement (it's impossible for only two of the three pairs to be in agreement). Therefore, the relative number of pairs in agreement takes one of the three values $\{0, 1/3, 1\}$. The group of three raters receives a full agreement credit (i.e. 1) only when they all classify the subject into the exact same category. They will receive no agreement credit when each classifies the subject into a category different from that of the other two raters, and will receive one third of a credit when only two of the three raters use the same category[8]. The average of all these agreement credits over all subjects yields the percent agreement p_a in the case of multiple raters.

The idea of adjusting the percent agreement for chance agreement finds a more compelling justification in the context of multiple raters. Let us consider an experiment where three raters classify subjects into one of two possible response categories. Because the number of categories is limited to 2, the three raters will never have the opportunity to classify a subject into three separate categories. At the minimum, two out of three raters are necessarily going to agree regardless of the way they rate. Consequently, some observed agreements are expected to occur by pure chance as a result of constraints imposed by the experimental conditions. Adjusting the estimated percent agreement for chance agreement becomes essential for dampening the negative influence of artificially-created situations of agreement. If the experimental design is a contributing factor to an agreement between raters, then such an agreement cannot reflect the raters' reliability.

2.4.2 *Computing Inter-Rater Reliability*

Multiple-rater reliability data can be presented in the form of a distribution of raters by category and subject (e.g. Table A.4 of appendix A), in the form of a distribution of subjects by category and rater (c.f. Table 2.12), or as a direct report

---

[7]For example 3 pairs (A,B), (A,C) and (B,C) can be formed from a group of 3 raters $\{$A, B, C$\}$.

[8]Note that Conger (1980) introduced the notion of g-Wise agreement as opposed to the pairwise agreement that is being discussed. The practical circumstances under which g-Wise agreement with $g \geq 3$ will be recommended are unclear.

of the categories into which the subjects were classified (e.g. Table A.3 of Appendix A). Table A.3 shows the raw reliability data of an experimental study aimed at detecting the coloration change on Stickleback fishes as reported by Rowland (1984). The 5 categories represent different intensity levels in the fish color displays. Table A.4 shows the distribution of raters by fish and category, while Table 2.12 shows the distribution of fishes by rater and color category. However, the techniques presented in this chapter require at the minimum the information contained in Table A.4 to compute Fleiss' generalized Kappa (c.f. Fleiss (1971)) as well Gwet's AC_1 coefficient (c.f. Gwet (2008a)). The computation of Conger's generalized coefficient (c.f. Conger (1980)) requires the information contained in both Tables A.4 and 2.12. The information in Table A.3 is the most complete, and is required for variance calculation as will be seen in chapter 5.

In their abstract forms, the two distribution tables A.4 and 2.12 are represented as shown in Tables 2.13 and 2.14 respectively. Table 2.13's "Total" column contains marginal totals that represent the number of raters r_i who scored subject i. Therefore, the missing ratings are accounted for in Table 2.13. Missing ratings are also taken into consideration in Table 2.14 where the "Total" column shows the count of subjects scored by each rater.

- Table 2.13 represents the distribution of r raters by participating subject and response category. For example, r_{ik} represents the number of raters who classified subject i into category k. In the "Total" column, r_i is the number of raters who rated subject i. If all r raters participating in the reliability study actually rate subject i, then r_i will equal r . *The column average $\bar{r}_{.k}$ (read r bar dot k)*[9] *is the mean number of raters who classified a subject into category k.*

- Table 2.14 contains the distribution of n subjects by rater and by response category, where n_{gk} is the count of subjects that rater g classified into category k. *The column average $\bar{n}_{.k}$ is the mean number of subjects that were classified into category k.* Note that n represents the total number of subjects rated by at least one rater. Subjects not rated by any rater would be excluded from analysis altogether.

Kappa was extended to the general case of three raters or more by a number of authors. Most generalized versions of Kappa are formulated as, Kappa = $(p_a - p_e)/(1-p_e)$, where p_a is the percent agreement, and p_e the percent chance agreement. While all generalized agreement coefficients share the same percent agreement except Krippendorff's alpha, they differ on their expression used to compute the percent chance agreement. The common percent agreement based on Table 2.13 is defined as

---

[9]The bar over letter r indicates the mean, and the dot on the left side of k indicates that the averaging is carried out across all subjects (the first subscript in r_{ik} always refers to the subject).

follows:

$$p_a = \frac{1}{n'} \sum_{i=1}^{n'} \sum_{k=1}^{q} \frac{r_{ik}(r_{ik} - 1)}{r_i(r_i - 1)}, \tag{2.4.1}$$

where n' is the number of subjects that were scored by two raters or more. Subjects that were rated by a single rater are not considered in the calculation of the percent agreement. In fact, the number of raters entering into the calculation of the percent agreement (i.e. n') is random. This randomness will decrease the precision with which the percent agreement is evaluated. Therefore, researchers should minimize the number of missing values during the conduct of a reliability experiment.

Table 2.12:
Distribution of Stickleback Fishes By Rater and Color Category

Rater	Color					Total
	1	2	3	4	5	
Rater 1	10	0	11	1	7	29
Rater 2	10	2	11	1	5	29
Rater 3	10	1	9	3	6	29
Rater 4	12	0	6	3	8	29
Average	1.448	0.103	1.276	0.276	0.897	29

Table 2.13: Distribution of r raters by participating subject and response category

Subject	Category					Total
	1	$\cdots$	k	$\cdots$	q	
1	r_{11}	$\cdots$	r_{1k}	$\cdots$	r_{1q}	r_1
$\vdots$		$\cdots$		$\cdots$	$\vdots$	$\vdots$
i	r_{i1}	$\cdots$	r_{ik}	$\cdots$	r_{iq}	r_i
$\vdots$		$\cdots$		$\cdots$	$\vdots$	$\vdots$
n	r_{n1}	$\cdots$	r_{nk}	$\cdots$	r_{nq}	r_n
Average	$\bar{r}_{\cdot 1}$	$\cdots$	$\bar{r}_{\cdot k}$	$\cdots$	$\bar{r}_{\cdot q}$	$\bar{r}$

Equation 2.4.1 represents the average of all pairwise agreement percentages. Although this equation has been used as a measure of the percent agreement of multiple raters numerous times (e.g. Fleiss, 1971), some authors have questioned its suitability (see Conger (1980) or Hubert (1977)). I nevertheless recommend its use.

Table 2.14: Distribution of n subjects by rater and response category

Rater	Category					Total
	1	$\cdots$	k	$\cdots$	q	
1	n_{11}	$\cdots$	n_{1k}	$\cdots$	n_{1q}	n_1
$\vdots$		$\cdots$		$\cdots$	$\vdots$	$\vdots$
g	n_{g1}	$\cdots$	n_{gk}	$\cdots$	n_{gq}	n_g
$\vdots$		$\cdots$		$\cdots$	$\vdots$	$\vdots$
r	n_{r1}	$\cdots$	n_{rk}	$\cdots$	n_{rq}	n_r
Average	$\overline{n}_{\cdot 1}$	$\cdots$	$\overline{n}_{\cdot k}$	$\cdots$	$\overline{n}_{\cdot q}$	$\overline{n}$

FLEISS' GENERALIZED KAPPA COEFFICIENT

To define the multiple-rater percent chance agreement, Fleiss (1971) considered a scenario where a rater selected randomly and with replacement from a pool of r raters, must rate a subject randomly selected from a pool of n subjects. *The probability to select a subject and a rater who classifies it into a category k is denoted by π_k,* and its value was estimated by Fleiss (1971) as,

$$\hat{\pi}_k = \frac{1}{n} \sum_{i=1}^{n} \frac{r_{ik}}{r_i}. \tag{2.4.2}$$

Note that subjects rated by a single rater are also used in the calculation of $\hat{\pi}_k$.

Under the assumption of independence where the knowledge of the rating from one rater does not affect that of the other (i.e. assigning a subject to a category is a random process), Fleiss defined the percent chance agreement[10] the probability that any pair of raters classify a subject into the same category. The resulting Fleiss' multiple-rater Kappa coefficient is defined as follows:

$$\widehat{\kappa}_{\mathrm{F}} = \frac{p_a - p_e}{1 - p_e}, \text{ where } p_e = \sum_{k=1}^{q} \hat{\pi}_k^2. \tag{2.4.3}$$

---

[10]Fleiss did not consider the treatment of missing values. Therefore, the version of the percent chance agreement presented here is more general than that of Fleiss.

CONGER'S GENERALIZED KAPPA COEFFICIENT

Conger (1980) criticized Fleiss' generalized Kappa for not reducing to Cohen's Kappa when the number of raters is two[11]. This criticism is justified since Fleiss' proposal intended to generalize Kappa and failed to do so in a rigorous way. To resolve this generalization problem, Conger (1980) adopted the same percent agreement p_a as Fleiss, but suggested to estimate the percent chance agreement by averaging all $r(r-1)/2$ Cohen-type pairwise percent chance agreement estimates (see equation 2.3.1). However, obtaining Conger's percent chance agreement by averaging all pairwise probabilities becomes time-consuming if the number of raters exceeds 3. Fortunately, a more efficient and direct alternative calculation method exits.

Let $p_{gk} = n_{gk}/n_g$ (obtained from Table 2.14) be the proportion of subjects that rater g classified into category k, and s_k^2 the sample variance[12] of the r proportions $p_{1k}, \cdots, p_{rk}$. This variance is given by,

$$s_k^2 = \frac{1}{r-1} \sum_{g=1}^{r} (p_{gk} - \overline{p}_k)^2,$$
(2.4.4)

where $\overline{p}_k$ is the mean value of the probabilities $(p_{1k}, \cdots, p_{rk})$. The multiple-rater Kappa $\widehat{\kappa}_C$ of Conger (1980) is given by[13],

$$\widehat{\kappa}_C = \frac{p_a - p_e}{1 - p_e}, \text{ where } p_e = \sum_{k=1}^{q} \overline{p}_k^2 - \sum_{k=1}^{q} s_k^2/r$$
(2.4.5)

GWET'S AC$_1$ COEFFICIENT

The AC$_1$ coefficient was suggested by Gwet (2008a) as a paradox-resistant alternative to Cohen's Kappa and is discussed in greater details in chapter 4. This coefficient relies on the same percent agreement of equation 2.4.1 as the generalized Kappa coefficients of FLeiss and Conger. As for the percent chance agreement, it is defined as the propensity for raters to agree on hard-to-score subjects[14], and is calculated by multiplying the probability to agree when the rating is random by the probability to select a hard-to-score subject.

---

[11]It should be pointed out that Fleiss' generalized statistic reduces instead to the π statistic of Scott (1955) when the number of raters is 2.

[12]Note that that Conger (1980) defined the variance s_k^2 using r in the denominator rather than $r-1$ as done here and commonly done in the statistical literature.

[13]Note that $\widehat{\kappa}_C$ designates both Cohen's and Conger's kappa. This should not create any confusion, since Cohen's kappa was defined for two raters, while Conger's was for three raters or more, and both coincide in the case of two raters.

[14]These subjects are rated randomly and any possible agreement they produce is considered to be due to pure chance. A more detailed discussion of this issue can be found in chapter 4.

Gwet's AC_1 coefficient is calculated as follows:

$$\widehat{\kappa}_{\mathrm{G}} = \frac{p_a - p_e}{1 - p_e}, \text{ where } p_e = \frac{1}{q(q-1)} \sum_{k=1}^{q} \widehat{\pi}_k (1 - \widehat{\pi}_k), \qquad (2.4.6)$$

where $\widehat{\pi}_k$ is given by equation 2.4.2.

BRENNAN-PREDIGER COEFFICIENT

The agrement coefficient recommended by Brennan and Prediger (1981) is the simplest of all chance-corrected coefficients. It is also based on the percent agreement of equation 2.4.1, and a percent chance agreement of $1/q$, which is the inverse of the number of categories.

$$\widehat{\kappa}_q = \frac{p_a - 1/q}{1 - 1/q}. \qquad (2.4.7)$$

The Brennan-Prediger percent chance agreement of $1/q$ assumes that when the rating of a subject is a random process, the subject would be assigned to any of the q categories with equal probability $1/q$. Two raters will then assign a subject to any of the same q categories with probability $q \times 1/q^2 = 1/q$, which explains why the percent chance agreement is $1/q$. The only problem I have noticed about the Brennan-Prediger coefficient is with this percent chance agreement that is calculated as if the subjects were all rated randomly, which is unlikely to be the case. This may lead to more severe chance correction than necessary.

KRIPPENDORFF'S ALPHA COEFFICIENT

A key aspect of Krippendorff's alpha coefficient (1970, 1978, 2004) is that it is solely based on subjects that are rated by two raters or more. All subjects rated by a single rater are excluded from all calculations. Another important aspect of this coefficient is its percent agreement that is different from that of the other agreement coefficients discussed in this section. Let p_a be the regular percent agreement of equation 2.4.1. The percent agreement p'_a associated with Krippendorff's alpha is given by,

$$p'_a = (1 - \varepsilon_n)p_a + \varepsilon_n, \qquad (2.4.8)$$

where $\varepsilon_n = 1/(n'\bar{r})$, n' is the number of subjects rated by two raters or more, and $\bar{r}$ the average number of raters to rate a subject (c.f. Table 2.13). Krippendorff's alpha coefficient is defined as follows:

$$\widehat{\alpha}_{\mathrm{K}} = \frac{p'_a - p_e}{1 - p_e}, \text{ where } p_e = \sum_{k=1}^{q} \widehat{\pi}_k^2, \qquad (2.4.9)$$

where $\hat{\pi}_k$ is given by,

$$\hat{\pi}_k = \frac{1}{n'} \sum_{k=1}^{n'} r_{ik}/\bar{r}. \tag{2.4.10}$$

Readers who are already familiar with the Krippendorff's alpha coefficient must have noticed that my formulation of it may appear startlingly different from what one may see anywhere else in the literature. Nevertheless, the results obtained with equation 2.4.9 or with those alternative and more complex formulations are rigorously identical. Moreover, equation 2.4.9 makes it easier to compare Krippendorff's alpha to other agreement coefficients, and to derive a simple expression for its variance as will be see in chapter 5.

Krippendorff's alpha coefficient is very similar to Fleiss' generalized Kappa, and both coefficients will generally be close. This will especially be true when no missing rating was produced by the experiment, and the number of raters is 5 or more.

The following example illustrates the calculation of the different agreement coefficients discussed in this section using Table 2.15 data.

Table 2.15: Classification of 12 subjects by 4 raters into 5 categories

Units	Rater1	Rater2	Rater3	Rater4
1	a	a		a
2	b	b	c	b
3	c	c	c	c
4	c	c	c	c
5	b	b	b	b
6	a	b	c	d
7	d	d	d	d
8	a	a	b	a
9	b	b	b	b
10		e	e	e
11			a	a
12			c	

Readers wanting to see more details about the different steps for calculating these agreement coefficients using Table 2.15 data, could download the Excel spreadsheet www.agreestat.com/book4/chapter2examples.xlsx, and use the worksheet labeled as "Example 2.4." This well-documented spreadsheet will walk you through the calculations step by step.

Example 2.4 _____

To illustrate the calculation of the various multiple-rater agreement coefficients presented ion this section, let us consider the data in Table 2.15, where 4 raters classified 12 subjects into 5 categories labeled as a, b, c, d, and e. This dataset contains missing ratings since Rater 3 for example did not rate subject 1. Table 2.17 represents Table 2.15 data in the form of a distribution of raters by subject and by category. It appears for example that two raters classified subject 11 into category a, and these are the only raters that rated subject 11. Table 2.16 on the other hand, represents Table 2.15 data in the form of a distribution of subjects by rater and by category. It follows from Table 2.16 that "Rater2" classified 4 subjects into category b.

Table 2.15 provides the most complete information about the outcome of this reliability experiment. It allows for the computation of all agreement coefficients discussed in this section. However, Table 2.17 alone provides insufficient information for computing Conger's Kappa, although it allows for the calculation of the other coefficients. But the use of both Table 2.16 and 2.17 will be sufficient to compute Conger's Kappa and the other coefficients.

- The regular percent agreement of equation 2.4.1 is given by $p_a = 0.8182$.

- Fleiss' percent chance agreement is $p_e = 0.2387$. Therefore, Fleiss' generalized Kappa is calculated from equation 2.4.3 as follows:

$$\widehat{\kappa}_F = (0.8182 - 0.2387)/(1 - 0.2387) = 0.7612.$$

- Conger's percent chance agreement is calculated from equation 2.4.5 as $p_e = 0.24212 - 0.03479/4 = 0.23343$. Therefore, Conger's generalized Kappa is calculated from equation 2.4.5 as,

$$\widehat{\kappa}_C = (0.8182 - 0.23343)/(1 - 0.23343) = 0.7628.$$

- Gwet's percent chance agreement defined by equation 2.4.6 is given by $p_e = 0.19032$. Therefore the AC_1 coefficient is,

$$\widehat{\kappa}_G = (0.8182 - 0.19032)/(1 - 0.19032) = 0.7754.$$

- The percent chance agreement associated with the Brennan-Prediger coefficient is $1/5 = 0.2$ since there are 5 possible categories into which a subject can be classified. This leads to a Brennan-Prediger coefficient of (c.f. equation 2.4.7),

$$\widehat{\kappa}_5 = (0.8182 - 0.2)/(1 - 0.2) = 0.7727.$$

- Krippendorff's percent chance agreement is given by $p_e = 0.30909$ and was calculated using only the 11 subjects that were rated by 2 raters or more. To calculate Krippendorff's percent agreement you need to first compute $\varepsilon = 1/(11 \times 3.6364) = 0.025$. The percent agreement is $p'_a = (1 - 0.025) \times p_a + 0.025 = (1 - 0.025) \times 0.8182 + 0.025 = 0.8227$. This yields a Krippendorff's alpha coefficient of,

$$\widehat{\alpha}_K = (0.8227 - 0.30909)/(1 - 0.30909) = 0.74342.$$

As it appears, the difference between both Fleiss and Conger coefficients is trivial. The only merit of Conger's coefficient is to be a more natural extension of Cohen's Kappa to the case of three raters or more. Its biggest disadvantage is to require more calculations. However, both coefficients get closer as the number of raters increases.

Table 2.16: Distribution of 12 subjects by rater and by category

Raters	a	b	c	d	e	Total
Rater1	3	3	2	1	0	9
Rater2	2	4	2	1	1	10
Rater3	1	3	5	1	1	11
Rater4	3	3	2	2	1	11
Average	2.3	3.3	2.8	1.3	0.8	10.2

Table 2.17: Distribution of 4 raters by subject and category

Units	a	b	c	d	e	Total
1	3	0	0	0	0	3
2	0	3	1	0	0	4
3	0	0	4	0	0	4
4	0	0	4	0	0	4
5	0	4	0	0	0	4
6	1	1	1	1	0	4
7	0	0	0	4	0	4
8	3	1	0	0	0	4
9	0	4	0	0	0	4
10	0	0	0	0	3	3
11	2	0	0	0	0	2
12	0	0	1	0	0	1
Mean	0.75	1.08	0.92	0.42	0.25	3.42

2.5 The Kappa Coefficient and Its Paradoxes

Any discussion regarding the Kappa coefficient will be incomplete without a word about the unexpected results it occasionally produces. Kappa often yields coefficients that are unexpectedly low when compared to the percent agreement. This problem has been referred to in the literature as the Kappa paradoxes. Feinstein and Cicchetti (1990) provides a detailed account of two such paradoxes. These authors made the following two statements:

- *"The first paradox of κ [kappa] is that if p_e [the percent chance agreement] is large, the correction process can convert a relatively high value of p_0* [15] *into a relatively low value of κ" (Feinstein & Cicchetti (1990, p. 544)*

- *"The second paradox occurs when unbalanced marginal totals produce higher values of κ than more balanced totals." (Feinstein & Cicchetti (1990, p. 545)*

This problem is discussed extensively by Gwet (2008a).

2.5.1   *Kappa's Dependency on Trait Prevalence*

On February 9, 2003 I received an e-mail from a researcher asking whether it would be possible to apply the AC_1 coefficient[16] to the data shown in Table 2.18. The motivation behind this request is presumably the failure of Kappa to provide a reasonable estimation of the extent of agreement between the two laboratories.

Table 2.18: Distribution of 125 subjects by laboratory and Category $(+/-)$

Test Laboratory	Reference Laboratory		Total
	$+$	$-$	
$+$	120	5	125
$-$	0	0	0
Total	120	5	125

A simple look at Table 2.18 reveals that the test and the reference laboratories agree almost perfectly about the scoring of the 125 participating subjects, with the exception of 5 subjects classified as positive and negative by the test and reference laboratories respectively. The exceptionally high agreement on one category is an indication of high prevalence of the positive trait in the subject population being tested. The Kappa coefficient associated with this data is obtained as follows:

---

[15]Note that p_0 in Feinstein-Cicchetti notation is the overall percent agreement denoted in this book by p_a.

[16]The AC_1 coefficient, which I recommended as an alternative to Kappa (see Gwet - 2008a), is discussed in greater details in chapter 4.

$$\left.\begin{aligned} p_a &= (120 + 0)/125 = 0.96, \\ p_e &= (125 \times 120 + 0 \times 5)/125^2 = 0.96 \end{aligned}\right\} \Rightarrow \widehat{\kappa}_{\mathrm{C}} = \frac{p_a - p_e}{1 - p_e} = 0.$$

Here is an example of a situation where a researcher would normally expect a near perfect agreement between observers, regardless of how it is measured. Yet Kappa yields a 0 coefficient, suggesting a total absence of agreement between laboratories. I want to make the following two comments:

(i) Regardless of how the notion of agreement between laboratories is defined in this particular instance, Kappa does not quantify it well. Therefore, this situation is a paradox.

(ii) The magnitude of the percent agreement p_a of 0.96 is as largely expected as the magnitude of the percent chance agreement of 0.96 is unexpected. This raises questions about the very nature of the concept being represented by the percent chance agreement p_e recommended by Cohen (1960). According to Cohen (1960), the inventor of the Kappa coefficient, p_e represents *"... the proportion of units for which agreement is expected by chance."* An examination of the expression of p_e suggests that it measures agreement probability under the following two assumptions:

- Both laboratories classify all 125 subjects randomly,
- Each laboratory's random classification is performed according to the observed marginal probabilities (1.0 and 0 for the test laboratory, and 0.96 and 0.04 for the reference laboratory).

Both conditions are unreasonable. First, only some of the subjects can be expected to be classified randomly, and certainly not all of them. But the second condition is likely the main cause of the paradox. The observed marginals indicate that the test laboratory classifies all subjects into the "+" category with certainty (i.e. with a probability of 1), while the reference laboratory classifies 96% of the subjects into the same category. Implementing a model for generating random ratings according to these probabilities will dramatically and artificially increase the percent of agreement by pure chance. The use of observed marginals to define chance agreement may not be reasonable if these marginals are very unbalanced toward one category. Moreover if all subjects are used to compute both p_a and p_e (as defined by Cohen -1960-) then the difference $p_a - p_e$ will not have a clear meaning (more on this topic in chapter 4).

The use of marginal probabilities as an objective means for quantifying the percent chance agreement p_e is questionable, and is a contributing factor to the

Kappa paradoxes. On this issue, Feinstein and Cicchetti (1990, p.548) say the following:

> *The reasoning makes the assumption that each observer has a relatively fixed prior probability of making positive or negative responses. The assumption does not seem appropriate, however for most clinical observers. If unbiased, the observers will usually respond to whatever is presented in each particular instance of challenge. The observers may develop a fixed prior probability if they know in advance that the challenge population is predominantly normal or abnormal, positive or negative - but there is no reason to assume that such probabilities will be established in advance if the observers are "blind" to the characteristics of the challenge population.*

This paradox problem is in my views not created by a high trait prevalence (which is generally unknown) as often suggested in the literature. Instead, it finds its origin in the way the researcher defines agreement by chance. In the current formulation of Kappa, all or most ratings associated with one category could be used in the calculation of p_e as if they were all assigned randomly. This may lead to a percent chance agreement that is higher than the overall percent agreement, producing a negative value for the Kappa coefficient. This problem is discussed extensively by Gwet (2008a). Regardless of what causes the Kappa paradoxes, they pose a serious underestimation problem in the extreme situations where the table is very unbalanced in its marginals.

Kraemer et al. (2002, p. 2114) attempted to defend the merit of Kappa and its paradoxical behavior in the situation illustrated in Table 2.18, by saying the following:

> *It is useful to note that $\kappa = 0$ indicates either that the heterogeneity of the patients in the population is not well detected by the raters or ratings, or that the patients in the population are homogeneous. Consequently, it is well known that it is very difficult to achieve high reliability of any measure (binary or not) in a very homogeneous population (P near 0 or 1 for binary measures). That is not a flaw in kappa ... or any other measure of reliability, or a paradox. It merely reflects the fact that it is difficult to make clear distinctions between the patients in a population in which those distinctions are very rare or fine. In such populations, 'noise' quickly overwhelms the 'signals'.*

This statement is very convoluted, and does not tell why a homogeneous population (i.e. high prevalence) should prevent two raters from agreeing about the classification of subjects, when they appear to have everything in common. Is Kappa measuring the extent of agreement among raters then ? Moreover, what is known in statistical science is not the difficulty to achieve high reliability of very homogeneous populations ($P = 0$, or $P = 1$), it is rather the difficulty to achieve high reliability of very heterogeneous populations (i.e. $P \approx 0.5$); it is the situation in which the variance will reach its maximum value.

2.5.2 *Kappa's Dependency on Marginal Homogeneity*

Feinstein and Cicchetti (1990) presented Tables 2.19 and 2.20 to illustrate the second Kappa paradox, which is characterized by a low Kappa value associated with good agreement among raters on marginal counts. These authors argue that good agreement on marginals should translate into a good interrater agreement[17]. The Kappa value associated with Table 2.19 data is $\widehat{\kappa}_C = 0.13$, which is twice smaller than the Kappa value of $\widehat{\kappa}_C = 0.26$ associated with Table 2.20 data. The point here is that observers the A and B in Table 2.20 should not be penalized when their marginal probabilities are identical to those in Table 2.19.

Table 2.19:
Distribution of 100 subjects by rater: symmetrical imbalance

Observer B	Observer A		Total
	Yes	No	
Yes	45	15	60
No	25	15	40
Total	70	30	100

Table 2.20:
Distribution of 100 subjects by rater: asymmetrical imbalance

Observer B	Observer A		Total
	Yes	No	
Yes	25	35	60
No	5	35	40
Total	30	70	100

The root cause of the second Kappa paradox is similar to that of the first Kappa paradox, which lies in the way the percent chance agreement is calculated. That is, to obtain Cohen's percent chance agreement p_e for Table 2.19, one must make the (strong and often unreasonable) assumption that the observed marginal probabilities - (0.7,0.3) for Observer A and (0.6,0.4) for Observer B - are fixed and predetermined "yes" and "no" classification propensities specific to each observer, which they will remain associated with whether they classify a subject randomly or not. A major implication of this assumption for Table 2.19 is the unduly high percent chance agreement on the "yes" category alone of $0.7 \times 0.6 = 0.42$, which will lead to a low Kappa value.

---

[17]Although reasonable, this statement could be disputable and may be inaccurate if the overall percent agreement p_a among raters is low.

I indicated in the beginning of this section that the use of three ordinal categories or more may create different types of disagreements, some potentially more serious than others. Researchers may want to consider the less serious disagreements as partial agreements and treat them accordingly. This problem has been resolved by weighting the agreement coefficients, and is briefly discussed in the next section for Kappa. A more detailed discussion of ordinal and interval ratings is presented in chapter 3.

2.6 Weighting the Kappa Coefficient

Tables 2.21 and 2.22 contain pregnancy type data collected from 100 women who entered an Emergency Room with a positive pregnancy test and a second condition, which is either abdominal pain or vaginal bleeding. After reviewing their medical records, three reviewers (also referred to as abstractors) classified them into one of the following three pregnancy categories: Ectopic Pregnancy (Ectopic), Abnormal Intrauterine pregnancy (ABN IUP), and Normal Intrauterine Pregnancy (NOR IUP).

The extent of agreement between abstractors 1 and 2 measured by the Kappa coefficient is given by : $\widehat{\kappa}_C(1,2) = (p_a - p_e)/(1 - p_e) = (0.89 - 0.4597)/(1 - 0.4597) = 0.7964$, and is identical to the extent of agreement[18] between abstractors 1 and 3. However, the clinician's objective in this chart review could be to know whether a given pregnancy is ectopic or intrauterine. That is, a disagreement over the nature of the intrauterine pregnancy (normal versus abnormal) may be of secondary importance. This fact suggests that abstractors 1 and 2 are more in agreement than abstractors 1 and 3 are. But the Kappa coefficient does not reflect this reality.

This example features a reliability experiment where certain disagreements are more serious than others. Those less serious disagreements such as abnormal versus normal intrauterine pregnancies are actually "partial" agreements that should be treated as such. To resolve this problem Cohen (1968) proposed the weighted Kappa coefficient that typically assigns a weight of 1 to the full (or diagonal) agreements, and assigns to the disagreements a weight whose magnitude decreases proportionally to their seriousness.

Cohen(1968) proposed the weighted Kappa in the context of two raters and q-item response categories. A set of weights w_{kl} ($k, l = 1, \cdots, q$) between 0 and 1 must be assigned to the q^2 cells of the contingency table similar to Table 2.7, and prior to collecting the ratings. This a-priori assignment of weights to cells aims at ensuring

---

[18]The overall percent agreement p_a and the percent chance agreement p_e are obtained as follows: $p_a = (13+20+56)/100 = 0.89$, and $p_e = (13/100)^2 + (27/100)(24/100) + (60/100)(63/100) = 0.4597$.

their independence from the observations, which will make them an integral part of the definitional formulation of the Weighted Kappa coefficient. For the classical unweighted Kappa of Cohen (1960) the weights are defined as $w_{kk} = 1$ for $k = 1, \cdots, q$, and $w_{kl} = 0$ if $k \neq l$. Once the weights are assigned, the weighted Kappa can be defined as follows:

$$\widehat{\kappa}'_{\mathrm{C}} = \frac{p'_a - p'_e}{1 - p'_e}, \tag{2.6.1}$$

where the weighted percent agreement p'_a, and weighted percent chance agreement p'_e are respectively given by:

$$p'_a = \sum_{k=1}^{q} \sum_{l=1}^{q} w_{kl} p_{kl}, \text{ and } p'_e = \sum_{k=1}^{q} \sum_{l=1}^{q} w_{kl} p_{k+} p_{+l}. \tag{2.6.2}$$

Cohen(1968) suggests that the weights could be assigned in an arbitrary fashion either by a group of experts or by a particular investigator. Two sets of weights that have been proposed in the literature are the "Linear Weights" defined for all cell (k, l) by $w_{kl} = 1 - |k - l|/(q - 1)$ and the "Quadratic Weight" defined by $w_{kl} = 1 - (k - l)^2/(q - 1)^2$.

Table 2.21: Distribution of 100 pregnant women by pregnancy type and by abstractor, for abstractors 1 and 2

Abstractor 1	Abstractor 2			Total
	Ectopic	ABN IUP	NOR IUP	
Ectopic	13	0	0	13
ABN IUP	0	20	7	27
NOR IUP	0	4	56	60
Total	13	24	63	100

Table 2.22: Distribution of 100 pregnant women by pregnancy type and by abstractor, for abstractors 1 and 3

Abstractor 1	Abstractor 3			Total
	Ectopic	ABN IUP	NOR IUP	
Ectopic	10	2	1	13
ABN IUP	2	21	4	27
NOR IUP	1	1	58	60
Total	13	24	63	100

Example 2.5 _____

Let us label the three response categories {Ectopic, ABN IUP, NOR IUP} of Tables 2.21 and 2.22 numerically as categories 1, 2, and 3. The following tables show the steps taken to compute the weighted Kappa coefficient based on Table 2.21 data and using both linear as well as quadratic weights.

Table 2.23: Linear and Quadratic Weights
for the Pregnancy Classification Example

	Linear Weights			Quadratic Weights		
	1	2	3	1	2	3
1	1.0	0.5	0.0	1.00	0.75	0.00
2	0.5	1.0	0.5	0.75	1.00	0.75
3	0.0	0.5	1.0	0.00	0.75	1.00

Table 2.24: Weighted Cell Proportions ($w_{kl}p_{kl}$)
of Table 2.17 using Linear and Quadratic Weights

	Linear Weights			Quadratic Weights		
	1	2	3	1	2	3
1	0.13	0.00	0.000	0.13	0.00	0.0000
2	0.00	0.20	0.035	0.00	0.20	0.0525
3	0.00	0.02	0.560	0.00	0.03	0.5600

Using equations 2.6.1 and 2.6.2 the weighted Kappa coefficient based on linear weights is given by $\widehat{\kappa}'_C = (0.945 - 0.6499)/(1 - 0.6499) = 0.8429$. The weighted percent agreement of 0.945 is obtained by summing all elements of Table 2.24 under the title "Linear Weights", while the weighted percent chance agreement of 0.6499 is obtained by summing all weighted expected cell proportions of Table 2.25. The weighted Kappa coefficient based on quadratic weights is given by $\widehat{\kappa}'_C = (0.9725 - 0.745)/(1 - 0.745) = 0.8922$.

The reader may want to verify that the weighted Kappa coefficients based on Table 2.22 data, using linear and quadratic weights are respectively given by 0.814 and 0.833, as opposed to 0.796 for the unweighted Kappa.

Table 2.25:
Weighted Expected Cell Proportions ($w_{kl}p_{k+}p_{l+}$)
of Table 2.17 using Linear and Quadratic Weights

	Linear Weights			Quadratic Weights		
	1	2	3	1	2	3
1	0.13	0.00	0.000	0.13	0.00	0.0000
2	0.00	0.20	0.035	0.00	0.20	0.0525
3	0.00	0.02	0.560	0.00	0.03	0.5600

While weighting Kappa addresses important issues in the assessment of the extent of agreement among raters, a more satisfying interpretation of the weighted Kappa coefficients is needed. An improved interpretation depends on the availability of a clear-cut definition of what the weight actually means. A more precise definition of the weight will also provide guidelines for developing alternative and more effective sets of weights, and to distinguish between a good and a bad set of weights. For example when a quadratic weight of 0.75 is assigned to cell (1,2), does it mean 75% of subjects in that cell could have been classified in one or more diagonal cells? These are outstanding issues that require further research.

I will further discuss the weighting of agreement statistics in a more general setting in chapter 3. I will among other things provide a more general formulation of the weighted Kappa that can handle missing ratings, be used with multiple raters, as well as with multiple-item measurement scales.

2.7   More Alternative Agreement Coefficients

In addition to the agreement coefficients that I have discussed in sections 2.3 and 2.4, a few other alternatives have been proposed in the literature that are worth mentioning. Our presentation of these inter-rater reliability coefficients will be short and references for further reading provided.

- Goodman and Kruskal (1954) proposed the following agreement coefficient:

$$\lambda = \frac{p_a - \underset{1 \leq k \leq q}{\text{Max}} \{\widehat{\pi}_k\}}{1 - \underset{1 \leq k \leq q}{\text{Max}} \{\widehat{\pi}_k\}},\tag{2.7.1}$$

where $\widehat{\pi}_k$ is the probability of classification into category k defined by equation 2.3.2 for a two-rater reliability experiment, or by equation 2.4.2 for a multiple-rater experiment. The λ (read "lambda") coefficient can be used for two raters with the percent agreement p_a of equation 2.3.1 and may be used for three raters or more with a percent agreement p_a of equation 2.4.1. Janson and Vegelius (1979) indicated however that the Goodman-Kruskal coefficient can sometimes yield unpredictable results.

- Perreault and Leigh (1989) have proposed an agreement coefficient generally denoted by I_r. It is calculated as follows:

$$I_r = \begin{cases} \sqrt{S} & if\ S \geq 0, \\ 0 & otherwise, \end{cases}\tag{2.7.2}$$

where $S = (p_a - 1/q)/(1 - 1/q)$ is the agreement coefficient recommended by Bennet et *al.* (1954) and is a special case of the coefficient recommended by Brennan and Prediger (1981). The symbol I_r used by Perreault et Leigh (1989) appears to stand for "Index of Reliability." I carefully reviewed the article written by Perreault and Leigh. It presents an excellent review of the various agreement coefficients that were current at the time it was written. However, I firmly believe that the mathematical derivations that led to the I_r coefficient were wrong, even though the underlying ideas are right. A proper translation of these ideas would inevitably have led to the Brennan-Prediger coefficient or to the percent agreement depending on the assumptions made. But it would certainly not have led to the square root of S.

Perreault and Leigh define I_r as the percent of subjects that a typical judge could code consistently given the nature of the observations. Note that I_r is an attribute of the typical judge, and therefore does not represent any aspect of agreement among the judges. Perreault and Leigh (1989) consider NI_r^2 (with N representing the number of subjects) to represent the number of reliable judgments on which judges agree. This cannot be true. To see this, note that I_r^2 is the probability that two judges both independently perform a reliable judgment. If both (reliable) judgments must lead to an agreement then they have to be associated with the exact same category. However the probability I_r^2 does not say which category was chosen and cannot represent any agreement among raters. Even if you decide to assume that any two reliable judgments must necessarily result into an agreement, then the judgments will no longer be independent. The probability for two judges to agree will now become equal to the probability for the first rater to perform a reliable judgment times the conditional probability for the second judge to perform a reliability judgment given that the first judge did. This second conditional probability cannot be evaluated unless there are additional assumptions.

A convenient way to address this problem is to first tie the reliability notion conveyed by I_r to the notion of agreement among judges. To this end, *we need to assume that I_r pre-identifies in the pool of all subjects, the specific sub-group of subjects on which all judges are reliable.* Furthermore, we need to make one of the following two assumptions:

(i) The judges always agree when they are reliable, and may agree or disagree when they are unreliable. That is reliability leads to automatic agreement, while unreliability leads to agreement only with a certain probability.

(ii) The judges agree only when they are reliable. Consequently they disagree whenever they are not both reliable. Here reliability and agreement are two identical concepts.

I_r is the probability that one judge performs a reliable judgment[19]. Under assumption (i), the number of reliable judgments on which judges agree will be NI_r (basically all reliable observations represent agreement). Now, for the remaining $N(1-I_r)$ non-reliable observations agreement occurs with a probability of $1/k$ as assumed by Brennan and Prediger (1981) and others. Consequently, the total number observations where agreement is expected is $NI_r + N(1-I_r)/k$ (note that this expression is very similar to that Perreault and Leigh, except that I_r is not squared). If you equate this to the observed frequency of agreement F_0 as Perreault and Leigh (1989) did, you will get the Brennan-Prediger coefficient. Under assumption (ii) the number of reliable judgments on which judges agree will still be NI_r, and there is no other agreement expected from the other subjects. This leads to I_r being equal to the percent agreement.

ALTERNATIVE GENERALIZATION OF SCOTT'S PI COEFFICIENT

The agreement coefficient that Fleiss (1971) recommended for multiple raters reduces to Scott's π coefficient in the case of two raters as previously indicated. If the objective is to generalize Scott's π coefficient from two raters to three raters or more, would Fleiss' proposal be a good generalization? There is no known procedure that formally generalizes Scott's coefficient to Fleiss'. However, I can use Conger's method that consists of averaging all pairwise chance-agreement probabilities to obtain the generalization needed. This method would lead to the following percent chance agreement:

$$p_e = \sum_{k=1}^{q} \bar{p}_k^2 + (1/2 - 1/r) \sum_{k=1}^{q} s_k^2, \qquad (2.7.3)$$

where s_k^2 is given by equation 2.4.4. This percent chance agreement is greater than Fleiss' version, and will generally yield a smaller agreement coefficient. However it represents an adequate generalization of Scott's π coefficient.

One would note that the second term of equation 2.7.3 measures the variability in raters' marginal probabilities. If the raters have the same marginals (i.e. the same propensity for classification into respective categories) then this second term will be negligible. If there are substantial disparities in raters' marginals, then this second term may inflate the magnitude of the percent chance agreement.

LIGHT'S GENERALIZED KAPPA COEFFICIENT

Light (1971) recommended an extension of Cohen's Kappa to the case of multiple raters by averaging all pairwise Cohen-type Kappa coefficients. For example, from a

---

[19]Note that performing a reliable judgment is equivalent to selecting a subject among those subjects pre-identified as being susceptible to reliable rating.

group of 4 raters A, B, C and D, one can create 6 pairs[20] of raters $\{(A, B), (A, C),$ $(A, D), (B, C), (B, D), (C, D)\}$. For each of the 6 pairs of raters, a Kappa coefficient can be computed as discussed in section 2.3. The average of all 6 Kappa coefficients yields Light's generalized Kappa coefficient.

Example 2.6 ──

Table 2.25, which is a dataset Conger (1980) first used in his article, summarizes the ratings of 4 raters A, B, C, and D who classified 10 subjects into one of the three categories $\{a, b, c\}$.

Table 2.26: Category membership data by rater and subject

Subject	Rater			
	A	B	C	D
1	a	a	a	c
2	a	a	b	c
3	a	a	b	c
4	a	a	c	c
5	a	b	a	a
6	b	a	a	a
7	b	b	b	b
8	b	c	b	b
9	c	c	b	b
10	c	c	c	c

Table 2.26 shows the Kappa coefficient for each of the 6 pairs of raters as well as their average, which is Light's generalized Kappa.

Table 2.27: Light's Kappa Calculation

Pair	(A, B)	(A, C)	(A, D)	(B, C)	(B, D)	(C, D)	**Light's Kappa**
Cohen's kappa	0.524	0.242	0.155	0.130	−0.014	0.565	**0.267**

Light's approach becomes computationally intensive if the number of raters is high. Moreover, averaging several pairwise Kappa coefficients will yield a measure with no clear meaning.

Note that Light's generalized Kappa is different from Conger's Kappa because the later coefficient uses pairwise averaging only to compute the percent chance agreement, while the former averages the pairwise Kappa coefficients.

────────────────────────────

[20]Note that the number of pairs of raters one can form from 4 raters equals the number of combinations C_4^2 of 2 out of 4, where $C_4^2 = 4!/(2!(4-2)!) = 6$.

BAK AND PABAK COEFFICIENTS

Byrt, Bishop, and Carlin (1993) proposed the Bias-Adjusted Kappa (BAK) in an effort to prevent Kappa from producing lower values when table marginals are balanced than when they are unbalanced. The same authors also proposed the Prevalence-Adjusted and Bias-Adjusted Kappa (PABAK) in an attempt to correct for the two paradoxes mentioned by Feinstein and Cicchetti (1990). As it turned out, the BAK statistic is nothing else than the π statistic of Scott (1955), while the PABAK is identical to the Brennan-Prediger statistic discussed earlier in this chapter.

Although Scott's π statistic is not sensitive to the marginal distributions, it remains nevertheless very sensitive to trait prevalence. The Brennan-Prediger statistic on the other hand behaves reasonably well under various conditions. The reader may see a detailed discussion of the merit of these statistics in Gwet (2008a).

2.8   Concluding Remarks

The focus of this chapter was the study of various agreement coefficients for measuring inter-rater reliability for two raters, and also to discuss some well-known extensions to the more general case of three raters or more. Only ratings that are of nominal type were considered. These are ratings, which cannot be ranked in any meaningful way and which are generally analyzed as labels that raters assigned to the subjects that are being rated. I provided a detailed discussion of the computational procedures needed to quantify each of the coefficients, and attempted to explain the purpose of each step. In particular, the notion of chance agreement was extensively discussed for all coefficients. While the intuition behind Kappa has always been a good one, I believe that it did not translate well into a formal equation. Cohen's formulation of Kappa has been proven flawed on numerous occasions as can be seen with the different paradoxes described in the literature. Nevertheless, this coefficient remains popular among researchers in the medical and social science fields. I do believe that it is about time for researchers in various fields to give full consideration to some alternative procedures that have been recently proposed in the literature, and which I briefly presented in this chapter, and will further discuss in subsequent chapters.

Also addressed in this chapter is the important and complex problem of missing ratings, which has inexplicably often been overlooked in the literature. I recommended an approach that uses all subjects rated by one rater or more. All subjects not rated at all must be excluded from the analysis. If the number of missing values is high then ignoring subjects that were not rated by all raters would result in a colossal waste of useful information, and possibly a substantial loss of precision in the calculations. This must be avoided. However, if the number of missing values is small then their impact on the different agreement coefficients is expected to be minimal.

Figure 2.8.1 shows a flowchart with the different agreement coefficients discussed in this chapter, their equation numbers, and the conditions under which they should be used. This may help practitioners quickly identify the specific agreement coefficient they want to use. These agreement coefficients were formulated differently according as the number of raters involved is two or three and more. This distinction was motivated by the different ways ratings are organized when the number of raters is two, and when it is three or more. Therefore, when looking for the right equation to use for computing the agreement coefficient, the first step must be to know the number of raters involved in the experiment. If that number is three or more, then you have six agreement coefficients to choose from. An equation number is associated with each coefficient for fast reference. I also added what I considered to be advantages or disadvantages for using each of the coefficients. If that number is two, then knowing what the number of categories used in the experiment would be the next step, before selecting one of the six agreement coefficients. I did not recommend a particular agreement coefficient nor did I conceal my preference for the AC_1 coefficient to be further discussed in chapter 4. Zhao et al. (2013) discuss a comparative study of various chance-corrected agreement coefficients that I found insightful in many aspects. The reader is encouraged to experiment with some of these coefficients and to compare their properties using a dataset one is familiar with.

Chapter 3 is devoted to ordinal and interval ratings, and special techniques for dealing with them will be discussed. Ordinal categories can be ordered from low to high, and disagreements on adjacent categories are often perceived as partial agreements. These partial agreements will be accounted for in the evaluation of inter-rater reliability. Interval data such as Temperature (e.g. 20^0F, 55^0F), or Year (e.g. 2002, 2009) in addition to being ordered from low to high, can produce meaningful intervals (e.g. 2002 to 2009 represents an interval of 7 years, or 20^0F to 55^0F represents a difference of 35^0F in temperature). The agreement coefficients discussed in this chapter will further be generalized in chapter 3 to provide an efficient approach for handling such data.

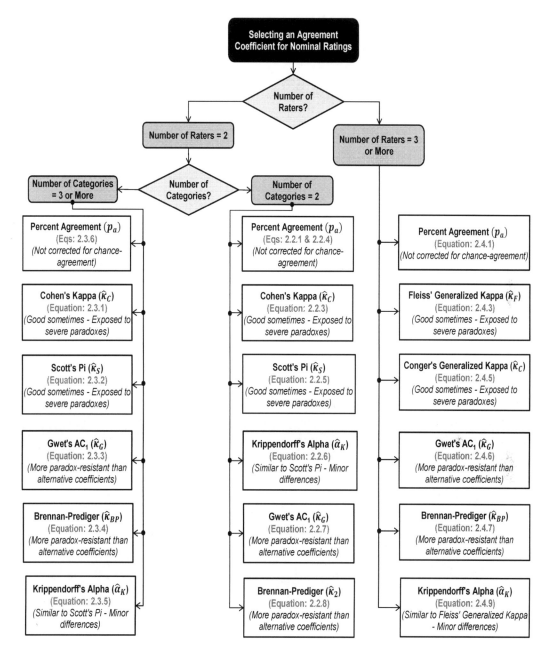

Figure 2.8.1: Choosing an Agreement Coefficient for Nominal Ratings

CHAPTER $\boxed{3}$

Agreement Coefficients for Ordinal, Interval, and Ratio Data

OBJECTIVE

The objective of this chapter is to extend the study of agreement coefficients to ordinal, interval, and ratio data. We will see that the approach recommended by Berry and Mielke (1988), and Janson and Olsson (2001) for ordinal and interval data reduces to the weighted Kappa proposed by Cohen (1968) when quadratic weights are used. Also extended to ordinal, interval, and ratio ratings are Scott's Pi coefficient (Scott, 1955), Brennan-Prediger statistic (see Brennan & and Prediger, 1981), Krippendorff's Alpha coefficient, and Gwet's AC_1. These extensions are first described for the simple situation of two raters and two response categories, before being generalized to the case of three raters or more. The little-known generalized Kappa of Conger (1980) is described. Several sets of predefined weights are presented in section 3.5, and provide different ways in which to calibrate partial agreements. Figure 3.6.1 represents a flow-chart showing which agreement coefficient to use (with reference to equation numbers) based on the number of raters and type of ratings.

CONTENTS

3.1 Overview

Cohen's Kappa coefficient discussed in chapter 2 is suitable only for the analysis of nominal ratings. With nominal ratings, raters classify subjects into categories that have no order structure. That is, two consecutive nominal categories are considered to be as different as the first and last categories. If categories can be ordered (or ranked) from the "Low" to the "High" ends, then the Kappa coefficient could dramatically understate the extent of agreement among raters. Consider an example where a group of adult men are classified twice into one of the categories "Underweight", "Normal", "Overweight", and "Obese" based on their Body Mass Index (BMI). The men are classified the first time using BMI values that are actually measured (i.e. the "Measured" approach). They are classified for the second time using self-reported BMI values (i.e. the "Self-Reported" approach). The problem is to evaluate the extent of agreement between the "Measured" and the "Self-Reported" approaches. Although Kappa may technically be used to evaluate the extent of agreement between the measured and self-reported approaches, we expect it to yield misleading results. The results will be misleading primarily because Cohen's Kappa treats any disagreement as total disagreement. Most researchers would consider the self-reported and measured approaches to be more in agreement if they categorize a participant into the "Overweight" and "Obese" categories, than if they categorize that same participant into the "Underweight" and "Obese" groups. Because it does not account for partial agreement, Kappa as proposed by Cohen (1960) is inefficient for analyzing ordinal ratings. Cohen (1968) proposed the weighted version of Kappa to fix this problem. But what is needed, is a systematic and logical approach for expanding agreement coefficients to handle ordinal as well as interval and ratio data.

Berry and Mielke (1988), Janson and Olsson (2001), as well as Janson and Olsson (2004) have proposed important extensions of Kappa to ordinal, interval, and ratio data[1]. These extensions even allow for the use of multivariate scores on subjects. While a single score determines the subject category membership, the multivariate score on the other hand is a vector of several scores, each being associated with one of the categories. The magnitude of one score associated with a category commensurate with the subject's likelihood of belonging to that category. Situations where a subject could potentially belong to many categories to some degree are common in practice. For example a patient may show symptoms for multiple diseases. Giving raters the option to classify such a patient into more than one categories could prove convenient

---

[1] Note that ordinal data can be ranked but the difference between 2 ordinal numbers may have no meaning. Interval data are ordinal data with the exception that the difference between 2 numbers has a meaning although the ratio of 2 numbers may not. With ratio type data however, all arithmetic operations are possible and are meaningful.

in some applications.

This chapter is devoted to the various extensions of several agreement coefficients to ordinal, interval, and ratio data[2]. While Berry and Mielke (1988) deserve credit for being among the first to introduce these ideas, I believe that Janson and Olsson (2001) formulated them with more clarity, in addition to further expanding them to handle missing ratings in Janson and Olsson (2004). Therefore, the current presentation is more in line with Janson and Olsson (2001). The reader will notice that the treatment of missing ratings presented in this chapter is substantially different from that of Janson and Olsson (2004), due to my desire to be more practical.

3.2 Generalizing Kappa in the Context of two Raters

Let us consider a simple inter-rater reliability experiment where two raters A and B must each classify 10 subjects into one of two possible categories $+$ (presence of a trait), and $-$ (absence of a trait). Table 3.1 shows the raw ratings as reported by the raters, and illustrates what will later be referred to as the raw representation of rating data. Table 3.2 on the other hand, offers an alternative method of reporting the same data that I refer to as the vector representation of ratings.

Table 3.1:
Raw Representation of Rating Data

Subject	Rater A	Rater B
1	$+$	$+$
2	$+$	$+$
3	$+$	$-$
4	$+$	$+$
5	$+$	$-$
6	$-$	$+$
7	$-$	$-$
8	$+$	$+$
9	$-$	$-$
10	$+$	$+$

Table 3.2:
Vector Representation of Rating Data

Subject	Rater A	Rater B	Squared Euclidean Distance
1	$(1,0)$	$(1,0)$	0
2	$(1,0)$	$(1,0)$	0
3	$(1,0)$	$(0,1)$	2
4	$(1,0)$	$(1,0)$	0
5	$(1,0)$	$(0,1)$	2
6	$(0,1)$	$(1,0)$	2
7	$(0,1)$	$(0,1)$	0
8	$(1,0)$	$(1,0)$	0
9	$(0,1)$	$(0,1)$	0
10	$(1,0)$	$(1,0)$	0
Total			6

---

[2]We assume here that the list of individual ratings that can be assigned to subjects is defined and known before the beginning of the experiment. Otherwise, you should use the intraclass correlation coefficients of chapters 7 through 10.

Vector $(1,0)$ for example, indicates that the rater has classified the subject into the first category (i.e. "+") and not into the second. For this reliability experiment each vector has 2 elements, one for each of the 2 categories "+" and "-". If a three-category measurement scale is used, then a three-dimensional vector such as $(0,1,0)$ will be associated with the raters and the subjects they classified into category 2. With this representation, the rater assigns not a single score to each subject, but rather a *Vector Score (or an Array Score)*. The rightmost column of Table 3.2 represents the discrepancy between rater A's and rater B's ratings measured by the Euclidean distance defined in the next paragraph.

THE EUCLIDEAN DISTANCE

Quantifying how far apart two vectors such as $(1,0)$ and $(0,1)$ are, has traditionally been accomplished with the Euclidean distance defined as $\sqrt{(0-1)^2 + (1-0)^2} = \sqrt{2}$. That is, the two vectors are $\sqrt{2}$ units apart. For two arbitrary vectors (a,b) and (c,d), the squared Euclidean distance is given by: $(c-a)^2 + (d-b)^2$. This definition indicates that two identical vectors have a distance of 0, which represents a perfect agreement between two raters when vector scores are used. The last column of Table 3.2 contains the squared Euclidean distances between the vector ratings associated with raters A and B. If an inter-rater reliability coefficient is expressed in the form of distances between the raters' respective vector ratings, then generalizing it to ordinal, interval or ratio data will be done in a natural way. This will be feasible since the Euclidean distance has always been used with interval and ratio data.

3.2.1 Calculating the Kappa Coefficient

Table 3.3 contains the distribution of the 10 subjects of Table 3.1 by rater and category. From this contingency table and from equations 2.2.1, 2.2.2, and 2.2.3 of chapter 2, it follows that the percent agreement is $p_a = (5+2)/10 = 0.7$, while the percent chance agreement is $p_e = (6 \times 7 + 4 \times 3)/100 = 0.42 + 0.12 = 0.54$. Consequently, Cohen's Kappa for raters A and B is given by:

$$\widehat{\kappa}_{\text{C}} = \frac{p_a - p_e}{1 - p_e} = (0.70 - 0.54)/(1 - 0.54) = 0.35.$$

Note that Kappa can alternatively be obtained as follows:

$$\widehat{\kappa}_{\text{C}} = 1 - \frac{\text{Average of the 10 squared distances of Table 3.2}}{\text{Average of the 100 squared distances of Table 3.4}}, \qquad (3.2.1)$$

$$= 1 - \frac{6/10}{92/100} = 1 - \frac{0.60}{0.92} = \frac{0.32}{0.92} = 0.35.$$

To create Table 3.4, each of the 10 vector scores of rater A (c.f. Table 3.2) must be paired with all 10 vector scores of rater B. This pairing process produces 100 pairs of vector scores from both raters. The squared Euclidean distance between the two vector scores of each pair is used to populate Table 3.4.

Equation 3.2.1 shows that Cohen's Kappa is also a function of the squared Euclidean distances between the vector scores of raters A and B. The fact that the Euclidean distance can be used with various data types paves the way for an extension of Kappa to ordinal, interval, or even ratio data.

Table 3.3:
Distribution of 10 subjects by Rater and Category

Rater B	Rater A		Total
	+	−	
+	5	1	6
−	2	2	4
Total	7	3	10

Table 3.4:
Squared Euclidean Distances between Rater A and Rater B's Vector Scores

Rater A	Rater B										Total
	$(1,0)$	$(1,0)$	$(0,1)$	$(1,0)$	$(0,1)$	$(1,0)$	$(0,1)$	$(1,0)$	$(0,1)$	$(1,0)$	
$(1,0)$	0	0	2	0	2	0	2	0	2	0	8
$(1,0)$	0	0	2	0	2	0	2	0	2	0	8
$(1,0)$	0	0	2	0	2	0	2	0	2	0	8
$(1,0)$	0	0	2	0	2	0	2	0	2	0	8
$(1,0)$	0	0	2	0	2	0	2	0	2	0	8
$(0,1)$	2	2	0	2	0	2	0	2	0	2	12
$(0,1)$	2	2	0	2	0	2	0	2	0	2	12
$(1,0)$	0	0	2	0	2	0	2	0	2	0	8
$(0,1)$	2	2	0	2	0	2	0	2	0	2	12
$(1,0)$	0	0	2	0	2	0	2	0	2	0	8
Total	6	6	14	6	14	6	14	6	14	6	92

3.2.2   Kappa: a Function of Squared Euclidean Distances

Let us consider a situation where two raters A and B must classify n subjects into one of two categories 1 or 2. Classifying a subject into one of these categories is equivalent to assigning a two-element vector to that subject. Let A_{ik} be a binary variable, which takes value 1 if rater A classifies subject i into category k (k could be 1 or 2), and will take value 0 otherwise. For rater A, categorizing subject i amounts to assigning a vector score (A_{i1}, A_{i2}) to i. This vector score will be labeled as A_i. Similarly, one can define vector $B_i = (B_{i1}, B_{i2})$ associated with rater B. The Kappa coefficient can then be represented as follows:

$$\widehat{\kappa}_C = 1 - \frac{\dfrac{1}{n}\sum_{i=1}^{n} d^2(A_i, B_i)}{\dfrac{1}{n^2}\sum_{i=1}^{n}\sum_{j=1}^{n} d^2(A_i, B_j)}, \tag{3.2.2}$$

where $d^2(A_i, B_j)$ represents the squared Euclidean distance from A_i to B_j. Equation 3.2.2 remains the same even if the number of categories q is greater than 2. In the case of q categories A_i and B_i become q-dimensional vectors. For example, the vector score associated with rater A and subject i will be given by:

$$A_i = (A_{i1}, \cdots, A_{ik}, \cdots, A_{iq}) \tag{3.2.3}$$

Equation 3.2.2 can still be used even if the raters assign one of three interval-type scores x_1, x_2 and x_3 rather than nominal-type scores. In this case, vector A_i will not be a three-element vector consisting of a single occurrence of 1 and two occurrences of 0. Instead, A_i will take a single value (either x_1 or x_2, or x_3 depending on which one is assigned to subject i). As previously seen, this coefficient is identical to the classical Kappa coefficient of Cohen (1960) if x_1, x_2, and x_3 are simply category labels.

When used with q interval data $(x_1, \cdots, x_k, \cdots, x_q)$, equation 3.2.2 leads to the following Kappa coefficient:

$$\widehat{\kappa}_C' = 1 - \frac{\sum_{k,l}^{q} p_{kl}(x_k - x_l)^2}{\sum_{k,l}^{q} p_{k+}p_{+l}(x_k - x_l)^2}, \tag{3.2.4}$$

where p_{kl} is the proportion of subjects to whom raters A and B assigned the scores x_k and x_l respectively, p_{k+} is the proportion of subjects to whom rater A assigned score x_k and p_{+l} the proportion of subjects to whom rater B assigned score x_l. This result is obtained from equation 3.2.2 by replacing the vector score A_i with the single interval score x_l $(l = 1, \cdots, q)$ that rater A assigned to subject i.

When dealing with interval data, and a complete dataset with no missing rating, then you may use equation 3.2.4 for calculating the Kappa coefficient. However, datasets in practice are often incomplete with some raters producing ratings on a limited number of subjects. Therefore, I am recommending a more general formulation of Kappa, whose objective is to ensure that the different proportions of subjects p_{kl}, p_{k+}, or p_{+l} are evaluated with respect to the appropriate number of scoring raters. For example, the proportion of subjects that raters A and B classified into categories k and l respectively, must be evaluated with respect to the subjects that both raters have scored. If a subject was scored by only one of the two raters, then it will be excluded from the calculation of that proportion. Not excluding those subjects will lead to an understatement of the Kappa coefficient. Let us consider the following quantities:

- Let $p'_{kl} = p_{kl}/p_{AB}$, where p_{AB} is the relative number of subjects scored by both raters A and B, and p_{kl} the relative number of subjects classified into categories k and l by raters A and B respectively.

- $p'_{k+} = p_{k+}/p_A$, where p_{k+} is the relative number of subjects that rater A classified into category k, and p_A the relative number of subjects that rater A has scored.

- $p'_{+l} = p_{+l}/p_B$, where p_{+l} is the relative number of subjects that rater B classified into category l, and p_B the relative number of subjects that rater B has scored.

- Any two categories k and l have a weight w_{kl} associated with them, and defined as follows:

$$
w_{kl} = \begin{cases} 1 - (x_k - x_l)^2/(x_{max} - x_{min})^2, & \text{if } k \neq l, \\ 1, & \text{if } k = l, \end{cases} \tag{3.2.5}
$$

where x_{max} and x_{min} are the largest and smallest scores respectively. The set of weights described by equation 3.2.5 is known in the literature as "Quadratic Weights."

How are these weights calculated when the scores are ordinal and alphabetic such as LOW, MEDIUM, HIGH? The commonly-used approach in this case, is to assign integer values 1,2, and 3 sequentially to categories according to their ascending order. That is 1, 2, and 3 will be assigned to LOW, MEDIUM, and HIGH respectively.

The Kappa coefficient for interval data when the number of raters is limited to two, has the following general form:

$$\widetilde{\kappa}'_{\mathrm{C}} = \frac{p_a - p_e}{1 - p_e}, \text{ where } p_a = \sum_{k,l}^{q} w_{kl} p'_{kl}, \text{ and } p_e = \sum_{k,l}^{q} w_{kl} p'_{k+} p'_{+l}, \quad (3.2.6)$$

Equation 3.2.6 describes what is known in the literature as the weighted Kappa coefficient of Cohen (1968). As suggested by Cohen (1968), when defining the weighted kappa, the researcher may well define a custom set of weights that may best described the experimental design. Later in this chapter, I will present alternative sets of weights that have been proposed in the literature.

The following example illustrates the calculation of the weighted and unweighted Kappa coefficients using a dataset that contains missing ratings.

Example 3.1 ───

Consider the rating dataset of Table 3.5 where two raters named Rater1 and Rater2 have classified 11 units into one of the three categories labeled as A, B, and C. As it appears some units where rated by only one of the two raters (units not rated by either rater must be excluded from analysis).

Table 3.5: Rating of 11 subjects by 2 Raters

Units	Rater1	Rater2
1	A	
2	B	C
3	C	C
4	C	C
5	B	B
6	B	
7	A	A
8	A	B
9	B	B
10	B	B
11		C

Table 3.6 shows the distribution of units by rater, and includes marginal totals and percentages. This summary table is convenient for experiments involving a large number of units or subjects.

Table 3.7 on the other hand, shows the quadratic weights associated with the three categories A, B, and C. These weights are assigned to the categories under the assumption that the ranking $A \rightarrow B \rightarrow C$ (i.e. C is ranked higher than B, which in turn is ranked higher than A) represents their correct ascending order. It follows from this table that all diagonal elements equal 1 and represent "full agreement," while off-diagonal elements have a weight of 0 or 0.75 representing "partial agreement." To compute these quadratic weights from equation 3.5, I initially assigned the numbers 1, 2, and 3 to the three categories A, B, and C respectively (note: if the categories are numeric, then these same numeric values must be used to compute the weights).

Table 3.6: Distribution of Subjects by Rater

Rater1	Rater 2				Total	Row %
	A	B	C	Missing		
A	1	1	0	1	3	27.3%
B	0	3	1	1	5	45.5%
C	0	0	2	0	2	18.2%
Missing	0	0	1	0	1	9.1%
Total	1	4	4	2	11	100%
Column %	9.1%	36.4%	36.4%	18.2%	110%	

The weighted Kappa is given by,

$$\widehat{\kappa}'_{\mathrm{C}} = \frac{0.9375 - 0.7194}{1 - 0.7194} = 0.7772.$$

Readers who want more details regarding these calculations may download the Excel workbook,

www.agreestat.com/book4/chapter3examples.xlsx,

which contains the "Example 3.1" worksheet with all the steps leading to the weighted Kappa. Note that if you replace quadratic weights with Identity weights where all diagonal elements equal 1, and all off-diagonal elements equal 0, then you will obtain the unweighted kappa of chapter 2. The unweighted kappa is given by,

$$\widehat{\kappa}_{\mathrm{C}} = \frac{0.75 - 0.3444}{1 - 0.3444} = 0.61864.$$

Table 3.7: Quadratic Weights for a three-Level Nominal Scale

	A	B	C
A	1	0.75	0
B	0.75	1	0.75
C	0	0.75	1

3.3   Agreement Coefficients for Interval Data: the Case of two Raters

The purpose of this section is to generalize several existing agreement coefficients so that they can be used for analyzing ordinal and interval, or ratio ratings. This generalization will be accomplished with the same approach used in section 3.2 to extend Cohen's kappa coefficient so that it can handle ratings of interval type. This approach consists of using the interval or ratio data to calculate the weights as in equation 3.2.5, which in turn are used in the weighted versions of the agreement coefficients. Among the coefficients discussed here are the Pi coefficient of Scott (1955), the Brennan-Prediger (BP) coefficient (see Brennan & Prediger, 1981), Krippendorff's alpha, and Gwet's AC_1 suggested by Gwet (2008a).

Assume that two raters A and B must assign one of q interval-type values $(x_1, \cdots, x_k, \cdots, x_q)$ to each subject.

- **Weighted Scott's Pi Coefficient**

  Let $\widehat{\kappa}'_s$ be the weighted Pi coefficient. This coefficient is defined as follows:

$$\widehat{\kappa}'_s = \frac{p_a - p_e}{1 - p_e}, \text{ where } p_a = \sum_{k,l}^{q} w_{kl} p'_{kl}, \text{ and } p_e = \sum_{k,l}^{q} w_{kl} \pi'_k \pi'_l, \qquad (3.3.1)$$

  where $\pi'_k = (p'_{k+} + p'_{+k})/2$, with p'_{k+} and p'_{+k} being defined as in section 3.2.2. Scott's coefficient is often used by researchers, although it shares the same weaknesses of Kappa. The paradoxes discussed in the previous chapter for Cohen's Kappa, will have a negative impact on Scott's Pi as well.

- **Weighted Brennan-Prediger Coefficient**

  Let $\widehat{\kappa}'_q$ be the weighted BP coefficient[3]. It is defined as,

$$\widehat{\kappa}'_q = \frac{p_a - p_e}{1 - p_e}, \text{ where } p_a = \sum_{k,l}^{q} w_{kl} p'_{kl}, \text{ and } p_e = \frac{1}{q^2} \sum_{k,l}^{q} w_{kl}. \qquad (3.3.2)$$

The BP coefficient has been extensively discussed by Brennan & Prediger (1981), and is known to be resistant to the paradoxes associated with Kappa

---

[3]Note that Brennan & Prediger (1981) discuss an unweighted agreement coefficient that can only handle nominal scores, and complete datasets with no missing ratings. I am proposing here an extension to interval data that can also handle missing ratings.

and Pi. Its percent chance agreement p_e may at times slightly overstate the propensity for raters to agree by pure chance (see Gwet 2008a).

- **Krippendorff's Alpha Coefficient**

Krippendorff (1970, 1978, 2004) has proposed an agreement coefficient known as alpha, which is often used by researchers in the area of content analysis. *For the purpose of calculating Krippendorff's alpha, only subjects rated by both raters are used. Subjects with missing ratings are excluded from the analysis altogether. Krippendorff's alpha accommodates missing ratings only in the case of raters or more.*

Let n be the number of subjects rated by both raters. Krippendorff's alpha is defined as follows:

$$\widehat{\alpha}'_{\mathrm{K}} = \frac{p_a^\star - p_e}{1 - p_e}, \text{ where } \begin{cases} p_a^\star = (1 - \varepsilon_n)p_a + \varepsilon_n, \ \varepsilon_n = 1/(2n), \\ p_a = \sum_{k,l}^{q} w_{kl}p_{kl}, \ p_e = \sum_{k,l}^{q} w_{kl}\pi_k\pi_l. \end{cases} \quad (3.3.3)$$

Note that $\pi_k = (p_{k+} + p_{+k})/2$, with p_{k+} and p_{+k} being defined as in section 3.2.2 (remember that for studies based on two raters only, all subjects with missing ratings must be removed from the dataset prior to calculating Krippendorff's alpha). One may observe that Krippendorff's alpha is very similar to the weighted Scott's Pi coefficient of equation 3.3.1. When there is no missing ratings, I expect both coefficients to yield values that are close. My formulation of Krippendorff's alpha is very different from what you will find else. It is nevertheless accurate and much simpler to implement than any other alternative formulation found in the literature.

- **Gwet's AC$_1$ Coefficient**

Let $\widehat{\kappa}'_{\mathrm{G}}$ be the weighted version of the AC$_1$ coefficient of Gwet (2008a) also referred to AC$_2$. This coefficient, which is discussed more extensively in chapter 4 is defined as follows:

$$\widehat{\kappa}'_{\mathrm{G}} = \frac{p_a - p_e}{1 - p_e}, \text{ where } \begin{cases} p_a = \sum_{k,l}^{q} w_{kl}p'_{kl}, \\ p_e = \frac{T_w}{q(q-1)} \sum_{k=1}^{q} \pi'_k(1 - \pi'_k), \end{cases} \quad (3.3.4)$$

where $\pi'_k = (p'_{k+} + p'_{+k})/2$, with p'_{k+} and p'_{+k} being defined as in section 3.2.2. T_w represents the total sum of all weight values w_{kl}.

The calculation of these coefficients is illustrated in the following example.

Example 3.2 _____

Let us consider the rating data of Table 3.5. I previously used that dataset to illustrate the calculation of the weighted kappa, and will now use it to compute the weighted Pi and BP coefficients.

Table 3.8 shows the coefficients Kappa, Pi, BP, and the percent agreement in their unweighted and weighted versions. The weighted versions of these coefficients use quadratic weights.

- Cohen's Kappa is, $\widehat{\kappa}_C = (0.9375 - 0.7194)/(1 - 0.7194) = 0.7772$.
- Gwet's AC_2 is, $\widehat{\kappa}_G = (0.9375 - 0.6309)/(1 - 0.0.6309) = 0.8307$.
- Scott's Pi is, $\widehat{\kappa}_S = (0.9375 - 0.7429)/(1 - 0.7429) = 0.7569$.
- Krippendorff's Alpha is, $\widehat{\alpha}_K = (0.9414 - 0.7578)/(1 - 0.7578) = 0.75806$.
- Brennan-Prediger coefficient is, $\widehat{\kappa}_3 = (0.9375 - 0.6667)/(1 - 0.6667) = 0.8125$.

You may find more details regarding these calculations in the "Example 3.2" worksheet of the Excel workbook,

www.agreestat.com/book4/chapter3examples.xlsx.

Table 3.8: Unweighted and Weighted Coefficients from Table 3.5 Data

Agreement Coefficient	Unweighted	Weighted
Cohen's Kappa	0.6186	0.7772
Gwet's AC_1/AC_2	0.6348	0.8307
Scott's Pi	0.6038	0.7569
Krippendorff's Alpha	0.6203	0.7581
Brenann-Prediger	0.625	0.8125
Percent Agreement	0.75	0.9375

Until now, I have discussed about various methods for calculating agreement coefficients for ordinal, and interval data when the number of raters is limited to two. In the next section, I will extend these methods to reliability studies that involve three raters or more. The focus will still be on Cohen's Kappa, Scott's Pi, and Brennan-Prediger coefficients.

3.4 Agreement Coefficients for Interval Data: the Case of three Raters or More

Equations (3.2.6), and (3.4.1) through (3.4.4) are useful for computing the extent of agreement between 2 raters using interval scores, but cannot provide a global measure of agreement among 3 raters or more. When an arbitrarily large number r

of raters must assign one of q possible interval scores to n subjects, a global inter-rater reliability coefficient is necessary and can be obtained.

Defining the Multiple-Rater Agreement Coefficient

A chance-corrected agreement coefficient between two raters labeled as g and h generally takes the following form:

$$\widehat{\kappa}(g, h) = \frac{p_a(g, h) - p_e(g, h)}{1 - p_e(g, h)} = 1 - \frac{1 - p_a(g, h)}{1 - p_e(g, h)}, \qquad (3.4.1)$$

which is the expression I previously used to extend Kappa to interval data following the approach of Janson and Olsson (2001). The generalization to the case of three raters or more can be accomplished as follows:

- First form all possible pairs (g, h) of raters out of the initial set of r raters. There is a total of $r(r-1)/2$ such pairs.

- Average separately the two expressions $\left[1 - p_a(g, h)\right]$ and $\left[1 - p_e(g, h)\right]$ across all $r(r-1)/2$ pairs of raters. This operation produces two averages, one for the numerator, and another one for the denominator.

- The generalized agreement coefficient is then obtained by replacing the pair-specific ratio $\left[1 - p_a(g, h)\right]/\left[1 - p_e(g, h)\right]$ of equation 3.4.1 with the ratio of the two averages calculated in the previous step.

This is the approach that Conger (1980) used to obtain the correct generalization of Cohen's Kappa to the case of three raters or more.

Consider an experiment involving 3 raters A, B, and C. The number of raters is $r = 3$, and $3 \times (3 - 1)/2 = 3$ pairs of raters can be formed out of that group of raters. These pairs are (A,B), (A,C), and (B,C). Therefore, I can compute agreement coefficients (using one of the equations 3.2.6, 3.3.1, or 3.3.2) separately for each of the three pairs. This produces a percent agreement p_a, and a percent chance agreement p_e for each of the pairs. Both quantities can then be used as described above to obtained the global agreement coefficient.

The procedure I just described is purely definitional. Its purpose is to explain how multiple-rater agreement coefficients are defined. In practice however, I would use a more efficient computational procedure to analyze the rating data. In the remaining portion of this section, I define Conger's and Fleiss' versions of the weighted Kappa, as well as the Brennan-Prediger coefficient for multiple raters.

Formulating the Multiple-Rater Agreement Coefficient

Let r_{ik} be the number of raters who assigned a particular score x_k to subject i (note that this could well be the number of raters who classified subject i into category k if categories are used in the study as opposed to numeric scores). The number of raters who has scored subject i is denoted by r_i. I will always assume that only the subjects scored by one rater or more will be included in the analysis. Likewise, q denotes the number of categories (or numeric scores) susceptible to be used by a rater. Researchers are expected to ensure that all categories or scores are are well chosen and have a reasonable chance of being used. Categories deemed unlikely to be used should not be part of any inter-rater reliability experiment.

Let n_{gk} be the number of subjects associated with rater g and score x_k, and n_g the number of subjects scored by rater g . The agreement coefficients are defined as follows:

- ### Conger's Kappa

  Conger's version of the generalized Kappa (Conger, A.J. 1980) is defined as follows:

$$\widehat{\kappa}_{\mathrm{C}} = \frac{p_a - p_e}{1 - p_e}, \quad \text{where} \quad \begin{cases} p_a = \dfrac{1}{n'} \displaystyle\sum_{i=1}^{n'} \sum_{k=1}^{q} \frac{r_{ik}\left(r_{ik}^{\star} - 1\right)}{r_i(r_i - 1)}, \\[2ex] p_e = \displaystyle\sum_{k,l} w_{kl}\left(\overline{p}_{+k}\overline{p}_{+l} - s_{kl}^2/r\right). \end{cases} \tag{3.4.2}$$

Note that n' is the number of subjects that were rated by two raters or more. The expressions $r_{ik}^{\star}$, $\overline{p}_{+k}$, p_{gk}, and s_{kl}^2 used in the calculation of the percent agreement and percent chance agreement are defined as follows:

$$r_{ik}^{\star} = \sum_{l=1}^{q} w_{kl}r_{il}, \quad \overline{p}_{+k} = \frac{1}{r}\sum_{g=1}^{r} p_{gk}, \tag{3.4.3}$$

$$p_{gk} = \frac{n_{gk}}{n_g}, \text{ and } s_{kl}^2 = \frac{1}{r-1}\left(\sum_{g=1}^{r} p_{gk}p_{gl} - r\overline{p}_{+k}\overline{p}_{+l}\right). \tag{3.4.4}$$

For a specific score x_k, agreement is determined not only by looking at the number of raters r_{ik} associated with subject i and score x_k, but also by looking at the other scores x_l that represent partial agreement with x_k. Two scores x_k and x_l (with $k \neq l$) are in partial agreement when the weight w_{kl} is nonzero. The contribution of scores other than x_k to the extent of agreement with respect to x_k is determined by the value of $r_{ik}^\star$, the weighted sum of the r_{il}'s for all categories $l = 1, \cdots, q$.

- **Brennan-Prediger**

The Brennan-Prediger agreement coefficient (Brennan & Prediger, 1981) is defined as follows:

$$\widehat{\kappa}_{\mathrm{Q}}' = \frac{p_a - p_e}{1 - p_e}, \text{ where } p_e = \frac{1}{q^2} \sum_{k,l} w_{kl}, \tag{3.4.5}$$

and p_a is defined as in equation 3.4.2.

- **Fleiss' Kappa**

Fleiss' Kappa (Fleiss, 1971)[4] is defined as follows:

$$\widehat{\kappa}_{\mathrm{F}}' = \frac{p_a - p_e}{1 - p_e}, \text{ where } p_e = \sum_{k,l} w_{kl} \pi_k \pi_l, \tag{3.4.6}$$

p_a is defined as in equation 3.4.2, and π_k is given by,

$$\pi_k = \frac{1}{n} \sum_{i=1}^{n} \frac{r_{ik}}{r_i}. \tag{3.4.7}$$

Note that Fleiss' version of kappa was not derived along the lines of Janson & Olsson(2001). It uses a percent chance agreement p_e, which is a straight generalization of its two-rater version. The only difference between the two-rater and the multiple-rater versions of Fleiss' kappa is the use of a different formulation for the π_k probabilities.

- **Krippendorff's Alpha Coefficient**

In the previous section, I introduced the alpha coefficient of Krippendorff (1970, 1978, 2004) in the case of two raters. The multiple-rater version of this coefficient will now be discussed. Once again, my formulation of the alpha coefficient is different from that of Krippendorff, although both formulations yield the exact same result. My formulation provides a much simpler and more efficient computational procedure, in addition to making it possible to derive a simple

---

[4]Fleiss (1971) proposed a generalized unweighted kappa coefficient that extended Kappa to three raters or more. Fleiss' Kappa only handles nominal data, and cannot accommodate missing ratings. I am extending it here to interval ratings, and to subjects with missing ratings.

variance estimator as shown in chapter 5. Furthermore, the comparison between the alpha coefficient and other multiple-rater chance-corrected agreement coefficients presented earlier in this chapter, will be considerable facilitated.

Note that for the purpose of calculating Krippendorff's alpha, all subjects rated by a single observer only or not rated at all must be excluded from the analysis altogether.

Let us introduce a few terms:

$\Rightarrow$ n' designates the number of subjects rated by 2 observers or more, and n the total count of subjects that participated in the reliability experiment.

$\Rightarrow$ r_i is the count of raters who scored subject i.

$\Rightarrow$ $\bar{r}$ is the average value of the r_i's. That is, the mean number of raters who scored a subject.

Let $\varepsilon_n = 1/(n'\bar{r})$. The alpha coefficient is defined as follows:

$$\widehat{\alpha}_{\mathrm{K}} = \frac{p_a - p_e}{1 - p_e}, \quad \text{where} \quad \begin{cases} p_a &= (1 - \varepsilon_n)p'_a + \varepsilon_n, \\ p'_a &= \frac{1}{n'} \sum_{i=1}^{n'} \sum_{k=1}^{q} \frac{r_{ik}(r^{\star}_{ik} - 1)}{\bar{r}(r_i - 1)}, \\ p_e &= \sum_{k,l} w_{kl} \pi_k \pi_l, \end{cases} \tag{3.4.8}$$

The $r^{\star}_{ik}$ and π_k quantities used to compute the percent agreement and percent chance agreement are given by,

$$r^{\star}_{ik} = \sum_{l=1}^{q} w_{kl} r_{il}, \text{ and } \pi_k = \frac{1}{n'} \sum_{i=1}^{n'} \frac{r_{ik}}{\bar{r}} \tag{3.4.9}$$

Krippendorff's alpha is in fact very similar to Fleiss' generalized Kappa $\widehat{\kappa}_{\mathrm{F}}$ presented earlier, especially when there is no missing ratings. Both coefficients differ in their treatment of missing ratings, and in the percent agreement p_a they are based upon.

- **Gwet's AC$_1$ Coefficient**

The AC$_2$ coefficient, which is the weighted version of Gwet's AC$_1$ coefficient (c.f. Gwet, 2008a) is discussed extensively in chapter 4. It is defined as follows:

$$\widehat{\kappa}_{G} = \frac{p_a - p_e}{1 - p_e}, \ \text{where} \ \begin{cases} p_a = \dfrac{1}{n'} \displaystyle\sum_{i=1}^{n'} \sum_{k=1}^{q} \dfrac{r_{ik}\left(r_{ik}^{\star} - 1\right)}{r_i(r_i - 1)}, \\[2ex] p_e = \dfrac{T_w}{q(q-1)} \displaystyle\sum_{k,l} \pi_k(1 - \pi_k). \end{cases} \tag{3.4.10}$$

Note that n' is the number of subjects that were rated by two raters or more, and r_i the number of raters who actually rated subject i. The expressions $r_{ik}^{\star}$, and π_k are defined as follows:

$$r_{ik}^{\star} = \sum_{l=1}^{q} w_{kl} r_{il}, \ \text{and} \ \pi_k = \frac{1}{n} \sum_{i=1}^{n} \frac{r_{ik}}{r_i}. \tag{3.4.11}$$

Once again, for a specific score x_k, agreement is determined by looking at all scores x_l that are in partial agreement with x_k in the sense that the weight w_{kl} associated with both scores is nonzero. The contribution of scores other than x_k to the extent of agreement with respect to x_k is determined by the value of $r_{ik}^{\star}$, the weighted sum of the r_{il}'s for all categories $l = 1, \cdots, q$.

Example 3.3

To illustrate the calculation of the five multiple-rater agreement coefficients presented in this section, I will consider the rating data of Table 3.9. One of the 5 scores 0.5, 1.0, 1.5, 2.0, and 2.5 is assigned to the subjects by the 4 raters labeled as L, K, W, and B. Since the ratings are of interval type, it is natural to use a weighted coefficient to analyze them. You may also have noticed that this data contains missing ratings. Subject "a.logan" for example was scored by raters K and W only.

Table 3.10 shows the quadratic weights used for calculating the different weighted agreement coefficients, and are calculated based on equation 3.2.5 and Table 3.9 numeric scores. I will only show the main results of this analysis. Those wanting to see detailed calculations, will find them in the "Example 3.3" worksheet of the Excel workbook,

www.agreestat.com/book4/chapter3examples.xlsx.

The weighted percent agreement, which is common to all weighted coefficients except to Krippendorff's alpha is given by $p_a = 0.9206$. Krippendorff's weighted percent agreement is given by $p_a = 0.9364$. However, all agreement coefficients have different percent chance agreement values. These agreement coefficients are given by,

- Conger's Weighted Kappa is, $\widehat{\kappa}_c = (0.9206 - 0.8314)/(1 - 0.8314) = 0.5290$.
- Brennan-Prediger Weighted Kappa is, $\widehat{\kappa}_4 = (0.9206 - 0.75)/(1 - 0.75) = 0.6823$.

- Fleiss' Weighted Kappa, $\widehat{\kappa}_C = (0.9206 - 0.8377)/(1 - 0.8377) = 0.5107$.
- Gwet's Weighted AC_1, $\widehat{\kappa}_G = (0.9206 - 0.6462)/(1 - 0.6462) = 0.7755$.
- Krippendorff's Alpha, $\widehat{\alpha}_K = (0.9364 - 0.8336)/(1 - 0.8336) = 0.6180$. Krippendorff's percent agreement is obtained as $p_a = (1 - 1/(16 \times 3.5)) \times 0.9353 + 1/(16 \times 3.5) = 0.9364$.

Table 3.9: Scores assigned to 16 subjects by 4 Raters

Subject	L	K	W	B
a.lycia	1	1.5	1	
a.milbe	2	2	2	2
a.hegon	0.5	1	1.5	1.5
a.oslar	1	1	1	1
a.viali	1	1	1	1.5
a.logan		1	2.5	
a.numit	2.5	2.5	2.5	2.5
a.saraa	1	1		1
a.sarat		1	2	1
a.mormo	1	1	0.5	1
a.celti	1.5	1.5	1.5	1.5
a.clyto	1	1.5	1	
a.hiann	1	1	1.5	
b.phile	1	2	2.5	2
b.alask		1	1.5	1
b.taad	0.5	0.5	0.5	0.5

Table 3.10: Quadratic Weights Associated with Table 3.9 Data

	0.5	1	1.5	2	2.5
0.5	1	0.9375	0.75	0.4375	0
1	0.9375	1	0.9375	0.75	0.4375
1.5	0.75	0.9375	1	0.9375	0.75
2	0.4375	0.75	0.9375	1	0.9375
2.5	0	0.4375	0.75	0.9375	1

As will often be the case, Gwet's AC_2 coefficient is higher than Brennan-Prediger coefficient, which in turn is higher than Conger's, Fleiss', and Krippendorff's. This is due to the tendency that the methods of Conger, Fleiss, and Krippendorff have to overstate the percent chance agreement.

3.5   More Weighting Options for Agreement Coefficients

I introduced and motivated the notion of weighting in section 2.6 of chapter 2 with the weighted Kappa coefficient of Cohen (1968). In the beginning of this chapter, I showed how the Janson-Olsson approach to interval data and the use of the Euclidean distance led to the quadratic weights. However, the researcher should not be restricted to quadratic weights when analyzing reliability data. Cohen (1968) even suggested the possibility of using custom weights if they are deemed more appropriate for a specific study. In this section, I will present a few additional sets of weights that the researcher may consider. Some of these weights have been suggested by various authors in the literature, others are proposed by us.

Ordinal Weights

I indicated earlier in this chapter that quadratic weights may be used with non-numeric ordinal data by first assigning integer values sequentially (i.e. 1, 2, 3, $\cdots$) to the ordinal scores following their ascending order. However, the choice of integer values is subjective, and the notion of subtraction used for calculating quadratic weights may not apply well to non-numeric ordinal ratings. Therefore, the researcher may consider *ordinal weights* defined as follows:

$$w_{kl} = \begin{cases} 1 - M_{kl}/M_{1q} & \text{if } k \neq l, \\ 1 & \text{if } k = l. \end{cases} \tag{3.5.1}$$

$M_{kl} = \#\{(i,j) : \min(k,l) \leq i < j \leq \max(k,l)\}$ represents the number of pairs (i,j) (with $i < j$), which can be formed with numbers between $\min(k,l)$ and $\max(k,l)$. Note that 1 and q are assumed to be the lowest and highest ranked categories. A straightforward way of calculating M_{kl} is to first assign integer values sequentially to the categories, and to use the following expression:

$$M_{kl} = \binom{\max(k,l) - \min(k,l) + 1}{2}, \tag{3.5.2}$$

which represents the number of combinations of 2 out of $\max(k,l) - \min(k,l) + 1$. This set of weights only uses the order structure of the ratings, and does not appeal to the notion of distance. The following example illustrates the calculation of ordinal weights.

Example 3.4 _____

Suppose that your reliability study consists of classifying subjects into 5 ordinal categories that are listed in ascending order as A, B, C, D, and E. The ordinal weights associated with these categories are given in Table 3.11. It appears that an A-B or

B-A disagreement carries a substantial weight of 0.9. But the ordinal weight decreases as the gap between 2 categories widens. To compute the ordinal weights of Table 3.11, note that $M_{max} = \binom{5-1+1}{2} = 10$. The weight 0.9 associated with categories A and B is labeled as w_{12} (1 is for A, and 2 is for B), and is calculated as $w_{12} = 1 - M_{12}/M_{max}$, where $M_{12} = \binom{2-1+1}{2} = 1$ following equation 3.15. Consequently, $w_{12} = 1 - 1/10 = 1 - 0.1 = 0.9$.

Table 3.11: Simple Ordinal Weights

	A	B	C	D	E
A	1.0	0.9	0.7	0.4	0.0
B	0.9	1.0	0.9	0.7	0.4
C	0.7	0.9	1.0	0.9	0.7
D	0.4	0.7	0.9	1.0	0.9
E	0.0	0.4	0.7	0.9	1.0

- The use of ordinal weights requires the categories to be at least of ordinal type. One should be able to rank all categories from the smallest to the largest.

- The actual values of the ratings do not affect the magnitude of ordinal weights. Only their ranks do. Note that these ordinal weights are not related to Krippendorff's ordinal distance (see Krippendorff, 2011) based on observed ratings, which become available only after the experiment.

Linear Weights

The linear weights are defined as follows:

$$
w_{kl} = \begin{cases} 1 - \dfrac{|x_k - x_l|}{\max_{i,j} |x_i - x_j|}, & \text{if } k \neq l, \\ 1, & \text{if } k = l, \end{cases} \tag{3.5.3}
$$

where $|\cdot|$ represents the absolute value function. The values taken by the linear weights depend on whether the ratings are of alphabetic or numeric type. If the ratings are alphabetic, then they are numbered sequentially from 1 to the number of categories, and these numbers are used to create the weights. If the ratings are already numeric, then these rating values should be used. Linear weights have been suggested in the literature (see Cohen, 1968), and have already been implemented in many software packages. The linear weights are generally smaller than the quadratic weights.

Radical Weights

For researchers who find quadratic and linear weights too large, I propose the use of *Radical weights*. The radical weights are defined as follows:

$$
w_{kl} = \begin{cases} 1 - \dfrac{\sqrt{|x_k - x_l|}}{\max\limits_{i,j} \sqrt{|x_i - x_j|}}, & \text{if } k \neq l, \\ \\ 1, & \text{if } k = l. \end{cases} \tag{3.5.4}
$$

The values taken by radical weights depend on whether the ratings are of alphabetic or numeric type. If the ratings are alphabetic, then they are numbered sequentially from 1 to the number of categories, and these numbers will be used to create the weights. If the ratings are already numeric, then these rating values are used for calculating the weights.

Ratio Weights

Ratio weights have been used (although in the form of distance functions) by Krippendorff (1970, 1978, 2004), and can be used with rating data of ratio type. This set of weights is defined as follows:

$$
w_{kl} = 1 - \frac{\left[(x_k - x_l)/(x_k + x_l)\right]^2}{\left[(x_{\text{Max}} - x_{\text{Min}})/(x_{\text{Max}} + x_{\text{Min}})\right]^2}, \tag{3.5.5}
$$

where x_k and x_l are two arbitrary scores, x_{Max} and x_{Min} are the maximum and minimum scores respectively. Ratio weights evaluate the differences between scores relative to their magnitudes. If these weights are used with non-numeric ordinal data, then one may need to assign integer values to the ratings before calculating the weights.

Circular Weights

Circular weights have also be used by Krippendorff (1970, 1978, 2004) in the form of a metric difference. These weights would be recommended if the rating represents the magnitude of an angle expressed in degrees or in radians. The endpoints in this case are generally considered to be close, and expected to be associated with large weights.

Let x_{Max} and x_{Min} be respectively the largest and smallest values on the scoring scale. For $U = x_{\text{Max}} - x_{\text{Min}} + 1$, the circular weights are defined as follows:

- If the sine function's argument is in degrees then,

$$w_{kl} = 1 - \frac{\left(\sin\left[180(x_k - x_l)/U\right]\right)^2}{M}, \tag{3.5.6}$$

where $M = \max\limits_{k,l} \left(\sin\left[180(x_k - x_l)/U\right]\right)^2$.

- If the sine function's argument is in radians then,

$$w_{kl} = 1 - \frac{\left(\sin\left[\pi(x_k - x_l)/U\right]\right)^2}{M}, \tag{3.5.7}$$

where $M = \max\limits_{k,l} \left(\sin\left[\pi(x_k - x_l)/U\right]\right)^2$.

Bipolar Weights

The bipolar weights, which behave like ratio weights at the center of the scale and like quadratic weights towards the ends, are defined as follows:

$$w_{kl} = \begin{cases} 1 - \dfrac{(x_k - x_l)^2}{M\left[(x_k + x_l) - 2x_{\text{Min}}\right]\left[2x_{\text{Max}} - (x_k + x_l)\right]}, & \text{if } k \neq l, \\ 1, & \text{if } k = l, \end{cases} \tag{3.5.8}$$

where M is defined by,

$$M = \max\limits_{k,l} \frac{(x_k - x_l)^2}{\left[(x_k + x_l) - 2x_{\text{Min}}\right]\left[2x_{\text{Max}} - (x_k + x_l)\right]}.$$

Example 3.5 _____

      To illustrate the magnitude of these different weights, let us consider a reliability experiment that consists of raters who assign one of the 5 scores $\{1, 2, 3, 4, 5\}$ to subjects. The associated weights are displayed in Tables 3.12 through 3.19. The main difference between these weights is the importance they assign to scores representing a disagreement. The researcher will have the responsibility to determine the set of weights appropriate for the study being conducted.

Table 3.12: Identity Weights

Score	Score				
	1	2	3	4	5
1	1	0	0	0	0
2	0	1	0	0	0
3	0	0	1	0	0
4	0	0	0	1	0
5	0	0	0	0	1

Table 3.13: Radical Weights

Score	Score				
	1	2	3	4	5
1	1	0.5	0.29	0.13	0
2	0.5	1	0.5	0.29	0.13
3	0.29	0.5	1	0.5	0.29
4	0.13	0.29	0.5	1	0.5
5	0	0.13	0.29	0.5	1

Table 3.14: Linear Weights

Score	Score				
	1	2	3	4	5
1	1	0.75	0.5	0.25	0
2	0.75	1	0.75	0.5	0.25
3	0.5	0.75	1	0.75	0.5
4	0.25	0.5	0.75	1	0.75
5	0	0.25	0.5	0.75	1

Table 3.15: Quadratic Weights

Score	Score				
	1	2	3	4	5
1	1	0.94	0.75	0.44	0
2	0.94	1	0.94	0.75	0.44
3	0.75	0.94	1	0.94	0.75
4	0.44	0.75	0.94	1	0.94
5	0	0.44	0.75	0.94	1

Table 3.16: Ordinal Weights

Score	Score				
	1	2	3	4	5
1	1	0.9	0.7	0.4	0
2	0.9	1	0.9	0.7	0.4
3	0.7	0.9	1	0.9	0.7
4	0.4	0.7	0.9	1	0.9
5	0	0.4	0.7	0.9	1

Table 3.17: Ratio Weights

Score	Score				
	1	2	3	4	5
1	1	0.75	0.44	0.19	0
2	0.75	1	0.91	0.75	0.59
3	0.44	0.91	1	0.95	0.86
4	0.19	0.75	0.95	1	0.97
5	0	0.59	0.86	0.97	1

Table 3.18: Circular Weights

Score	Score				
	1	2	3	4	5
1	1	0.62	0	0	0.62
2	0.62	1	0.62	0	0
3	0	0.62	1	0.62	0
4	0	0	0.62	1	0.62
5	0.62	0	0	0.62	1

Table 3.19: Bipolar Weights

Score	Score				
	1	2	3	4	5
1	1	0.86	0.67	0.4	0
2	0.86	1	0.93	0.75	0.4
3	0.67	0.93	1	0.93	0.67
4	0.4	0.75	0.93	1	0.86
5	0	0.4	0.67	0.86	1

The numbering of these categories is arbitrary and may be replaced with more meaningful numbers. If for example the 5 category levels {1,2,3,4,5} were obtained by categorizing a continuous score using ranges of values, then the range middle points may produce a more efficient scoring system than the arbitrary numbers $\{1, 2, 3, 4, 5\}$. Two consecutive categories need not be a single point apart. One pair of two consecutive categories could represent a higher level of partial agreement than another pair of consecutive categories, and this should be reflected in the scoring system.

There is no formal rule that can be used for deciding which set weights should be used in a particular inter-rater reliability study. The researcher needs to determine how much each type of disagreement (or partial agreement) should impact the agreement coefficient, and select the set of weights accordingly.

In order to visualize the impact that the different weighting schemes may have on the inter-rater reliability coefficient, let us consider the ratings shown in Table 3.20. These ratings were collected during an experiment where three raters classified 10 subjects into one of the five possible categories labeled as 1, 2, 3, 4, and 5.

Table 3.20: Rating of 10 Subjects by 3 Raters

Subject	Rater 1	Rater 2	Rater 3
1	3	4	5
2	4	5	3
3	3	3	3
4	2	3	1
5	4	4	4
6	4	2	1
7	5	4	5
8	3	3	5
9	2	3	4
10	5	5	5

Figure 3.5.1 for example shows two curves. The black curve represents the raters' unweighted percent agreement with respect to each subject, while the gray curve represents the raters' weighted percent agreement with respect to each subject based on quadratic weights. Note that the percent agreement of equation 3.4.2 for example is the average of all subject-level percent agreement values for subjects rated by two raters or more. These subject-level percent agreement values were calculated separately here to construct figures 3.5.1 through 3.5.6.

It appears that quadratic and bipolar weights tend to increase agreement considerably, while radical and circular apply a more moderate adjustment. The researcher may look at all these graphs and determine which weights will best represent the best strategy to account for partial agreements.

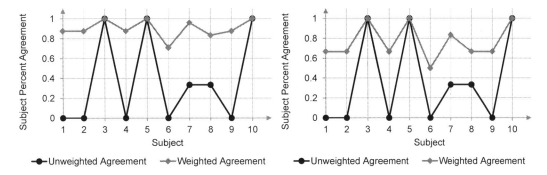

Figure 3.5.1: Unweighted and Weighted Percent Agreement - Quadratic Weights -

Figure 3.5.2: Unweighted and Weighted Percent Agreement - Linear Weights -

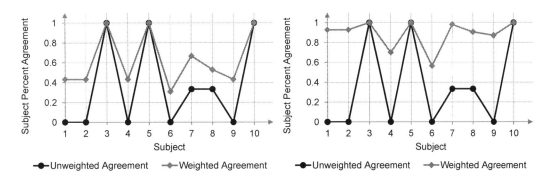

Figure 3.5.3: Unweighted and Weighted Percent Agreement - Radical Weights -

Figure 3.5.4: Unweighted and Weighted Percent Agreement - Ratio Weights -

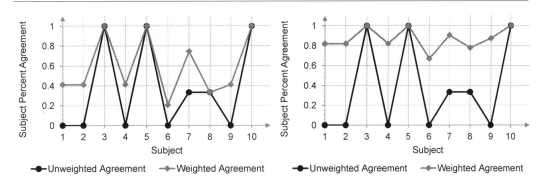

Figure 3.5.5: Unweighted and Weighted Percent Agreement - Circular Weights -

Figure 3.5.6: Unweighted and Weighted Percent Agreement - Bipolar Weights -

3.6   Concluding Remarks

There are two objectives that I wanted to achieve in this chapter: (1) To present the method of Janson and Olsson (2004) that provides a systematic way to extend any chance-corrected agreement coefficient to analyze ratings that are of ordinal or interval types, (2) To present the weighted version of several agreement coefficients that can handle missing ratings, and can use various sets of predefined and custom weights. The Janson-Olsson method made it possible to obtain weighted versions of Cohen's kappa, Scott's Pi, Conger's kappa, Gwet's AC_1, Brennan-Prediger coefficient, or Krippendorff's alpha.

The notion of weighted agreement coefficient introduced by Cohen (1968) has proved useful in many applications. It is indeed understandable that some "slight" disagreements would reveal a common view that two raters have about a particular subject's condition, while other disagreements may indicate a wide gap in the perception the two raters have about the same subject. Therefore, it became necessary to have a agreement coefficient that can incorporate these different degrees of disagreement to provide a more accurate representation of the "true" extent to which the views of the different raters converge. Weighting in this sense is an essential technique when the ratings present an ordinal structure at the minimum. Cohen (1968) confined himself to the case of two raters, and the Kappa coefficient. I extended the presentation of weighted coefficients in this chapter to the more general situation involving three raters or more.

The different weighted agreement coefficients are presented separately for two-rater and multiple-rater inter-rater reliability experiments. This is done for convenience since input ratings are generally organized differently in both situations. When the number of raters is three or more, all weighted agreement coefficients use the same weighted percent agreement except Krippendorff's alpha, whose weighted percent agreement is based on a slightly different expression. The difference between Krippendorff's alpha and Fleiss' generalized kappa remains negligible.

I also presented several predefined sets of weights that you may use with your agreement coefficients of choice. As previously mentioned, there is no recipe for selecting the optimal set of weights. However, all weights aim at incorporating some partial agreements into the calculation of the agreement coefficient. The extent to which you want partial agreements to impact the agreement coefficient can help decide which weight is appropriate. Perfect agreements are assigned a full weight of 1, and partial agreements a smaller weight. If some partial agreements are near as important as the perfect agreements then these partial agreements may be assigned a weight of 0.9 for example. Total disagreements receive a weight of 0. I presented Figures 3.5.1 to 3.5.6 to show how the different sets of weights treat partial agreements. An examination of these figures may help the researcher decide which set of weights is more appropriate for a particular analysis.

Although the weighted agreement coefficients can be used with ratings of interval and even of ratio type, one should remember that chance-corrected agreement coefficients can be used only when the inter-rater reliability experiment produces a limited number of predetermined ratings. Weighted or not, the chance-corrected agreement coefficients cannot handle ratings that belong to a continuum or are unknown prior to the experiment being conducted. In this particular situation, one needs to use intraclass correlation coefficients that are discussed in the third part of this book.

Figure 3.6.1 shows a flowchart describing the conditions under which different weights and weighted agreement coefficients are used. It appears that knowing the data type associated with your ratings is essential for selecting the correct set of weights, and the correct equation for calculating the agreement coefficient. For example if your ratings are purely ordinal, and cannot be treated as interval or ratio data, then the choice of weights that can be used is limited to ordinal weights. The other weights require some arithmetic operations such as subtraction, or division which may not carry any meaning when performed on ordinal ratings. I did not recommend a particular agreement coefficient, even though I discussed the strengths and weaknesses of many of them, and did not conceal my preference for the AC_2 coefficient. The reader is encouraged to experiment with some of these coefficients and to compare their properties.

Zhao et al. (2013) have attempted to compare various chance-corrected agreement coefficients, and the conditions under which one might be preferred over alternatives. I found this study insightful to some extent, provided one is willing to adopt the framework used for comparing the coefficients. Note that Zhao et al. (2013) have studied exclusively the magnitude of the different indexes, and did not attempt to validate them. They did not ask whether the different coefficients were even measuring what they are supposed to measure. For example they included in their analysis the Perreault & Leigh's coefficient (c.f. Perreault & Leigh - 1989), which is the only index I vehemently reject, because it was obtained following a false mathematical derivation as I mentioned in chapter 1.

Chapter 4 discusses in great details the notions of agreement, and chance agreement, and how they are used to derive two chance-corrected agreement coefficients: (i) Aickin's Alpha, and (ii) Gwet's AC_1. All assumptions and underlying models are discussed at length. The discussions in chapter 4 do not start with a description of computation procedures. Instead, the very concept of inter-rater reliability is defined in a formal way within a particular theoretical framework. Statistical methods are then described showing how the coefficients can be computed using observed ratings.

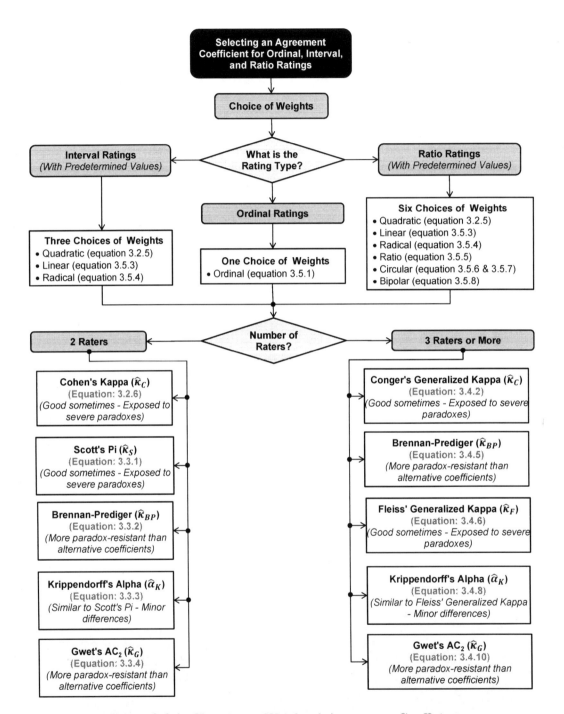

Figure 3.6.1: Choosing a Weighted Agreement Coefficient

CHAPTER $\boxed{4}$

Constructing Agreement Coefficients: AC_1 and Aickin's α

OBJECTIVE

This chapter presents a detailed discussion of two paradox-resistant alternative agreement coefficients named the AC_1 and Aickin's α (not to be confounded with Krippendorff's α of the previous chapter) proposed by Gwet (2008a) and Aickin (1990) respectively. These two agreement coefficients will be constructed step by step, from the definition of the theoretical construct to the formulation of the coefficient. All intermediary steps, which include the underlying statistical model, and the subject and rater population parameters will be spelled out. This chapter focuses particularly on the AC_1 coefficient, and aims at providing a detailed account of its real meaning, its advantages, and possible limitations. Also discussed is Gwet's AC_2, the extension of AC_1 to ordinal, interval and ratio ratings

CONTENTS

"There is no true value of any characteristic, state, or condition that is defined in terms of measurement or observation. Change of procedure for measurement (change in operational definition) or observation produces a new number $\cdots$. There is no such thing as a fact concerning an empirical observation."

- Edwards Deming (1900-1993) -

4.1   Overview

In this chapter, I discuss two particular agreement coefficients: (1) the AC_1 statistic proposed by Gwet (2008a) as a paradox-resistant alternative to the unstable Kappa coefficient, and (2) the alpha (α) coefficient of Aickin[1] (1990), an inter-reliability statistic based on a clear-cut definition of the notion of "extent of agreement among raters." I present the reader with a clear view of a step-by-step construction of an agreement coefficient, and will conduct an elaborate discussion of the underlying assumptions. Both coefficients differ from Kappa mainly in the way the percent chance agreement is calculated. As a matter of fact, the notion of chance agreement is pivotal in the study of chance-corrected agreement coefficients. Understanding it well is essential for developing effective agreement coefficients. The poor statistical properties of Kappa for example stem precisely from the inadequate approach used to evaluate the percent chance agreement.

Several authors have justified the Kappa coefficient on the ground that it represents the difference between the observed percent agreement (p_a) and the percent chance agreement[2] (p_e), which is normalized by its maximum value ($1 - p_e$) so that the coefficient is confined within the $(0, 1)$ interval. The problem is that this whole operation describes something that may not even be remotely close to what raters actually do. My views on this are more in line with Grove et al. (1981)   who while talking about what diagnosticians in the medical field actually do said this: *"They assign the easy cases or textbook cases, to diagnoses with little or not error; they may guess or diagnose randomly on the others. If one knew which cases were textbook cases, one could them separately; but that is a difficult matter."* I strongly believe that the distinction between textbook and non-textbook cases is the crux of the matter. Confronting this issue head-on is as important and difficult as it is inevitable, and how it is approached might decide how good or bad the agrement coefficient will turn out to be.

Grove et al. (1981) describes Kappa's percent chance agreement in the following

---

[1]Not to be confounded with Krippendorff's alpha, which is an entirely different coefficient discussed in the previous chapters.

[2]Chance agreement here stands for agreement when two raters assign ratings to subjects randomly.

terms: "When in doubt on a nontextbook case, each rater mentally flips a biased coin, with the probability of getting heads (giving the diagnosis) equal to his own base rates ..." This characterization of Kappa's percent chance agreement is likely too generous because Kappa's percent chance agreement does not behave near as well. The problem stems from the first 3 words "When in doubt" of this quote. In fact, there nothing considered to be an integral part of kappa, which suggests that its expression for chance-agreement probability applies only when the raters are in doubt. Kappa expression does not incorporate an estimate of the nontextbook or uncertain cases.

The Kappa and Pi coefficients rely on a percent chance agreement or chance-agreement probability expression that is valid only under the improbable assumption that all ratings are known to be independent even before the experiment had been carried out. To justify the two expressions used to evaluate the chance-agreement probabilities of Kappa and Pi, the reasoning was that if the processes by which two raters classify a subject are statistically independent, then the probability that they agree is the product of the individual probabilities of classification into the category of agreement. However, raters often rate the same subjects, and are therefore expected to produce ratings that are dependent with possibly a few exceptions when they are in doubt.

Throughout this chapter, I consider that independence occurs when a nondeterministic[3] rating (generally associated with hard or nontextbook cases) is assigned to a subject that is hard to rate. Nondeterministic ratings may be expected on a small fraction of subjects only, and certainly not on the whole subject sample or population. The AC_1 of Gwet(2008a), and the alpha of Aickin (1990) are based upon the more realistic assumption that only a portion of the observed ratings will potentially lead to agreement by chance. The difficulty to overcome will be to estimate the percent of subjects that are associated with a nondeterministic rating.

When I started working on an alternative to the Kappa coefficient, I was unaware of Aickin's work. I learned about it only after the publication in Gwet (2008a), of the ideas to be discussed here. I then discovered that the framework I proposed was made more general by allowing the group of textbook subjects to be specific to each rater instead of being unique for all raters as Aickin assumed. Moreover, my conceptual definition of the extent of agreement among raters differ from Aickin's. That is both coefficients do not quantify the same concept. Aickin's alpha coefficient for two raters represents the portion of the entire population of subjects that both raters are expected to classify identically for cause, as opposed to classifying them identically by chance. To see what Gwet's AC_1 for two raters conceptually represents,

---

[3]The process of rating a subject is considered *nondeterministic* if it has no apparent connection with the subject's characteristics.

imagine that all subjects to be classified into identical categories by pure chance are first identified, then removed from the population of subjects. This operation creates a new trimmed population of subjects where agreement by chance would be impossible. The AC_1 coefficient is the relative number of subjects in the trimmed subject population upon which the raters are expected to agree. AC_1 and alpha coefficients both represent a probability of agreement for cause, which are calculated with respect to two different reference subject populations. Although it is limited to two raters only, I have found Aickin's proposal useful and decided to include it into the discussions.

Among Kappa's strengths is a genuine attempt to correct the percent agreement for chance agreement, and the simplicity with which this was done. Among its limitations are the paradoxes described by Feinstein and Cicchetti (1990), where Kappa would yield a low value when the raters show high agreement. In this chapter I propose the AC_1 coefficient, which has some similarities with Kappa in its formulation and its simplicity, in addition to being paradox-resistant. The alpha coefficient is also close to Kappa in its form. But unlike Kappa and AC_1, the alpha coefficient is computation-intensive with its iterative procedure. AC_1 and alpha both share the same feature of being paradox-resistant.

4.2 Gwet's AC_1 and Aickin's α for two Raters

This section describes the procedures for computing the AC_1 and α coefficients in the case of two raters classifying a sample of n subjects into one of q possible categories. The calculation of these coefficients will also be illustrated in a numerical example.

4.2.1 The AC_1 Statistic

Let us consider a two-rater reliability experiment based on a q-level nominal measurement scale. As previously indicated, rating data resulting from such an experiment could be conveniently organized in a contingency table such as Table 2.7 in chapter 2. The AC_1 coefficient denoted[4] by $\widehat{\gamma}_1$ is defined as follows:

$$\widehat{\gamma}_1 = \frac{p_a - p_e}{1 - p_e}, \ \text{with } p_a = \sum_{k=1}^{q} p_{kk}, \ p_e = \frac{1}{q-1} \sum_{k=1}^{q} \pi_k(1 - \pi_k), \tag{4.2.1}$$

---

[4]I use $\widehat{\gamma}_1$ (read "gamma hat one") to designate the value of AC_1 estimated from observed ratings taken on a sample of subjects. Its estimand γ_1 is the AC_1 value based on the entire subject population. Later in this chapter, I will use the symbol $\widehat{\gamma}_2$ to designate AC_2, which the weighted version of AC_1.

where $\pi_k = (p_{k+} + p_{+k})/2$. Note that p_{k+} and p_{+k} represent the relative number of subjects assigned to category k by raters A and B respectively. The symbol p_{kk} is the relative number of subjects classified into category k by both raters. While π_k represents the probability for a randomly-selected rater to classify a randomly-selected subject into category k, the chance-agreement probability p_e is a product of the following two quantities:

- The probability that two raters agree given that the subject being rated is nontextbook and was therefore assigned a nondeterministic rating. This conditional[5] probability is $1/q$ since nondeterministic ratings are considered random with equal chance for all q categories.

- The propensity for a rater to assign a nondeterministic rating, which is estimated by the ratio: $\sum_{k=1}^{q} \pi_k(1 - \pi_k)/(1 - 1/q)$. More will be said about this expression later in this chapter. What is important to retain from this expression is that a distribution of subjects that is skewed towards a few categories will lower the nondeterministic rating propensity.

Section 4.4 contains a more detailed discussion of the theory behind this statistic. Gwet (2008a) also provides examples and theoretical results related to the AC$_1$ statistic.

4.2.2 Aickin's α-Statistic

The alpha statistic $\widehat{\alpha}_A$ of Aickin (1990) is defined as follows:

$$\widehat{\alpha}_A = \frac{p_a - p_e}{1 - p_e}, \ \text{where} \ p_e = \sum_{k=1}^{q} p_{k|H}^{(A)} \cdot p_{k|H}^{(B)}, \tag{4.2.2}$$

and $p_{k|H}^{(A)}$ represents the probability for rater A to classify into category k, a subject known to be hard to classify (i.e. a nontextbook subject). The final classification of this particular group of hard-to-classify subjects involves guesswork and will be random. The percent agreement p_a is the same as that of equation 4.2.1. The main difference between Kappa and alpha lies in the way the percent chance agreement is calculated. While Kappa's percent chance agreement includes all ratings, Aickin's only uses ratings associated with hard-to-classify subjects. Aickin's theory from which the alpha coefficient is derived, is discussed in section 4.3.

---

[5]The condition here being the nondeterministic nature of the ratings, which will lead any resulting agreement to be considered chance agreement.

Because the group of hard-to-classify subjects is not identifiable, there is no simple expression for obtaining the probabilities $p_{k|H}^{(A)}$ and $p_{k|H}^{(B)}$. To solve this problem, Aickin (1990) proposed an iterative algorithm based on the following system of 3 equations:

$$\hat{\alpha}^{(t+1)} = \frac{p_a - p_e^{(t)}}{1 - p_e^{(t)}}, \quad where \; p_e^{(t)} = \sum_{k=1}^{q} p_{k|H}^{A(t)} \cdot p_{k|H}^{B(t)}, \tag{4.2.3}$$

$$p_{k|H}^{A(t+1)} = \frac{p_{k+}}{\left(1 - \hat{\alpha}^{(t)}\right) + \hat{\alpha}^{(t)} p_{k|H}^{B(t)} \Big/ p_e^{(t)}}, \quad for \; k = 1, \cdots, q, \tag{4.2.4}$$

$$p_{k|H}^{B(t+1)} = \frac{p_{+k}}{\left(1 - \hat{\alpha}^{(t)}\right) + \hat{\alpha}^{(t)} p_{k|H}^{A(t)} \Big/ p_e^{(t)}}, \quad for \; k = 1, \cdots, q. \tag{4.2.5}$$

This iterative process is initiated with the marginal probabilities p_{k+} and p_{+k} as starting values for the varying probabilities $p_{k|H}^{A(t)}$ and $p_{k|H}^{B(t)}$. That is, $p_{k|H}^{A(0)} = p_{k+}$, and $p_{k|H}^{B(0)} = p_{+k}$. Therefore, the initial alpha value $\hat{\alpha}^{(0)}$ when $t = 0$ is identical to the classical Kappa statistic. The next alpha value $\hat{\alpha}^{(1)}$ when $t = 1$ is calculated from $\hat{\alpha}^{(0)}$ and the other probability values according to the above equations. The iterative process stops when the difference between two consecutive Alpha values $\hat{\alpha}^{(t+1)}$ and $\hat{\alpha}^{(t)}$ decreases below a predetermined small number such as 0.001, which represents a threshold below which you consider two coefficients to be identical for all practical purposes.

4.2.3   Example

I now want to illustrate the calculation of the AC_1 and α agreement coefficients with a practical example. To compute the α coefficient, Aickin recommends to add a pseudo-count[6] of 1 to the total count of subjects, and to distribute it uniformly among all cells to avoid convergence problems with the iterative algorithm. If your experiment uses 3 categories, your table will have 9 cells. Therefore, distributing a pseudo-count of 1 uniformly across cells increases each cell count by $1/9 = 0.11$ approximately. Cells with no subject would now have 0.11 subject allowing Aickin's algorithm to run smoothly.

Example 4.1 _____

To illustrate the calculation of AC_1 and alpha coefficients, let us consider the reliability data of Table 4.1. This data represents the distribution of human subjects suffering from back pain, by pain type, and observing clinician.

---

[6]A "pseudo-count" is an integer value primarily used for changing artificially a cell count value from being 0 to being negligible. Zero-count cells are known to be problematic to probability-based computing systems, but cannot be eliminated unless they represent events known to be impossible.

Table 4.1:

Ratings of Spinal Pain by Clinicians 1 and 2, and Pain Type

Clinician 1	Clinician 2		
	Derangement Syndrome	Dysfunctional Syndrome	Postural Syndrome
Derangement Syndrome	55	10	2
Dysfunctional Syndrome	6	4	10
Postural Syndrome	2	5	6

Cohen's Kappa for this data is given by $\widehat{\kappa}_{\mathrm{C}} = (0.65 - 0.4835)/(1 - 0.4835) = 0.3224$. The AC_1 coefficient on the other hand is $\widehat{\gamma}_1 = (0.65 - 0.257725)/(1 - 0.257725) = 0.5285$. As for Aickin's Alpha, after 10 iterations I obtained $\widehat{\alpha}_{\mathrm{A}} = (0.65 - 0.4121)/(1 - 0.4121) = 0.4047$, and the final "marginal" probabilities related to hard-to-classify subjects are given by $(p_{1|\mathrm{H}}^{(\mathrm{A})}, p_{2|\mathrm{H}}^{(\mathrm{A})}, p_{3|\mathrm{H}}^{(\mathrm{A})}) = (0.5993437, 0.2442839, 0.1563717)$ for clinician A, and by $(p_{1|\mathrm{H}}^{(\mathrm{B})}, p_{2|\mathrm{H}}^{(\mathrm{B})}, p_{3|\mathrm{H}}^{(\mathrm{B})}) = (0.5321665, 0.2274873, 0.2403553)$ for clinician B.

The Kappa, alpha, and AC_1 statistics of example 4.1 are respectively given by $0.322, 0.405$, and 0.529. Kappa represents less than half the magnitude of the percent agreement probability $p_a = 0.65$. This dramatic reduction in the magnitude of the percent agreement is a result of Kappa's unduly high chance-agreement correction. AC_1 on the other hand represents more than 80% of the value of the percent agreement, because of a less severe correction for chance agreement. I will explain in the next few sections that Aickin's alpha coefficient measures a dimension of raters' agreement that is different from what Kappa and AC_1 measure. Therefore, a direct comparison between Aickin's alpha and other coefficients may be inappropriate.

While AC_1 and Kappa represent agreement probabilities based on the pool of subjects from which the Hard-to-classify ones have been removed, alpha on the other hand represents the probability of "for-cause" agreement[7] based on all subjects. Because the reference population for evaluating alpha is bigger, $\widehat{\alpha}_{\mathrm{A}}$ will generally be lower than AC_1 unless the group of subjects does not have those special subjects that may lead to an agreement by chance. Conceptually, Aickin's alpha would be smaller that both Kappa and AC_1. In practice however, Aickin's alpha often exceeds Kappa because of Kappa's excessive chance-agreement correction in some situations.

The next two sections 4.3 and 4.4 deal with the theoretical foundations of the alpha and AC_1 statistics and require some limited abstract thinking. Our primary objective in these two sections is to answer the following question: "*If we knew eve-*

---

[7]A "for-cause" agreement is an agreement situation where both raters classified a subject into the same category for a reason, as opposed to doing it by pure chance.

rything about all subjects and raters of interest (including the ratings that the raters would assign to each subject, and the raters' skill level), how would we evaluate inter-rater reliability?" This hypothetical situation will lead to the creation of a theoretical framework. But carrying out a real experiment based on a sample of subjects instead of the whole subject population, always results in a loss of information about non-participating subjects. Only the use of special estimation procedures will compensate for these gaps in our knowledge. The result will be a statistical procedure that is susceptible to sampling errors. These errors also known as statistical errors, are discussed in chapter 5 using the techniques of inferential statistics.

Although both sections 4.3 and 4.4 discuss the motivation behind the formulation of AC_1, and that of alpha, they are not essential for using equations 4.2.1 and 4.2.2 in practice with experimental data. Practitioners not interested in this inquiry could skip these two sections without the chapter's readability[8] being affected, and continue with section 4.5 that is devoted to the AC_1 coefficient for multiple raters.

4.3   Aickin's Theory

Aickin's (1990) problem was to define a construct α (without a hat) that measures the extent of agreement between two raters A and B in a way that solely reflects the similarities in their knowledge, experience, and judgment. That is α should be insensitive to those agreements that may occur by pure chance, a possibility that cannot be ignored when using discrete measurement scales. Although there could be more than one way of defining such a parameter, Aickin proposed the following definition:

> *"The α parameter is defined as the fraction of the entire subject population made up of subjects that the two raters A and B classified identically for cause, rather than by chance."*

Without providing an explicit definition of the notion of for-cause agreement, Aickin considers that this type of agreement is reached on subjects that are easy to score, also known as textbook subjects in the terminology of Grove et al. (1981). A subject is considered easy to score when both raters have a strong opinion regarding its membership category. Disagreement as well as chance agreement on the other hand, are assumed to occur only on subjects that are difficult to classify. Any agreement on the hard-to-classify subjects is considered chance agreement. Aickin's theory consists of dividing the target population of subjects into two subpopulations. These are the subpopulation of Hard-To-Score subjects (or H-subjects), and the subpopulation of Easy-to-Score subjects (or E-subjects). Table 4.2 shows an abstract

---

[8]We nevertheless highly recommend the reading of these two sections for an ind-depth understanding of the concepts.

representation of the distribution of N population subjects broken down by rater and subpopulation in a two-level measurement scale study, as Aickin envisioned it.

In Table 4.2, $N_{11}^{(\mathrm{H})}$ for example represents the count of H-subjects in the study population expected to be classified into category 1 by both raters. Likewise, $N_{21}^{(\mathrm{H})}$ is the count of population H-subjects expected to be classified into categories 2 and 1 by raters A and B respectively. More generally, the subject population contains N subjects, $N_{kl}^{(\mathrm{H})}$ of which are expected to be H-subjects and to be classified into categories k and l by raters A and B respectively. $N_k^{(\mathrm{E})}$ $(k = 1, 2)$ of the N population subjects are expected to be E-subjects that both raters will classify into the same category k. All cells of Table 4.2 that are colored in black do not contain any population subjects in Aickin's model.

Table 4.2:

Distribution of N Population Subjects by Rater, Subpopulation, and Response Category.

Rater A		Rater B				Total	
		Hard Subjects		Easy Subjects		Total	
		1	2	1	2		
Hard	1	$N_{11}^{(\mathrm{H})}$	$N_{12}^{(\mathrm{H})}$	■	■	$N_{1+}^{(\mathrm{H})}$	N_{H}
Subjects	2	$N_{21}^{(\mathrm{H})}$	$N_{22}^{(\mathrm{H})}$	■	■	$N_{2+}^{(\mathrm{H})}$	
Easy	1	■	■	$N_1^{(\mathrm{E})}$	0	$N_1^{(\mathrm{E})}$	N_{E}
Subjects	2	■	■	0	$N_2^{(\mathrm{E})}$	$N_2^{(\mathrm{E})}$	
Total		$N_{+1}^{(\mathrm{H})}$	$N_{+2}^{(\mathrm{H})}$	$N_1^{(\mathrm{E})}$	$N_2^{(\mathrm{E})}$	N	
		N_{H}		N_{E}			

Aickin's α coefficient is then defined as follows:

$$\alpha = \frac{N_{\mathrm{E}}}{N},$$

(4.3.1)

where $N_{\mathrm{E}} = N_1^{\mathrm{E}} + N_2^{\mathrm{E}}$ is the population count of E-subjects. Note that even if the total count N of population subjects is known, the number N_{E} of population E-subjects will be unknown. After selecting a sample of n subjects for an inter-rater reliability study and rating them, the sub-sample of E-subjects will still be non-identifiable. Therefore, a direct estimation of the α coefficient is not feasible. To solve this problem, Aickin (1990) postulated a statistical model (to be presented in the next subsection) that governs the classification probabilities, and that incorporates α as a model parameter.

Some Remarks about Aickin's Theory

- The raters are assumed to always agree on E-subjects, a disagreement being possible on H-subjects only. Moreover, any such agreement is considered to be for cause.

- Hard-to-score (resp. Easy-to-score) subjects have their hardness (resp. their easiness) intimately tied to both raters' knowledge. Consequently, the configuration of Table 4.2 is specific to the pair of raters being studied, and both raters share the same Hard-to-score, and Easy-to-score subjects.
  This second assumption is the most restrictive in Aickin's theory. In practice two raters are seldom expected to have the same knowledge and skill level. Some subjects that one rater considers hard to score may prove easy to score for another.

4.3.1 *Aickin's Probability Model*

Let the probabilities P_{kl}, $P_{k|\text{H}}^{(\text{A})}$, and $P_{l|\text{H}}^{(\text{B})}$ be defined as follows:

P_{kl} = Probability that raters A and B classify a randomly selected
subject into categories k and l respectively,

$P_{k|\text{H}}^{(\text{A})}$ = Probability that rater A classifies an H-subject into category k,

$P_{l|\text{H}}^{(\text{B})}$ = Probability that rater B classifies an H-subject into category l.

In statistical jargon, $P_{k|\text{H}}^{(\text{A})}$ is referred to as the conditional probability that rater A classifies a randomly chosen subject into category k given that the subject was selected from the H-subject sub-population. Aickin's model is based on the following representation for the probability P_{kl} :

$$P_{kl} = (1-\alpha)P_{k|\text{H}}^{(\text{A})}P_{l|\text{H}}^{(\text{B})} + \alpha \left(\frac{d_{kl}P_{k|\text{H}}^{(\text{A})}P_{l|\text{H}}^{(\text{B})}}{\sum\limits_{k=1}^{q}P_{k|\text{H}}^{(\text{A})}P_{k|\text{H}}^{(\text{B})}} \right), \text{ where } d_{kl} = \begin{cases} 1 & \text{if } k = l, \\ 0 & \text{otherwise.} \end{cases} \quad (4.3.2)$$

This equation can be seen as a direct application of the Bayes' rule[9] in probability theory. The ratio in parentheses represents the conditional probability that both raters classify a subject into the same category k, given that it is an E-subject. In equation 4.3.2, $1 - \alpha$ represents the probability of selecting an H-subject and α that of selecting an E-subject. It should also be noted that checking the validity of such a model may not be a simple task.

By multiplying both sides of equation (4.3.2) by d_{kl} and by summing, one obtains the following:

$$\alpha_A = \frac{\sum_{k=1}^{q} P_{kk} - \sum_{k=1}^{q} P_{k|H}^{(A)} P_{k|H}^{(B)}}{1 - \sum_{k=1}^{q} P_{k|H}^{(A)} P_{k|H}^{(B)}}. \qquad (4.3.3)$$

Equation 4.3.3 shows that the α coefficient has a form similar to that of Kappa, with the important exception that the percent chance agreement is computed based on H-subjects only. That is, only the portion of the subject population where the assumption of independence is expected to be satisfied is used to compute the percent chance agreement. This provision surely protects Aickin's coefficient against the paradoxes associated with Kappa.

4.3.2   *Estimating α from a Subject Sample*

Using the n sample subjects that participated in the inter-rater reliability experiment, the α coefficient is estimated by $\hat{\alpha}_A$ defined by equation (4.2.2) where the probabilities $P_{k|H}^{(A)}$ $(k = 1, \cdots, q)$ would be replaced with their sample-based counterparts $p_{k|H}^{(A)}$. However, a direct calculation of $\hat{\alpha}$ is impossible due to the unknown probabilities $p_{k|H}^{(A)}$ $(k = 1, \cdots, q)$, and $p_{l|H}^{(B)}$ $(l = 1, \cdots, q)$. Aickin (1990) proposed to use the maximum likelihood estimates based on the system of three equations defined by equations (4.2.3), (4.2.4), and (4.2.5). The first equation of this system is a version of equation (4.3.3), the second and third equations are obtained by summing both sides of equation (4.3.2) over k and l respectively.

---

[9]The Bayes' rule stipulates that the probabilities $P(F)$ and $P(G)$ of any two events F and G are related as follows: $P(F) = P(G)P(F/G) + (1 - P(G))P(F/\overline{G})$, where $\overline{G}$ is the complement event of G and $P(F/G)$ the conditional probability of F given G.

4.4   Gwet's Theory

Unlike Aickin's alpha coefficient, which is defined as the probability that two raters A and B agree for cause, Gwet's AC_1 (see Gwet, 2008(a)) is defined as the probability that two raters agree given that the subjects being rated are not suscept-ible to agreement by pure chance. This definition is more in line with the goal set by Cohen (1960) for Kappa. Cohen wanted Kappa to represent "... the proportion of agreement after chance agreement is removed from consideration ..." The two let-ters A and C in "AC_1 statistic" stand for Agreement Coefficient, while subscript 1 indicates that only total agreement between the two raters (i.e. diagonal elements) is considered as agreement[10]. Another inter-rater reliability coefficient named the AC_2, which considers certain types of disagreements as partial agreements (also referred to as "second-level agreement") is discussed later in this chapter.

A key conceptual difference between AC_1 and alpha lies on the pool of subjects used as basis for computing the coefficients. Aickin's alpha is based on all subjects, while Gwet's AC_1 is based on the sub-population of subjects obtained after removing from the initial population all subjects that may lead to chance agreement. Although Gwet's model has some similarities with Aickin's, the following differences should be mentioned:

- In Aickin's model, any H-subject is hard to score not just for one rater, but for both. Likewise any E-subject will be easy to score for both raters. In Gwet's model, each rater has his/her own group of E-subjects, and his/her own group of H-subjects. Therefore, some of rater A's E-subjects will be rater B's H-subjects, and vice-versa (see Table 4.3).

- In both Gwet's and Aickin's models, any agreement involving an H-subject (with either rater) is by definition considered as agreement by chance. In Gwet's model however, all population H-subjects that would lead to an agreement by chance - assuming they are identifiable - must be removed from the pool of sub-jects before computing the relative number of for-cause agreement subjects. In Aickin's model, the relative number of for-cause agreement subjects is calcula-ted with respect to the entire subject population.

---

[10]This will also be referred to as first-level agreement throughout the book; hence the use of subscript "1."

Table 4.3:

Distribution of Population Subjects by Sub-Population of H- and E-Subjects, by Rater, and by Response Category (1,2)

Rater A		Rater B				Total	
		Hard Subjects		Easy Subjects		Total	
		1	2	1	2		
Hard	1	N_{11}^{HH}	N_{12}^{HH}	N_{11}^{HE}	N_{12}^{HE}	N_{1+}^{H}	$N_{\mathrm{HH}+}$
Subjects	2	N_{21}^{HH}	N_{22}^{HH}	N_{21}^{HE}	N_{22}^{HE}	N_{2+}^{HH}	
Easy	1	N_{11}^{EH}	N_{12}^{EH}	N_{11}^{EE}	0	N_{1+}^{E}	$N_{\mathrm{E}+}$
Subjects	2	N_{21}^{EH}	N_{22}^{EH}	0	N_{22}^{EE}	N_{2+}^{E}	
Total		N_{+1}^{H}	N_{+2}^{H}	N_{+1}^{E}	N_{+2}^{E}	N	
		$N_{+\mathrm{H}}$		$N_{+\mathrm{E}}$			

Table 4.3 shows the configuration of the study population of N subjects from which a subject sample will be selected. The quantity N_{12}^{EH} for example, is the count of subjects identified as E-subjects for rater A and as H-subjects for rater B, and expected to be classified into categories 1 and 2 by raters A and B respectively. As previously indicated, subjects identified as E-subjects for both subjects can only lead to an agreement for cause. No disagreement is possible on E-subjects. Hence the two cells with 0 frequency seen in Table 4.3.

Let γ_1 be the construct associated with the AC_1 coefficient. It represents the ideal quantity that AC_1 will approximate with the rating data collected from a reliability experiment. If all the information shown in Table 4.3 was known for all subjects of interest (not just those in an experimental sample), then the AC_1 statistic would be free of sampling errors and would be identical to the theoretical construct γ_1, defined for a general number q of categories as follows:

$$\gamma_1 = \frac{\sum_{k=1}^{q} N_{kk}^{\mathrm{EE}}}{N - \left(\sum_{k=1}^{q} N_{kk}^{\mathrm{HH}} + \sum_{k=1}^{q} N_{kk}^{\mathrm{HE}} + \sum_{k=1}^{q} N_{kk}^{\mathrm{EH}} \right)}, \qquad (4.4.1)$$

where the denominator represents the count of population subjects on which no agreement between raters can be reached by pure chance[11]. Note that under the current setting, Aickin's alpha coefficient would be defined as follows:

$$\alpha_{\mathrm{A}} = \frac{1}{N} \sum_{k=1}^{q} N_{kk}^{\mathrm{EE}}. \tag{4.4.2}$$

Aickin excludes chance-agreement subjects from the count of agreement subjects in the coefficient's numerator, but does not exclude them from the reference population in the denominator. Therefore, Gwet's AC_1 coefficient, which excludes chance-agreement subjects from consideration entirely is expected to be higher than Aickin's alpha coefficient.

COMPARING γ_1 AND α_{A}

I am not an advocate of Aickin's alpha coefficient for one reason: by excluding subjects that are susceptible to chance agreement from the numerator while leaving them in the denominator, Aickin makes it difficult if not impossible for its coefficient to reach the perfect value of 1. This is particularly the case when "Hard" subjects are present in the subject population. Consequently, Aickin's alpha coefficient could be artificially low for some subject populations.

The rationale that led to equation 4.4.1 can be looked at this way: Cohen (1960) stated an attractive property that he expected his agreement coefficient to satisfy, but ended up formulating Kappa in a way that did not satisfy it. Here is what Cohen (1960) said on page 40 (second paragraph): "The coefficient κ ... is the proportion of agreement after chance agreement is removed from consideration." The denominator in equation 4.4.1 aims at removing chance agreement from consideration before computing the proportion of agreement, by subtracting from the subject population all subjects susceptible to lead to an agreement by pure chance. The formula Cohen ended up developing was rather based on the following false assumption he made on page 38: "A certain amount of agreement is to be expected by chance, which is readily determined by finding the joint probabilities of the marginals." But Kappa does not attempt to quantify that "certain amount" of agreement expected by chance. The motive for not doing it is unknown to me. The joint probabilities of the marginals will hardly help quantify chance agreement, which by the way will occur only on an unknown proportion of subjects, and not on all of them.

---

[11]This denominator may include some disagreements as well as some agreement for cause. Only subjects causing agreement by chance are removed.

4.4.1   *The Probabilistic Model*

Although equation 4.4.1 provides a definitional expression for AC_1, it is useless for computing it since "Hard" and "Easy" subjects cannot be identified. What is needed is a probabilistic model that links observed ratings to the theoretical concepts of "Hard" and "Easy" subjects. Although Table 4.3 shows only two response categories for illustration purposes, I assume here that the rater must classify subjects into one of q possible response categories labeled as $k = 1, \cdots, q$.

Let us consider the following events:

- $\mathcal{R}$: The selected subject is an H-subject *(i.e. one of the two raters or both will perform a nondeterministic rating when classifying this subject).*

- A: Both raters A and B agree on the classification of the selected subject.

- $\mathcal{C} = A \cap \mathcal{R}$: Represents an agreement by chance *(i.e. the selected subject is an H-subject, and both raters A and B agree about its classification).*

For any two categories k and l, a simple application of the Bayes' rule suggests the following equation:

$$P_{kl} = P(\mathcal{C})P_{kl|\mathcal{C}} + P(\overline{\mathcal{C}})P_{kl|\overline{\mathcal{C}}}. \tag{4.4.3}$$

where $\overline{\mathcal{C}}$ is the event "No Chance Agreement," the complementary event of $\mathcal{C}$. Since $P(\mathcal{C}) = P(\mathcal{R})P(A|\mathcal{R})$ I propose the following statistical model for the join classification probability:

$$P_{kl} = P(\mathcal{R})\frac{d_{kl}}{q^2} + \left(1 - P(\mathcal{R})/q\right)P_{kl|\overline{\mathcal{C}}}, \tag{4.4.4}$$

where $d_{kl} = 1$ if $k = l$ and $d_{kl} = 0$ if not. Equation 4.4.4 stems from the fact that $P(\mathcal{C})P_{kl|\mathcal{C}} = P(\mathcal{R})P(A/\mathcal{R})P_{kl|\mathcal{C}}$, where the probability $P(A/\mathcal{R})$ of agreement given a random rating is $1/q$ and $P_{kl|\mathcal{C}} = d_{kl}/q$. Some authors (e.g. Groves et al. (1981) among others) have suggested that under the assumption of random rating, it may be inappropriate to assign equal probability $1/q$ to all categories. Some of these authors even recommended using the observed marginal probabilities. I do not recommend this. My view on this issue is that if a rater believes that one categpry is more likely than the others to be the correct one, then that category must be selected and the rating process should not even be considered random at all. Why would rater rate H-subjects the same way she rates E-subjects?

By multiplying both sides of equation 4.4.4 by d_{kl} and by summing over k and l one obtains:

$$\sum_{k=1}^{q} P_{kk} = P(\mathcal{R})/q + \left(1 - P(\mathcal{R})/q\right)\gamma_1.$$

Consequently γ_1 can be expressed as follows:

$$\gamma_1 = \frac{P_a - P(\mathcal{R})/q}{1 - P(\mathcal{R})/q}, \text{ where } P_a = \sum_{k=1}^{q} P_{kk}. \tag{4.4.5}$$

To be able to compute γ_1 from observed ratings, I need to compute the probability $P(\mathcal{R})$ of random rating, which represents the proportion of Hard-to-Score subjects for all raters combined.

4.4.2 *Quantifying the Probability $P(\mathcal{R})$ of Selecting an H-Subject*

Since H-subjects are rated randomly, they are expected to be distributed uniformly across categories. Conversely, subjects uniformly distributed across categories are not necessarily H-subjects. But for the purpose of estimating $P(\mathcal{R})$, I made the following assumption:

> *Subjects distributed more uniformly distributed across categories are more likely to contain H-subjects.*

Therefore, $P(\mathcal{R})$ is essentially a degree of uniformity of the distribution of subjects across categories. If the distribution of This assumption led to the following expression:

$$P(\mathcal{R}) = \frac{\sum_{k=1}^{q} \pi_k(1 - \pi_k)}{1 - 1/q}, \tag{4.4.6}$$

where π_k is the probability that a randomly selected subject is classified into category k by a rater (also selected randomly among raters).

To evaluate the degree of uniformity of the subject distribution across the q categories, consider the q variables $X_1, \cdots, X_k, \cdots, X_q$ where X_k is defined for a randomly-selected rater and a randomly-selected subject as follows:

$$X_k = \begin{cases} 1, & \text{if the rater classifies the subject into categpry } k, \\ 0, & \text{otherwise.} \end{cases} \tag{4.4.7}$$

These variables are independent Bernoulli trials where π_k is the probability of success associated with variable X_k. The sum of these variables $S_q = X_1 + \cdots + X_k + \cdots + X_q$ follows a Poisson binomial distribution whose variance is,

$$\sigma_q^2 = \sum_{k=1}^{q} \pi_k(1 - \pi_k). \tag{4.4.8}$$

when the subjects are uniformly distributed then σ_q^2 reaches its maximum value of $\sigma_{q.Max}^2 = 1 - 1/q$ (i.e. $\pi_k = 1/q$ for all $k = 1, \cdots, q$), and reaches its minimum value $\sigma_{q.Min}^2 = 0$ when all subjects are systematically classified into a single category (i.e. $\pi_{k_0} = 1$ for some category k_0). Hence $P(\mathcal{R})$ is the ratio of σ_q^2 to its maximum value. Equation 4.4.6 can also be justified using the chi-square distance between the observed subject distribution and the uniform distribution, from the family of quadratic distances on probabilities whose theoretical foundations were thoroughly studied by Lindsay et al. (2008).. The numerator of equation 4.4.6 would be the observed distance, and the denominator its maximum value.

One way to verify how well equation (4.4.6) works it to simulate a population of subjects similar to what is described in Table 4.3, to define the "true" inter-rater reliability according to equation 4.9, and to study the statistical properties of the coefficient given by equation 4.1. This verification was done by Gwet (2008a), and the results were very satisfactory.

Formulating γ_1 Relative to Model 4.4.4

It follows from equations (4.4.5) and (4.4.6) that the γ_1 construct may be rewritten as follows:

$$\gamma_1 = \frac{P_a - P_e}{1 - P_e}, \text{ where } P_e = \frac{1}{q-1} \sum_{k=1}^{q} \pi_k(1 - \pi_k). \tag{4.4.9}$$

Equation 4.4.9 shows that the γ_1 statistic has a form similar to that of Kappa, with the same percent agreement probability P_a and a different percent chance agreement P_e. To understand how P_e measures chance agreement, let us consider the simple situation where the number of categories is limited to 2. Then $P_e = 2\pi_1(1 - \pi_1)$ where π_1 is the probability that classify a subject is classified into category 1. If $\pi_1 = 1$ (i.e. all subjects are classified into category 1), then the percent chance agreement is 0. Intuitively, one can see that if all subjects are systematically classified into one category, then the raters must know what they are doing. An agreement under these conditions is not achieved as a result of pure chance, and the rating process is considered deterministic. On the other hand, if $\pi_1 = 1/2$ (i.e. a randomly selected subject has the same chance to be classified into either category), then $P_e = 0.5$. Again, if the subjects are equally distributed across the categories, then the uniform distribution of subjects matches the configuration that would be obtained if all subjects were H-subjects. The relative number of subjects on the diagonal will then be 50%, which equals P_e.

4.5   Calculating AC$_1$ for three Raters or More

Section 4.4 introduced the AC$_1$ coefficient as an abstract construct, the objective being to present an explicit formulation of the concept it represents. This goal was achieved by assuming the hypothetical situation where all subjects of interest as well as their categorization by each of the raters are known. The known includes the raters' knowledge, as well as the group of subjects they consider hard or easy to score. This theoretical framework does not provide the concrete pathway for quantifying the extent of agreement among raters in a practical setting where only observed ratings assigned to subjects are known. Ratings observed during a reliability experiment must be used with valid estimation methods to obtain the concrete value of an agreement coefficient.

An inter-rater reliability experiment is generally based on a sample of n subjects that represents only a fraction of the larger population subjects of interest. The resulting sample-based AC$_1$ coefficient is denoted by $\widehat{\gamma}_1$ (the hat indicating that it is an approximation of the fixed and unknown abstract γ_1 of equation 4.5.9). When the number of raters is limited to two then equation 4.2.1 is the coefficient that practitioners would use since it provides a good approximation of the population parameter γ_1 of equation 4.5.1 as shown by Gwet (2008a). However, when the number of raters is 3 or more, a different expression becomes necessary for practitioners to estimate the agreement coefficient.

AC$_1$ Statistic for three Raters or More, and for Nominal Scores

Generalizing AC$_1$ to the case of three raters or more and to multiple categories amounts to finding generalized versions of the percent agreement and percent chance agreement p_a and p_e. The percent agreement p_a used for AC$_1$ is the same as the one used with Kappa as well as with other chance-corrected agreement coefficients discussed in the past few chapters. This percent agreement was previously defined in chapter 2 (see equation 2.9 for example). The remaining problem is to find the percent chance agreement that can be used with AC$_1$ when the number of raters is 3 or more.

Although equation (4.4.9) was derived for the simpler case of two raters, it suggests a natural way for generalizing the percent chance agreement to the more general case of three raters or more. It consists of replacing π_k with its sample-based estimated value, which can handle three raters or more. This was already done by Fleiss (1971) while generalizing Kappa to three raters or more. Using Fleiss' approach to the π_k probabilities leads to the multiple-rater version of the AC$_1$ coefficient given by:

$$\hat{\gamma}_1 = \frac{p_a - p_e}{1 - p_e}, \ where \begin{cases} p_a = \frac{1}{n'} \sum_{i=1}^{n'} \sum_{k=1}^{q} \frac{r_{ik}(r_{ik} - 1)}{r_i(r_i - 1)}, \\ p_e = \frac{1}{q-1} \sum_{k=1}^{q} \pi_k(1 - \pi_k), \\ and \ \pi_k = \frac{1}{n} \sum_{i=1}^{n} \frac{r_{ik}}{r_i}. \end{cases} \tag{4.5.1}$$

In equation 4.5.1, q is the number of categories, r_{ik} is the count of raters who classified subject i into category k, r_i is the count of raters who rated subject i, n is the total count of subjects, and n' the count of subjects who were rated by two raters or more.

On the Percent Chance Agreement

In section 4.4, the percent chance agreement was defined as the probability that two raters agree about the rating of an H-subject. Generalizing this probability by replacing the two-rater version of the classification probability π_k with a multiple-rater version as suggested in the previous paragraph leads to the multiple-rater version of the percent chance agreement of equation 4.5.1. However, p_e as formulated in equation 4.5.1 does not appear to have an intuitive interpretation. Does it represent the probability that two randomly chosen raters agree about the rating of an H-subject? Or something else? This issue can be resolved using the same method Conger (1980) used to generalize Kappa to multiple raters. That is, p_e would be generalized by averaging all pairwise percent chance agreement values. *The resulting percent chance agreement can then be seen as the probability that two raters randomly selected from the pool of r raters agree on the rating of an H-subject.*

One can form $r(r-1)/2$ pairs of raters out of a pool of r raters. For each pair, a percent chance agreement similar to that shown in equation 4.2.1 can be calculated. Averaging all such pairwise percent chance agreement values will lead to a multiple-rater chance-agreement probability defined as follows:

$$p'_e = p_e - (1/2 - 1/r) \sum_{k=1}^{q} s_k^2/(q-1), \tag{4.5.2}$$

where p_e is defined as in equation 4.5.1, and s_k^2 is the variance of the p_{gk}'s (over all raters g) with $p_{gk} = n_{gk}/n$ being the relative number of subjects that rater g classified into category k. However, our investigation has revealed that the two expressions p'_e and p_e of the percent chance agreement generally yield estimates that are very close. Consequently, I recommend the use of the simpler expression p_e of equation 4.5.1.

Example 4.2 _____

To illustrate the calculation of AC_1 for multiple raters, let me consider Table 4.4 data obtained from an experiment where 4 raters classified 12 subjects into 5 possible categories labeled as a, b, c, d, and e. A look at Table 4.4 reveals that each of the 4 raters only rated some of the 12 subjects. Therefore, using this data will also show how the handling of missing ratings is done when computing the AC_1 coefficient.

Table 4.4: Rating Data from 4 Raters and 12 Subjects

Subject	Rater1	Rater2	Rater3	Rater4
1	a	a		a
2	b	b	c	b
3	c	c	c	c
4	c	c	c	c
5	b	b	b	b
6	a	b	c	d
7	d	d	d	d
8	a	a	b	a
9	b	b	b	b
10		e	e	e
11			a	a
12			c	

Table 4.5 shows the percent agreement, percent chance agreement, and various agreement coefficients based on five methods discussed in this chapter as well as in the previous chapters. The percent agreement is 0.818 for all coefficients except for Krippendorff's alpha whose percent agreement is 0.805. Each agreement coefficient has a different value for the percent chance agreement p_e. The AC_1 coefficient is 0.7754, and represents the highest values of all five coefficients studied in this example.

Table 4.5: Inter-Rater Reliability Coefficients for Table 4.4 Data

Method	Percent Agreement (p_a)	Percent Chance Agreement (p_e)	Coefficient
Conger Kappa	0.818	0.2334	0.7628
Gwet AC_1	0.818	0.1903	0.7754
Fleiss Kappa	0.818	0.2387	0.7612
Krippendorff	0.805	0.2400	0.7434
Brennan-Prediger	0.818	0.2	0.7727

If you want to see all the details regarding these calculations, you may download the Excel workbook,

www.agreestat.com/book4/chapter4examples.xlsx,

and look at the "Example 4.2" worksheet. It shows all the steps from the input data leading up to the ultimate coefficient values.

4.6 AC$_2$: the AC$_1$ Coefficient for Ordinal and Interval Data

The AC$_1$ statistic is developed primarily for nominal data, and is expected to be ineffective for evaluating the extent of agreement among raters on ordinal, or interval measurement scales. It is because when using ordinal or interval ratings, some disagreements are known to be more serious than others, and only agreement coefficients that assign different weights to different types of agreement are desirable. In this section, I extend the AC$_1$ statistic to ordinal, interval, and ratio data based on the same techniques used in chapter 3 to extend Kappa to interval data. This generalized AC$_1$ coefficient is named AC$_2$, and is essentially a weighted version of AC$_1$ with the weights being used to account for partial agreements. The simpler case involving two raters only will be treated first, and will next be generalized to the more complex situation of three raters or more.

4.6.1 *AC$_2$ for Interval Data and two Raters*

Let us consider a reliability experiment where two raters must each assign an interval-type rating to each of the n subjects in the subject sample. Assume also that one of the q scores labeled as $x_1, x_2, \cdots, x_q$ can be assigned to subjects. Note that if these scores are alphabetic and ordinal at the same time, then they are typically treated as interval data where each score x_k is replaced with its rank. Suppose for example that the alphabetic scale is made up of the scores {LOW, MEDIUM, HIGH}. For the purpose of analysis, these scores would be replaced with the ranks 1, 2, and 3. One may use numbers other than the ranks for a more accurate representation of scores that are not equally-spaced. Numeric scores on the other hand, are used as reported.

Table 4.6 shows the raw scores of 12 subjects produced by two raters named "Rater1" and "Rater2." These two raters had to assign one of the scores {0.5, 1, 1.5, 2, 2.5} to each of the 12 subjects participating in the experiment. This rating scale is numeric, and its values will be used in the analysis as reported. Moreover, this dataset contains some missing ratings ("Rater1" did not score subject 1, and "Rater2" did not score subject 9).

The AC_2 statistic for interval data is defined as follows:

$$\widehat{\gamma}_2 = \frac{p_a - p_e}{1 - p_e}, \text{ where} \begin{cases} p_a = \sum_{k,l}^{q} w_{kl} p'_{kl}, \\ \\ p_e = \frac{T_w}{q(q-1)} \sum_{k=1}^{q} \pi_k (1 - \pi_k). \end{cases}$$

(4.6.1)

The various terms in equation 4.6.1 are defined as follows:

- q is the number of scores used in the experiment,
- w_{kl} is the weight associated with the two categories k and l,
- $p'_{kl} = p_{kl}/\theta$, where p_{kl} is the relative number of subjects that raters 1 and 2 scored as x_k and x_l respectively, and θ the relative number of subjects scored by both raters (i.e. subjects with no missing rating).
- T_w is the sum of all weights w_{kl} associated with all categories.
- π_k is the probability that a rater assigns score x_k to a subject, and is calculated as $\pi_k = (p'_{k+} + p'_{+k})/2$. Note that $p'_{k+} = p_{k+}/\theta_1$ with θ_1 being the relative number of subjects that rater 1 has scored, and p_{k+} the relative number of subjects that rater 1 scored as x_k. Likewise, $p'_{+k} = p_{+k}/\theta_2$ with θ_2 being the relative number of subjects that rater 2 has scored, and p_{+k} the relative number of subjects that rater 2 scored as x_k.

Table 4.6: Scores assigned to 12 subjects by raters 1 and 2.

Subject	Rater1	Rater2
1		1
2	1.5	1.5
3	2	2
4	1	1
5	0.5	0.5
6	2	2.5
7	0.5	1
8	0.5	0.5
9	0.5	
10	0.5	0.5
11	2	0.5
12	1.5	2

Equation 4.6.1 is obtained from the AC_1 coefficient, and its derivation follows the general approach of chapter 3. The percent agreement p_a is the weighted sum of

the individual classification probabilities p'_{kl}, which are adjusted for missing values. To make sense of the percent chance agreement p_e, note that it can be rewritten as follows,

$$p_e = \left\{ \sum_{k,l} \left(\frac{w_{kl}}{q^2} \right) \right\} \times P(\mathcal{R}),$$

$P(\mathcal{R})$ being the likelihood of random rating of equation 4.4.6. The term in brackets is the weighted probability that both raters agree.

The following example illustrates the AC$_2$ coefficient using the rating data of Table 4.6.

Example 4.3 _____

In this example, you want to compute the extent of agreement between two raters named Rater1 and Rater2 using the ratings reported in Table 4.6. Since this data is numeric and can be considered of interval type, you want to use weighted agreement coefficient to perform the analysis.

Table 4.7 shows the distribution of the 12 subjects of Table 4.6 by rater and by score, and includes the distribution of missing values, as well as marginal totals and percentages. Table 4.8 on the other hand, shows the weighted agreement coefficients calculated using six methods and the quadratic weights. The coefficients used are Cohen's kappa, Gwet's AC$_2$, Scott's Pi, Krippendorff's alpha, Brennan-Prediger, and the percent agreement not corrected for chance agreement.

Table 4.7: Distribution of 12 subjects by rater and score.

Rater1	Rater2							
	0.5	1	1.5	2	2.5	Missing	Total	Percent
0.5	**3**	1	0	0	0	1	5	41.7%
1	0	**1**	0	0	0	0	1	8.3%
1.5	0	0	**1**	1	0	0	2	16.7%
2	1	0	0	**1**	1	0	3	25%
2.5	0	0	0	0	**0**	0	0	0%
Missing	0	1	0	0	0	0	1	8.3%
Total	4	3	1	2	1	1	12	100%
Percent	33.3%	25%	8.3%	16.7%	8.3%	8.3%	100%	

Table 4.8: Agreement coefficients associated with Table 4.6 ratings

Method	Coefficient	Method	Coefficient
Cohen's Kappa	0.6600	Krippendorff's α	0.6737
Gwet's AC_1	0.7643	Brenann-Prediger	0.7000
Scott's Pi	0.6596	Percent Agreement	0.9250

4.6.2 AC_2 for Interval Data and for three Raters or More

When an arbitrarily large number r of raters must score n subjects based on q interval-type scores, the AC_1 coefficient of equation 4.5.1 must be weighted to account for the ordering and the distance between scores. This will allow for the some "minor" disagreements to be treated as partial agreements by assigning to them weights that are smaller than those associated with full agreements. The weighted version of AC_1, named AC_2 is more efficient, is denoted by $\widehat{\gamma}_2$, and is defined for a given set of weights (w_{kl}) as follows:

$$\widehat{\gamma}_2 = \frac{p_a - p_e}{1 - p_e}, \ where \begin{cases} p_a = \dfrac{1}{n'} \sum_{i=1}^{n'} \sum_{k=1}^{q} \dfrac{r_{ik}(r_{ik}^{\star} - 1)}{r_i(r_i - 1)}, \\[2mm] p_e = \dfrac{T_w}{q(q-1)} \sum_{k=1}^{q} \pi_k(1 - \pi_k). \end{cases} \tag{4.6.2}$$

The different terms in equation 4.6.2 are defined as follows:

- n' is the number of subjects that are scored by two raters of more, and q the number of different score values that raters can use to score the subjects.

- r_i is the number of raters who actually scored subject i, and r_{ik} the number of raters who assigned the k-th score x_k to subject i. The term $r_{ik}^{\star}$ on the other hand, represents the weighted count of raters who assigned to subject i, the k-th score x_k or any score in partial agreement[12] with the k-th score. More formally, $r_{ik}^{\star}$ is defined as,

$$r_{ik}^{\star} = \sum_{l=1}^{q} w_{kl} r_{il}. \tag{4.6.3}$$

---

[12] A score x_l is in partial agreement with the k-th score x_k if the weight w_{kl} associated with these two scores is nonzero.

- T_w is the summation of all weights w_{kl} associated with all q scores, and π_k is the propensity for assigning score x_k to a subject, and is calculated as shown in equation 4.5.1.

The only difference between the unweighted and weighted AC$_1$ of equations 4.5.1 and 4.6.2 is the use of the weighted rater count $r_{ik}^{\star}$ and the summation of weights T_w. The two expressions become identical if identity weights (i.e. weights where all diagonal elements are 1, and all off-diagonal elements are 0) are used with equation 4.6.2. For this reason, equation 4.6.2 is often used with the appropriate set of weights to compute both the AC$_1$ and the AC$_2$ coefficients. Both terms AC$_1$ and AC$_2$ will sometimes be used interchangeably for that same reason.

Consider Table 4.9 that contains data from a reliability experiment where 5 observers score 20 units on a 4-point numeric scale based on the values $\{0, 1, 2, 3\}$. This data is used in the next example to illustrate the calculation of AC$_2$ and other weighted coefficients.

Table 4.9: Scores assigned by 5 observers to 20 experimental units

Unit	Obs1	Obs2	Obs3	Obs4	Obs5
1	1	1	2		2
2	1	1	0	1	
3	2	3	3	3	
4		0	0		0
5	0	0	0		0
6	0	0	0		0
7	1	0	2		1
8	1		2	0	
9	2	2	2		2
10	2	1	1	1	
11		1	0	0	
12	0	0	0	0	
13	1	2	2	2	
14	3	3	2	2	3
15	1	1	1		1
16	1	1	1		1
17	2	1	2		2
18	1	2	3	3	
19	1	1	0	1	
20	0	0	0		0

Example 4.4 _____

To illustrate the calculation of the AC_2 statistic for 3 raters or more, let us consider the reliability data of Table 4.9. This data will be treated as interval data because the possible scores 0, 1, 2, and 3 can be ranked from small to large, and the difference between any two scores is assumed to have a practical meaning. The scores associated with each experiment must be carefully interpreted prior to deciding whether to treat them as nominal, ordinal or interval data.

Table 4.10 shows the distribution of subjects by rater and by score value. The numbers in the rightmost column (labeled as "Total") are not identical; an indication that some observers scored more units than others. Observer 4 for example scored only 10 units, while observer 3 scored all 20. Table 4.11 on the other hand, shows the quadratic weights used in the calculation of the weighted agreement coefficients. The quadratic weight associated with the scores (1,0) for example is $1-(1-0)^2/3^2 = 1-1/9 = 0.8889$, where 3 is the maximum difference between scores.

Table 4.12 shows the different values associated with the unweighted and weighted agreement coefficients. It appears that accounting for partial agreements with the use of quadratic weights increases the AC_1 coefficient from its unweighted value 0.502 to its weighted value of 0.8224.

Table 4.10: Distribution of 20 subjects by rater and score.

		Score			
Rater	0	1	2	3	Total
Obs1	4	9	4	1	18
Obs2	6	8	3	2	19
Obs3	8	3	7	2	20
Obs4	3	3	2	2	10
Obs5	4	3	3	1	11
Average	5	5.2	3.8	1.6	15.6

Table 4.11: Quadratic Weights Associated with Scores $\{0, 1, 2, 3\}$

	0	1	2	3
0	1	0.8889	0.5556	0
1	0.8889	1	0.8889	0.5556
2	0.5556	0.8889	1	0.8889
3	0	0.5556	0.8889	1

Table **4.12**: Weighted Agreement Coefficients for Table 4.9 Rating Data

Coefficient	Unweighted	Weighted
Conger's Kappa	0.4762	0.7435
Gwet's AC_1	0.5021	0.8224
Fleiss' Kappa	0.4651	0.7305
Krippendorff's α	0.4817	0.7468
Brenann-Prediger	0.4933	0.7980
Percent Agreement	0.6200	0.9439

4.7   Concluding Remarks

The primary objective of this chapter was to present a theoretical framework for investigating the notion of agreement among raters, and to introduce the AC_1 statistic as a robust alternative agreement coefficient to Kappa, Pi, or Krippendorff's alpha. I wanted to have an in-depth discussion about the relationship between the computational procedures and the concept of agreement for the purpose of justifying the different approaches. I wanted the reader to see why some computational procedures are formulated the way they are, and to see what their limitations may be. The whole framework developed in this chapter is based on the notion of E-subjects or easy subjects also known as textbook subjects, and on the notion of H-subjects or hard subjects that are expected to be rated randomly and susceptible to produce agreement among raters by pure chance. Because of the difficulty to tease apart the subpopulations of E- and H-subjects, it is often necessary to make assumptions in order to obtain a definitive formulation of the computational procedures.

All agreement coefficients discussed in the past few chapters were developed around the percent agreement p_a, which is corrected for chance agreement using various strategies. Agreement by pure chance is perceived by most researchers as false agreement that if left untreated may artificially increase the estimated extent of agreement among raters. Therefore, correcting the percent agreement for chance agreement aims at dampening down the adverse effect of spurious agreements on the agreement coefficients, and the false sense of uniformity in the ratings they convey. An agreement by pure chance does not reflect any leveling in raters' knowledge and skills.

While adjusting for chance agreement is necessary, not all adjustment methods are expected to bring the percent agreement closer to the "true" extent of agreement among raters. Kappa, and Pi are known to behave as well as other alternative coefficients only when the percent agreement is around 0.5. The BP coefficient's performance appears to be superior to that of Kappa and Pi. However, the fixed percent chance agreement of 0.5 used by BP sometimes indicates a propensity for chance agreement that exceeds what would be expected from the data. This artificially reduces the magnitude of the inter-rater reliability coefficient.

Improving inter-rater reliability coefficients requires one to define a construct and to formulate the operational definition that shapes it, possibly through statistical modeling. Aickin (1990) proposed the approach discussed in section 4.3. His approach led to an agreement coefficient with good statistical properties, and is based on the notion of "Hard-to-score Subjects" who are assigned nondeterministic ratings. Among the disadvantages of Aickin's alpha coefficient are its time-consuming iterative computation procedure, and its magnitude that cannot reach the maximum value of 1. Gwet's approach, which led to the AC_1 coefficient is discussed in section 4.4. It also uses the notion of "Hard-to-score Subjects" that produce agreement by chance. While Aickin's alpha represents the relative number of "Easy-to-score Subjects" with respect to the total number of subjects, Gwet's AC_1 represents the relative number of "Easy-to-score Subjects" with respect to the group of subjects left after removing H-subjects. That is, if the raters agree on all H-subjects then the AC_1 coefficient will be 1, and Aickin's alpha will still be the proportion of E-subjects in the population. In fact alpha takes the maximum value of 1 only if there is no H-subject in the subject population. For Aickin (1990) the very existence of H-subjects makes it impossible to obtain a perfect agreement even if there is no observed disagreement. For Gwet (2008), only an observed disagreement (on an H-subject) would make it impossible to obtain the maximum agreement coefficient of 1.

When special types of disagreements represent a certain level of agreement (or partial agreement), the AC_2 coefficient introduced in section 4.6, provides a more accurate assessment of the inter-rater reliability. This is achieved by assigning a weight to each pair of scores, downweighting the pairs that represent little agreement while upweighting those representing substantial agreement. Although we have only considered a few types of weights in this chapter, practitioners could consider different weights to serve different purposes, provided the weights used in the analysis are defined prior to the reliability experiment.

Agreement Coefficients and Statistical Inference

OBJECTIVE

This chapter describes several approaches for evaluating the precision associated with the inter-rater reliability coefficients of the past few chapters. Although several factors ranging from the misreporting of ratings to deliberate misstatements by some raters, could affect the precision of Kappa, AC_1 or any other agreement coefficient, the focus is placed on the quantification of sampling errors. These errors stem from the discrepancy between the pool of subjects we want our findings to apply to (i.e. the target subject population), and the often smaller group of subjects that actually participated in the inter-rater reliability experiment (i.e. the subject sample). The sampling error is measured in this chapter by the variance of the inter-rater reliability coefficient. The concept of variance will be rigorously defined, and associated computation methods described. Numerous practical examples are presented to illustrate the use of these precision measures.

CONTENTS

> *Without theory, experience has no meaning,* $\cdots$ *Without theory, one has*
> *no questions to ask. Hence without theory, there is no learning.*
> - Edwards Deming (1900-1993) -

5.1   The Problem

Tables 5.1 and 5.2 are two representations of hypothetical rating data that Conger (1980) used as examples to illustrate the Kappa coefficient. The ratings are those of 4 raters $R1$, $R2$, $R3$, and $R4$ who each classified 10 subjects into one of 3 possible categories a, b, or c. Applied to this data, Fleiss' generalized Kappa (see equation 2.11 of chapter 2) yields an inter-rater reliability of $\widehat{\kappa}_{\text{F}} = 0.247$. To interpret the meaning of this empirical number, and to understand its real value, the researcher may need answers to some of the following fundamental questions:

▶ Is 0.247 a valid number ? Does it quantify the actual phenomenon the researcher wants to measure ? Can the notion of "extent of agreement among raters" be framed with rigor for researchers to have a common understanding of its most important aspects ?

▶ Can we demonstrate the validity of an observed sample-based agreement coefficient by measuring how close it is to a theoretical construct representing the "extent of agreement among raters ?"

▶ The Kappa coefficient of 0.247 is based on a single sample of 10 subjects and 4 raters. Are the 10 participating subjects sufficient in number to prove the reliability of a newly-developed classification system ? Assuming the number 0.247 measures what it is supposed to measure, how accurate is it ? Moreover, will the 4 raters of the study be the only ones to use the classification system ? How would a different group of raters affect inter-rater reliability ?

Asking those questions leads you straight to the domain of inferential methods. These methods allow a researcher to use information gathered from the observed portion of the subject universe of interest, and to project findings to the whole universe (including its unobserved portion). Several inferential methods ranging from crude guesswork to the more sophisticated mathematical modeling techniques have been used to tackle real-world problems. The focus in this chapter will be on the methods of statistical inference, which are based on the sampling distribution of the agreement coefficients of interest.

Several authors have stressed out the need to have a sound statistical base for studying inter-rater reliability problems. For example Kraemer (1979), or Kraemer et al. (2002) emphasize the need to use Kappa coefficients to estimate meaningful population characteristics. Likewise, Berry and Mielke Jr. (1988) mentioned the need for every measure of agreement to have a statistical base allowing for the implementation of significance tests. The analysis of inter-rater reliability data has long suffered from the absence of a comprehensive framework for statistical inference since the early works of Scott (1955) and Cohen (1960). This problem stems from the initial and modest goal the pioneers set to confine agreement coefficients to a mere descriptive role. Cohen (1960) saw Kappa as a summary statistic that aggregates rating data into a measure of the extent of agreement among observers who participated in the reliability study. Variances and standard errors proposed by various authors approximate the variation of agreement coefficients with respect to hypothetical and often unspecified sampling distributions. But without a comprehensive framework for statistical inference, standard errors are difficult to interpret, and hypothesis testing, or comparison between different agreement coefficients difficult to implement.

Table 5.1:

Categorization of 10 subjects into 3 groups $\{a, b, c\}$

Subjects	Raters			
	$R1$	$R2$	$R3$	$R4$
1	a	a	a	c
2	a	a	b	c
3	a	a	b	c
4	a	a	c	c
5	a	b	a	a
6	b	a	a	a
7	b	b	b	b
8	b	c	b	b
9	c	c	b	b
10	c	c	c	c

Table 5.2:

Distribution of 4 Raters by Subject and Category

Subjects	Categories			Total
	a	b	c	
1	3	0	1	4
2	2	1	1	4
3	2	1	1	4
4	2	0	2	4
5	3	1	0	4
6	3	1	0	4
7	0	4	0	4
8	0	3	1	4
9	0	2	2	4
10	0	0	4	4

The number of statistical techniques developed to address various practical problems is very large. Determining which ones apply to our particular problem, requires some efforts. The researcher must first and foremost develop a clear understanding of the reliability experiment's main objective. The following two objectives are often of interest:

▶ The researcher wants to understand the process by which raters assign subjects to categories. One may want to know what factors affect the classification and to what degree. Here, no particular group of subjects and no particular group of raters is of interest. The only thing that matters is the scoring process.

Each individual score is seen as a sample[1] from the larger set of all possible scores that can be assigned to any particular subject. During a given reliability experiment, each rater may have to provide several scores (or score samples) from different subjects. The score in this context is analyzed in its abstract form with no reference to a particular group of subjects and raters. Although the number of different scores that a rater can assign to a subject (i.e. the size of the population of scores) may be finite, the fact that the analysis does not target any specific group of subjects nor any particular group of raters led statisticians to refer to this approach as "infinite population inference". Infinity for all practical purposes simply means no reference is made to a specific group of subjects or raters, therefore to the number of samples that can be generated. Agresti (1992) recommends this inferential approach that also uses a theoretical statistical model as an effective way to study the relationship between raters' scores and the factors affecting them. These techniques represent a particular form of statistical inference, but are out of the scope of this book. Readers interested in this problem may also want to look at Shoukri (2010) or von Eye and Mun (2006)

▶ The framework of inference developed in this chapter assumes that the researcher has a target group of subjects and a target group of raters of interest. These two target groups are generally bigger than what the researcher can afford to include in the reliability experiment. A psychiatrist at a hospital may want the reliability study to only target his group of patients and the group of raters who may be called upon to use a newly-developed diagnosis procedure. If the group of patients is small, the researcher may conduct a census[2] of the patient population, in which case there will be no need for statistical inference since the statistics produced will match the population parameters. If on the other hand, the large size of the patient population could lead to a costly census that the researcher cannot afford, then a more affordable option is to survey a subgroup of patients. In this case, the results will be projected only to the predefined finite population of patients the participating subjects were selected from. Note that the same reasoning applies to the population of raters. That is, statistical inference may be required for the subject population, the rater population, or for both populations. This inferential approach is referred to as "Finite Population Inference[3]", and will be the focus in this chapter.

---

[1]A sample (or a score population sample) in this context is a single observation randomly generated by an often unspecified scoring process, which will be specific to each rater.

[2]A census refers to the participation of all subjects of interest in the study

[3]This framework for statistical inference was invented by a Polish mathematician named Jersey Neyman(1934) and is widely used in large-scale social and business survey projects. Key references related to this topic include Cochran (1977), and Särndal et al. (2003)

5.2 Finite Population Inference in Inter-Rater Reliability Analysis

Let us consider a reliability study that aims at quantifying the extent of agreement among raters with respect to a given scoring method. We assume that R raters form the rater universe named $\mathcal{U}_{\mathcal{R}}$, and are of interest as potential users of the classification method being tested. Likewise, N subjects forming a subject universe named $\mathcal{U}_{\mathcal{S}}$ are of interest after each of them had been identified as a possible candidate to be scored by one of the R raters. The researcher will ideally want to claim that all R raters can rate all N subjects with a high level of agreement. The raters in the rater population of inference, and subjects in the subject population of inference are labeled as follows:

$$\mathcal{U}_{\mathcal{S}} = \{1, \cdots, i, \cdots, N\},$$
$$\mathcal{U}_{\mathcal{R}} = \{1, \cdots, g, \cdots, R\}.$$

Although some of the R raters and some of the N subjects will not participate in the actual reliability experiment, the researcher still wants the experimental results to be applicable to them. One approach for making this feasible is to start by defining inter-rater reliability, the percent agreement and percent chance agreement with respect to these two populations. If the target numbers of subjects (N) and raters (R) are small then all subjects and raters can be included into the reliability experiment at a reasonable cost. If these numbers are large however, the cost of including all raters and subjects of interest into the study will become prohibitive. A solution to this cost problem is often to randomly select a subset of n subjects from the subject population $\mathcal{U}_{\mathcal{S}}$ and another subset of r raters from the rater population $\mathcal{U}_{\mathcal{R}}$. The two subsets referred to as the *"Rater sample"* (denoted by $s_r^\star$) and the *"Subject sample"* (denoted by s_n) define the participants in the inter-rater reliability experiment. In the notation $s_r^\star$, letter s indicates that the group of units (subjects or raters) represents a sample (not a population), the star ($\star$) indicates that the sample unit is the rater, and r represents the count of raters in the sample. On the other hand s_n (s without the star) represents a sample of n subjects.

Each time an inter-rater reliability experiment is based on a group of subjects or a group of raters that is smaller than the one being targeted, there is a loss of information that will subject resulting agreement coefficients to errors due to sampling (also known as *"Sampling Errors"*). Quantifying this sampling error and using it in all decisions involving the inter-rater reliability, are among the most fundamental goals of statistical inference. If the reliability experiment involves all N subjects and all R raters of interest then no sampling error will be associated with the resulting agreement coefficients, and there will be no need for inference.

5.2.1   *Defining the Notion of Sample*

Some researchers with background in the social or medical sciences tend to refer to each individual subject as a population sample, and to see a group of n subjects as n subject population samples, the same way one would see 10 blood drops in a medical facility as 10 blood samples. However, the selection of an entire group of n subjects as a whole and the selection of an entire rater group as a whole are the most fundamental building blocks in finite population inference. Consequently, the group of n subjects will be referred to as one sample of subjects of size n, while the whole group of r raters will be seen as one sample of raters of size r.

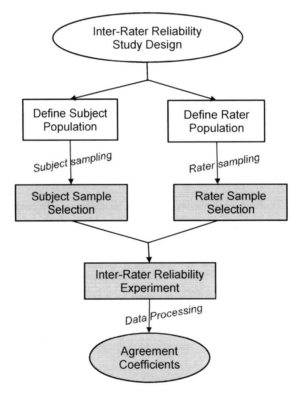

Figure 5.2.1: The Random Process Leading to the Agreement Coefficients

Note that our ultimate goal is to obtain the sampling distribution of the sample-based agreement coefficient. But the magnitude of the agreement coefficient is determined by both the rater and the subject samples, as well as the respective populations they were selected from (see Figure 5.2.1 - shaded areas represent what is observable in the process). Therefore the sampling distribution of the agreement coefficient is essentially determined by the selection probability of the whole subject and rater samples. Individual subjects and individual raters have a marginal importance in the inference. Only whole samples are relevant.

For the sake of fixing ideas, let us label all r sample raters and all n sample subjects with numbers as follows:

$$s_r^\star = \{1, \cdots, g, \cdots, r\}, \text{ and } s_n = \{1, \cdots, i, \cdots, n\}.$$

The framework of finite population inference requires that both samples s_n and $s_r^\star$ be selected randomly. The random selection of both groups induces a randomization process, which will define the probabilistic structure of statistical inference.

In a target population of N subjects for example, the total number of samples of size n that one may form is the number of combinations[4] of N objects taken n at a time, and is denoted by C_N^n. Likewise C_R^r, which is the number of combinations[5] of R raters in groups of r, equals the total count of rater samples of size r one can form from a population of R raters. Note that the researcher will have considerable flexibility in the way the subjects and raters are included in the samples as long as the selection process is random. For example one may decide that all subjects will have an equal chance of being selected for participation in the reliability study, in which case all C_N^n samples of subjects will have the same chance ($p = 1/C_N^n$) of being retained. This is the simple random sampling design. However, the researcher may also decide that one particular subject i_0 has to be part of any participating group for a reason. Such a design will assign a 0 selection probability to all samples not comprising subject i_0. In this case not all samples have the same selection probability. This is a complex sampling design. In this chapter, we will confine ourselves to the simple random sampling design where all samples have the same selection probability.

5.2.2 The Notion of Parameter in Finite Population Inference

Let i be an arbitrary population subject, and k one of the q response categories into which a rater may classify subject i. If all R raters in the target population were to score subject i, then R_{ik} would be the count of population raters to classify subject i into category k. Likewise $P_{ik} = R_{ik}/R_i$ would be the percent of population raters to classify subject i into category k, where R_i is the count of population raters who rated subject i. The population percent of raters π_k to classify (a subject) in category k is given by:

$$\pi_k = \frac{1}{N} \sum_{i=1}^{N} P_{ik}. \tag{5.2.1}$$

---

[4]Note that $C_N^n = \binom{N}{n} = N!/[n!(N-n)!]$ where $N! = N \times (N-1) \times \cdots \times 1$ is N factorial. Moreover, C_N^n can be calculated with MS Excel using the function " $= \mathsf{COMBIN}(N, n)$"

[5]i.e. $C_R^r = \binom{R}{r} = R!/(r!(R-r)!)$

For the sake of clarity, let us consider Fleiss' generalized weighted Kappa as an example. The percent agreement and Fleiss' percent chance agreement (Fleiss, 1971), calculated at the population level are respectively denoted by P_a and P_e (the P's are capitalized to indicate that the probabilities are evaluated based on the entire population, and not restricted to the samples), and defined as follows:

$$P_a = \frac{1}{N} \sum_{i=1}^{N} \sum_{k=1}^{q} \frac{R_{ik}(R_{ik}^{\star} - 1)}{R_i(R_i - 1)}, \quad \text{and } P_e = \sum_{k,l}^{q} w_{kl} \pi_k \pi_l, \tag{5.2.2}$$

where $R_{ik}^{\star}$ is the weighted count of raters who classified subject i into any category linked[6] to k through weighting (i.e. the sum of all $w_{kl} r_{il}$ across all values of l). For a researcher using Fleiss' generalized Kappa coefficient, the parameter of interest κ_{F} for the purpose of inference is defined as,

$$\kappa_{\mathrm{F}} = \frac{P_a - P_e}{1 - P_e}. \tag{5.2.3}$$

All the quantities P_{ik}, π_k, P_e, P_a or κ_{F} are population parameters to be estimated from the subject and rater samples. We generally use capital Latin letters or Greek letters for population parameters, while sample-based estimated values of these parameters use small Latin letters, or capital Latin letters with a hat on the top. For example, $p_{ik} = r_{ik}/r_i$ is the estimated percent of raters who classified subject i into category k, with r_i being the number of sample raters who rated subject i. Similarly, the estimated values of P_a and P_e respectively denoted by p_a and p_e are defined as follows:

$$p_a = \frac{1}{n} \sum_{i=1}^{n} \sum_{k=1}^{q} \frac{r_{ik}(r_{ik}^{\star} - 1)}{r_i(r_i - 1)}, \quad p_e = \sum_{k,l}^{q} w_{kl} \widehat{\pi}_k \widehat{\pi}_l, \tag{5.2.4}$$

where $r_{ik}^{\star}$ is the weighted count of sample raters who classified subject i into a category related to k through the weights, $\widehat{\pi}_k$ is the average of the n values p_{ik} $(i = 1, \cdots, n)$, and represents an estimated value of π_k. For simplicity of notations, we will often use π (without a hat) in place of $\widehat{\pi}$. The estimated value of the Fleiss' agreement coefficient of equation 5.2.3 is denoted by $\widehat{\kappa}_{\mathrm{F}}$ and given by:

$$\widehat{\kappa}_{\mathrm{F}} = \frac{p_a - p_e}{1 - p_e}. \tag{5.2.5}$$

The rater and subject samples must be selected in such a way that the estimated coefficient $\widehat{\kappa}_{\mathrm{F}}$ is as close as possible to its unknown population counterpart κ_{F}. Investigating the relationship between the sample-based $\widehat{\kappa}_{\mathrm{F}}$ and the population-based

---

[6]Two categories k and l are linked if the corresponding agreement weight w_{kl} takes a non-zero value. That is a classification of a subject into these categories is seen as partial agreement.

κ_{F} is a key goal of statistical inference. Note that justifying the particular form that the population-based coefficient takes (e.g. equation 5.3)) is not an integral part of the finite population inference framework. This latter task is accomplished with the use of statistical models as shown in chapter 4.

For Gwet's AC_1 or AC_2, the associated population parameters will be respectively γ_1 and γ_2. Their sample-based estimates, respectively denoted by $\widehat{\gamma}_1$ and $\widehat{\gamma}_2$, are defined in chapter 4. Their variances are discussed in the next few sections.

5.2.3   *The Nature of Statistical Inference*

Three distinct activities generally define what is known as statistical inference. These are,

▶ *Point estimation of a population parameter,*

▶ *Interval estimation of a population parameter,*

▶ *Test of hypothesis.*

Point estimation is about obtaining a single number as our best approximation of a population parameter using the subject and rater samples. For example p_a will often be our best sample-based approximation of the population parameter P_a. However, the estimation p_a is subject to a sampling error, which may be large. To deal with this error, some researchers will use interval estimation, which provides a range of values in the form of an interval, expected to include the "true" value of the parameter with a high level of confidence. Hypothesis testing on the other hand, determines whether or not a conjecture about the magnitude of a population parameter is consistent with observed ratings. For example the hypothesis that "The Kappa coefficient (at the population level) is greater than 0.20" may or may not be consistent with the ratings observed on a subject sample. Hypothesis testing is a procedure that leads to the rejection or the non rejection of hypotheses.

The inferential procedures of point estimation, interval estimation or hypothesis testing are all built from the sampling distribution of the sample-based agreement coefficients. For example, the overall percent agreement p_a is a function of the subject sample s_n, and the rater sample $s_r^\star$. Consequently, each pair of samples $(s_n, s_r^\star)$ will lead to a different percent agreement value $p_a(s_n, s_r^\star)$. All $C_{\text{N}}^n \times C_{\text{R}}^r$ such pairs of samples lead to a series of $C_{\text{N}}^n \times C_{\text{R}}^r$ values $p_a(s_n, s_r^\star)$, which forms the sampling distribution of p_a upon which statistical inference is built. Expectations, standard errors, and variances are calculated using that discrete sampling distribution. When the subject and rater samples are both generated by a random sampling process, the inference is said to be unconditional. If the subjects are selected randomly and all raters of interest included in the study as participants without sampling, then the inference will be conditional upon the specific group of participating raters. Although not common in practice, the situation where only raters are subject to random sampling will lead to inference conditionally on the subject sample.

5.3   Conditional Inference

This section deals with inferential procedures pertaining to reliability experiments where either the subjects or the raters are selected randomly, but noth both. That is if the subjects participating in the reliability study are selected randomly from the subject population, then no rater other than those participating in the study will be of interest. Likewise, if the participating raters are randomly selected from a larger rater population, then all subjects of interest will be included in the study. Section 5.3.1 is devoted to the situation where the subject sample is randomly selected from a bigger subject population, but all raters of interest participate in the reliability experiment. Therefore, the statistical error associated with the agreement coefficient will solely be due to the sampling of subjects.

5.3.1   *Inference Conditionally Upon the Rater Sample*

The researcher may decide that only the r participating raters in the rater sample $s_r^\star$ will be of interest, and no effort will be made to project the results beyond that group of raters. The rater sample $s_r^\star$ in this context, is identical to the rater population for the purpose of analysis. Here is a situation where any inter-rater reliability coefficient $\widehat{\kappa}$ will solely be a function of the subject sample. Each subject sample s_n among the C_N^n possible samples will yield a specific agreement coefficient $\widehat{\kappa}(s_n)$. Therefore, there are C_N^n possible values for the agreement coefficient, which provide the sampling distribution needed for statistical inference. This inferential procedure will be carried out conditionally upon the specific rater sample $s_r^\star$, and will be referred to as the *Conditional Inference on the Rater Sample* or the *Statistical Inference Conditionally upon the Rater Sample.*

By definition, the "true" or "Population", or "Exact" variance of an agreement coefficient $\widehat{\kappa}$ is the straight variance of all sample-based $\widehat{\kappa}\big(s_n^{(b)}\big)$ values taken on each of the C_N^n possible subject samples. It is given by:

$$V\big(\widehat{\kappa}(s_n)|s_r^\star\big) = \sum_{b=1}^{C_N^n} P\big(s_n^{(b)}\big)\Big[\widehat{\kappa}\big(s_n^{(b)}\big) - \overline{\overline{\kappa}}\Big]^2, \qquad (5.3.1)$$

where $s_n^{(b)}$ is the bth subject sample, $\overline{\overline{\kappa}}$ is the average of all C_N^n possible values that can be taken by the agreement coefficient $\widehat{\kappa}\big(s_n^{(b)}\big)$, and $P\big(s_n^{(b)}\big)$ the probability of selecting the specific sample $s_n^{(b)}$.

Evaluating the variance of an agreement coefficient using equation 5.3.1 is an impossible task. Not only will it be a tedious process to select all possible subject samples of size n out of the target population of N subjects, but implementing equation 5.3.1 would also require each of the N population subjects to have been scored by all raters, which is almost never the case. Consequently the exact variance of the agreement coefficient must be approximated based on a single subject sample and a single rater sample, which is all practitioners have at their disposal. The mathematical formulas used to compute these approximations, are referred to in the statistical literature as *Variance Estimators* as opposed to "Exact" variances such as equation (5.3.1). Gwet (2008a) suggested variance estimators for the AC_1, Kappa, Pi, and Brennan-Prediger (BP) agreement coefficients. These results are summarized here, and then expanded to accommodate the missing ratings, as well as the use of weights. As in the previous chapters, we will treat two-rater and multiple-rater experiments separately for the sake of clarity.

5.3.1A ESTIMATED VARIANCES IN TWO-RATER RELIABILITY EXPERIMENTS

In an inter-rater reliability experiment involving two raters A and B (i.e. $r = 2$), the ratings are often summarized as shown in Table 2.7 of chapter 2, where n_{kl} represents the count of subjects that raters A and B classified into categories k and l respectively, and $p_{kl} = n_{kl}/n$ the corresponding percentage. Moreover, $p_{k+} = n_{k+}/n$ and $p_{+k} = n_{+k}/n$ represent raters' A and B marginal classification probabilities respectively. As Fleiss (1971) suggested, $\pi_k = (p_{k+} + p_{+k})/2$ is interpreted as the probability that a randomly selected rater would classify a randomly selected subject into category k. If you are using interval data, then k might represent an interval score x_k instead.

Two-Rater Variances of the Unweighted and Weighted AC_1

Let $\widehat{\kappa}_G$ denote the AC_1 statistic[7]. It follows from chapter 4 that $\widehat{\kappa}_G = (p_a - p_e)/(1-p_e)$ where p_a, and p_e are the percent agreement and percent chance agreement respectively. Assuming that $f = n/N$ is the sampling fraction (i.e. the fraction of the target population that was sampled)[8],

▶ When there is no missing rating, and the ratings are organized in a contingency table, then the variance of the unweighted AC_1 coefficient proposed by Gwet

---

[7]We will use $\widehat{\kappa}_G$ as the generic notation for Gwet's AC_1 and AC_2 coefficients. The unweighted $\widehat{\kappa}_G$ will refer to the AC_1, while the weighted $\widehat{\kappa}_G$ will refer to AC_2.

[8]In many studies the size of the subject population N is unknown, in which case one should set $f = 0$. This amounts to assuming that the sampling fraction is negligible for all practical purposes.

(2008a) is given by:

$$v(\widehat{\kappa}_G) = \frac{1-f}{n(1-p_e)^2}\left\{p_a(1-p_a) - 4(1-\widehat{\kappa}_G)\left(\frac{1}{q-1}\sum_{k=1}^{q}p_{kk}(1-\widehat{\pi}_k) - p_a p_e\right)\right.$$

$$\left. + 4(1-\widehat{\kappa}_G)^2\left(\frac{1}{(q-1)^2}\sum_{k=1}^{q}\sum_{l=1}^{q}p_{kl}\left[1-(\pi_k+\pi_l)/2\right]^2 - p_e^2\right)\right\}, \quad (5.3.2)$$

▶ When there is no missing rating, and the ratings are organized in a contingency table, then the variance of the weighted AC_1 (also known as AC_2) is given by:

$$v(\widehat{\kappa}_G) = \frac{1-f}{n(1-p_e)^2}\left\{\sum_{k,l}^{q}p_{kl}\left[w_{kl} - 2\frac{(1-\widehat{\kappa}_G)T_w}{q(q-1)}\left(1-(\pi_k+\pi_l)/2\right)\right]^2\right.$$

$$\left. - \left[p_a - 2(1-\widehat{\kappa}_G)p_e\right]^2\right\}, \quad (5.3.3)$$

where T_w is the summation of all agreement weights. Note that equation 5.3.2 is a special case of equation 5.3.3 used with identity set of weights (i.e. weights were all diagonal elements are 1 and all off-diagonal elements are 0).

▶ If your data contains missing ratings (i.e. some subjects were rated by single rater, as opposed to being rated by both raters), then it becomes more convenient to analyze the raw ratings rather than a summary contingency table to avoid any loss of information. The following more general variance expression can be used to calculate the variance of the unweighted as well as the weighted AC_1 with the presence or absence of missing ratings,

$$v(\widehat{\kappa}_G) = \frac{1-f}{n}\frac{1}{n-1}\sum_{i=1}^{n}(u_i - \overline{u})^2, \quad (5.3.4)$$

where n is the number of subjects rated by at least one rater, and f the sampling fraction. Moreover, $u_i = a_i - 2(1-\widehat{\kappa}_G)e_i$, with a_i and e_i being defined as,

$$a_i = \frac{\varepsilon_i/\theta_2}{1-p_e}\sum_{k=1}^{q}\sum_{l=1}^{q}w_{kl}\left(\delta_{kl}^{(i)} - p'_{kl}\right), \text{ and } e_i = \frac{T_w}{q(q-1)(1-p_e)}\sum_{k=1}^{q}\pi_k b_k^{(i)},$$

where $\varepsilon_i = 1$ if both raters rated subject i, and $\varepsilon_i = 0$ otherwise. $\delta_{kl}^{(i)} = 1$ if raters A and B classified subject i into categories k and l respectively, $\delta_{kl}^{(i)} = 0$ otherwise. θ_2 is the percent of subject that are rated by both raters. $p'_{kl} = p_{kl}/\theta_2$, $b_k^{(i)} = \left(b_{+k}^{(i)} + b_{k+}^{(i)}\right)/2$ where,

$$b_{k+}^{(i)} = -(\varepsilon_{i\cdot}/\theta_A)\left(\delta_{k+}^{(i)} - p'_{k+}\right), \text{ and } b_{+k}^{(i)} = -(\varepsilon_{\cdot i}/\theta_B)\left(\delta_{+k}^{(i)} - p'_{+k}\right).$$

Note that $\varepsilon_{i\cdot} = 1$ (resp. $\varepsilon_{\cdot i} = 1$) if rater A (resp. rater B) scored subject i and will be 0 otherwise. Furthermore, θ_A (resp. θ_B) is the percent of subjects that rater A (resp. rater B) has scored, while $p'_{k+} = p_{k+}/\theta_A$ and $p'_{+k} = p_{+k}/\theta_B$.

Two-Rater Variances of the Unweighted and Weighted Scott's π Coefficient

Scott's π statistic (Scott, 1955) is given by $\widehat{\kappa}_S = (p_a - p_e)/(1 - p_e)$, where p_e is Scott's percent chance agreement of equation 2.6 in chapter 2.

▶ When there is no missing rating, and the ratings are organized in a contingency table then the variance of the unweighted Scott's coefficient proposed by Gwet (2008a) is given by:

$$
\begin{aligned}
v(\widehat{\kappa}_S) &= \frac{1-f}{n(1-p_e)^2} \Bigg\{ p_a(1-p_a) - 4(1-\widehat{\kappa}_S)\bigg(\sum_{k=1}^{q} p_{kk}\pi_k - p_a p_e \bigg) \\
&\quad + 4(1-\widehat{\kappa}_S)^2 \bigg(\sum_{k=1}^{q}\sum_{l=1}^{q} p_{kl}\Big[(\pi_k + \pi_l)/2\Big]^2 - p_e^2 \bigg) \Bigg\},
\end{aligned} \tag{5.3.5}
$$

▶ When there is no missing rating, and the ratings are organized in a contingency table, then the variance of the weighted Scott's coefficient is given by,

$$
\begin{aligned}
v(\widehat{\kappa}_S) &= \frac{1-f}{n(1-p_e)^2} \Bigg\{ \sum_{k,l}^{q} p_{kl}\Big[w_{kl} - (1-\widehat{\kappa}_S)(\overline{\pi}_k + \overline{\pi}_l) \Big]^2 \\
&\quad - \Big[p'_a - 2(1-\widehat{\kappa}_S)p'_e \Big]^2 \Bigg\},
\end{aligned} \tag{5.3.6}
$$

where p'_a and p'_e are defined as,

$$
\begin{aligned}
p'_a &= \sum_{k,l} w_{kl} p_{kl}, \;\; p'_e = \sum_{k,l} w_{kl}\pi_k\pi_l, \;\; \overline{\pi}_k = (\overline{p}_{+k} + \overline{p}_{k+})/2, \\
\overline{p}_{+k} &= \sum_{l=1}^{q} w_{kl}p_{+l}, \;\; \text{and} \;\; \overline{p}_{l+} = \sum_{k=1}^{q} w_{kl}p_{k+}.
\end{aligned} \tag{5.3.7}
$$

▶ If your data contains missing ratings (i.e. some subjects were rated by single rater, as opposed to being rated by both raters), then it becomes more convenient to analyze the raw ratings rather than a summary contingency table to avoid any loss of information. The following more general variance expression can be used to calculate the variance of the unweighted as well as the weighted $\widehat{\kappa}_S$ with the presence or absence of missing ratings,

$$
v(\widehat{\kappa}_S) = \frac{1-f}{n} \frac{1}{n-1} \sum_{i=1}^{n} (u_i - \overline{u})^2, \tag{5.3.8}
$$

where n is the number of subjects rated by at least one rater, and f the sampling fraction. Moreover, $u_i = u_{1i} + u_{2i}$, where u_{1i} and u_{2i} are defined as follows:

$$u_{1i} = \frac{\varepsilon_i/\theta}{1 - p_e} \sum_{k,l}^{q} w_{kl} \big(\delta_{kl}^{(i)} - p'_{kl} \big), \text{ and } u_{2i} = 2 \frac{1 - \widehat{\kappa}_S}{1 - p_e} \sum_{k=1}^{q} \pi_k^* b_k^{(i)},$$

where $b_k^{(i)}$ is defined as earlier in this sub-section, $\pi_k^* = (\overline{\pi}_{k+} + \overline{\pi}_{+k})/2$, $\overline{\pi}_{k+}$ and $\overline{\pi}_{+l}$ are defined as follows:

$$\overline{\pi}_{k+} = \sum_{l=1}^{q} w_{kl} \pi'_l, \text{ and } \overline{\pi}_{+l} = \sum_{k=1}^{q} w_{kl} \pi'_k, \tag{5.3.9}$$

and $\pi'_k = (p'_{k+} + p'_{+k})/2$.

Two-Rater Variances of the Unweighted and Weighted Cohen's Kappa

The Kappa coefficient (Cohen, 1960) is given by $\widehat{\kappa}_C = (p_a - p_e)/(1 - p_e)$, where p_e is Cohen's percent chance agreement (see equation 2.5 of chapter 2).

▶ When there is no missing rating, and the ratings are organized in a contingency table then the variance of the unweighted Cohen's kappa coefficient is given by,

$$\begin{aligned} v(\widehat{\kappa}_C) \quad &= \frac{1-f}{n(1-p_e)^2} \Bigg\{ p_a(1-p_a) - 4(1 - \widehat{\kappa}_C) \Bigg(\sum_{k=1}^{q} p_{kk} \widehat{\pi}_k - p_a p_e \Bigg) \\ &+ 4(1 - \widehat{\kappa}_C)^2 \Bigg(\sum_{k=1}^{q} \sum_{l=1}^{q} p_{kl} \big[(p_{Al} + p_{Bk})/2 \big]^2 - p_e^2 \Bigg) \Bigg\}. \end{aligned} \tag{5.3.10}$$

This expression was initially published by Gwet (2008a), and is mathematically equivalent to equation 13 of Fleiss et al. (1969), assuming no finite population correction (i.e. the sampling fraction f is 0).

▶ When there is no missing rating, and the ratings are organized in a contingency table, then the variance of the weighted Cohen's kappa coefficient is given by,

$$\begin{aligned} v(\widehat{\kappa}_C) \quad &= \frac{1-f}{n(1-p_e)^2} \Bigg\{ \sum_{k,l}^{q} p_{kl} \Big[w_{kl} - (1 - \widehat{\kappa}_C)(\overline{p}_{+k} + \overline{p}_{l+}) \Big]^2 \\ &- \Big[p'_a - 2(1 - \widehat{\kappa}_C) p'_e \Big]^2 \Bigg\}. \end{aligned} \tag{5.3.11}$$

While p'_a is defined as in equation 5.3.7, p'_e however is defined differently and is given by,

$$p'_e = \sum_{k,l}^{q} w_{kl} p_{k+} p_{+l}.$$

▶ If your data contains missing ratings (i.e. some subjects were rated by single rater, as opposed to being rated by both raters), then it becomes more convenient to analyze the raw ratings rather than a summary contingency table to avoid any loss of information. The following more general variance expression can be used to calculate the variance of the unweighted as well as the weighted kappa (see equation 3.6 of chapter 3) with the presence or absence of missing ratings:

$$v(\widehat{\kappa}_{\mathrm{C}}) = \frac{1-f}{n}\frac{1}{n-1}\sum_{i=1}^{n}(u_i - \overline{u})^2, \tag{5.3.12}$$

where n is the number of subjects rated by at least one rater, and f the sampling fraction. Moreover $u_i = u_{1i} + u_{2i}$, where u_{1i} and u_{2i} are defined as follows:

$$u_{1i} = \frac{\varepsilon_i/\theta}{1-p_e}\sum_{k,l}^{q} w_{kl}\big(\delta_{kl}^{(i)} - p'_{kl}\big),$$

and,

$$u_{2i} = \frac{1-\widehat{\kappa}_{\mathrm{C}}}{1-p_e}\left(\sum_{k=1}^{q}\overline{p}_{+k}b_{k+}^{(i)} + \sum_{k=1}^{q}\overline{p}_{k+}b_{+k}^{(i)}\right).$$

Two-Rater Variances of the Unweighted and Weighted Brennan-Prediger Coefficient

The generalized G-index, also referred to as the Brennan-Prediger (BP) coefficient is given in its unweighted version by $\widehat{\kappa}_{\mathrm{BP}} = (p_a - 1/q)/(1 - 1/q)$.

▶ When there is no missing rating, and the ratings are organized in a contingency table then the variance of the unweighted BP coefficient is given by,

$$v(\widehat{\kappa}_{\mathrm{BP}}) = \frac{1-f}{n(1-1/q)^2}p_a(1-p_a). \tag{5.3.13}$$

▶ When there is no missing rating, and the ratings are organized in a contingency table, then the variance of the weighted B-P coefficient is given by,

$$v(\widehat{\kappa}_{\mathrm{BP}}) = \frac{1-f}{n(1-p_e)^2}\left(\sum_{k,l}^{q} w_{kl}^2 p_{kl} - p_a'^2\right) \tag{5.3.14}$$

▶ If your data contains missing ratings (i.e. some subjects were rated by single rater, and not by both), then it becomes more convenient to analyze the raw ratings rather than a summary contingency table to avoid any loss of information. The following more general variance expression can be used to calculate the variance of the unweighted as well as the weighted kappa (see equation 3.8 of chapter 3) with the presence or absence of missing ratings:

$$v(\widehat{\kappa}_{\text{BP}}) = \frac{v(p_a)}{(1 - p_e)^2}, \tag{5.3.15}$$

where $v(p_a)$ is the variance of the percent agreement p_a, given by:

$$v(p_a) = \frac{1-f}{n} \frac{1}{n-1} \sum_{i=1}^{n} a_i^2, \text{ where } a_i = \varepsilon_i/\theta \sum_{k,l} w_{kl}\left(\delta_{kl}^{(i)} - p'_{kl}\right). \tag{5.3.16}$$

Without missing ratings equation 5.3.15 would be equivalent to equation 5.3.14, which in turn is equivalent to equation 5.3.13 if used with identity weights (i.e. the diagonal element is 1, and the off-diagonal element 0).

Two-Rater Variance of the Unweighted and Weighted Krippendorff's $\widehat{\alpha}_{\text{K}}$

Krippendorff's alpha coefficient denoted by $\widehat{\alpha}_{\text{K}}$ is based solely on subjects that were rated by both raters. All subjects with a missing rating are downright excluded from analysis. For the purpose of calculating Krippendorff's alpha, n always represents the count of subjects rated by both raters. This coefficient is given by $\widehat{\alpha}_{\text{K}} = (p_a - p_e)/(1 - p_e)$, where $p_a = (1 - \varepsilon_n)p'_a + \varepsilon_n$, $\varepsilon_n = 1/(2n)$, p'_a and p_e are given by,

$$p'_a = \sum_{k,l}^{q} w_{kl}p_{kl}, \text{ and } p'_e = \sum_{k,l}^{q} w_{kl}\pi_k\pi_l. \tag{5.3.17}$$

$p_{kl} = n_{kl}/n$ is the relative number of subjects that raters A and B classified into categories k and l respectively. Moreover, $\pi_k = (p_{k+}+p_{+k})/2$ where p_{k+} = proportion of subjects that rater A classified into category k, and p_{+l} = proportion of subjects that rater B classified into category l.

The standard error of the weighted Krippendorff's alpha coefficient is obtained as the square root of its variance, which is defined as follows:

$$v(\widehat{\alpha}_{\text{K}}) = \frac{1-f}{n(1-p'_e)^2}\left\{\sum_{k,l}^{q} p_{kl}\left[(1 - \varepsilon_n)w_{kl} - (1-\alpha_{\text{K}})(\overline{p}_k + \overline{p}_l)\right]^2 \right.$$
$$\left. - \left[(1 - \varepsilon_n)p_a - 2(1-\alpha_{\text{K}})p'_e\right]^2\right\}, \tag{5.3.18}$$

Since Krippendorff's alpha does not deal with missing ratings when the number of raters is limited to 2, the above variance expression is the only one needed. It can be used for computing the unweighted Krippendorff's coefficient using identity weights.

Two-Rater Variances of the Unweighted and Weighted Percent Agreement

The weighted percent agreement p'_a is given by,

$$p'_a = \sum_{k=1}^{q} \sum_{l=1}^{q} w_{kl} p_{kl}. \tag{5.3.19}$$

Used with identity weights, this expression will yield the regular unweighted percent agreement known in the literature.

▶ When there is no missing rating, and the ratings are organized in a contingency table, then the variance of the weighted percent agreement is given by,

$$v(p'_a) = \frac{1-f}{n} \left(\sum_{k=1}^{q} \sum_{l=1}^{q} w_{kl}^2 p_{kl} - p_a'^2 \right). \tag{5.3.20}$$

▶ If your data contains missing ratings (i.e. some subjects were rated by single rater, and not by both), then it becomes more convenient to analyze the raw ratings rather than a summary contingency table to avoid any loss of information. The following more general variance expression can be used to calculate the variance of the unweighted as well as the weighted kappa (see equation 3.8 of chapter 3) with the presence or absence of missing ratings:

$$v(p'_a) = \frac{1-f}{n} \frac{1}{n-1} \sum_{i=1}^{n} a_i^2, \text{ where } a_i = (\varepsilon_i/\theta) \sum_{k,l} w_{kl} \left(\delta_{kl}^{(i)} - p'_{kl} \right). \tag{5.3.21}$$

Without missing ratings equation 5.3.21 would be equivalent to equation 5.3.20.

Example 5.1

Let us consider the inter-rater reliability data of Table 2.6 in chapter 2, representing the distribution of patients with back pain classified into 3 pain categories by two clinicians 1 and 2. This inter-rater reliability experiment is based on a sample of 102 participating patients randomly selected from a bigger population of patients of interest suffering from back pain. However no clinicians other than the two who participated in the experiment is of interest. Consequently the observed extent of agreement will not apply to a larger group of clinicians. The variance recommended in this situation must be conditional on the specific pair of participating clinicians.

Table 5.3:
Distribution (p_{kl}) of Patients with Back Pain by Pain Category and Clinician

Category	Category - Clinician 2 -			p_{k+}	π_k
Clinician 1	DER	DYS	POS		
DER	0.21569	0.09804	0.01961	0.33333	0.31373
DYS	0.05882	0.26471	0.10784	0.43137	0.42157
POS	0.01961	0.04902	0.16667	0.23529	0.26471
p_{+k}	0.29412	0.41176	0.29412	1	1

Table 5.4:
Agreement Coefficients and Associated Variances for Table 2.6 Data

Statistics	Estimations				
	p_a	p_e	Coefficient	Variance	Standard Error
$\widehat{\kappa}_G$	0.6471	0.3269	0.4757	0.00495	0.070
$\widehat{\kappa}_S$	0.6471	0.3462	0.4602	0.00535	0.073
$\widehat{\kappa}_C$	0.6471	0.3449	0.4613	0.00534	0.073
$\widehat{\kappa}_{BP}$	0.6471	0.2500	0.4706	0.00504	0.071
$\widehat{\alpha}_K$	0.6488	0.3462	0.4628	0.00530	0.073

Table 5.3 contains various probabilities used in the variance calculations, while Table 5.4 shows the variances associated with the agreement coefficients. The standard error, which represents the square root of the variance is the precision measure that is used most in practice.

A standard error of 0.070 associated with an AC_1 coefficient of 0.4757 should be interpreted as follows: *"Our best estimate of the extent of agreement between clinicians 1 and 2 based on the AC_1 statistic and a sample of 102 patients is 0.4757. Its margin of error of 0.14 (i.e. 2 × 0.070) indicates that our best estimate may be off by 0.14, more or less."* In other words the "True" extent of agreement, which is based on all subjects in our target population could be as low as 0.3350 and as high as 0.6163.

Example 5.1 indicates that the margin of error associated with an agreement coefficient could be substantial. The following 3 important factors could contribute to its magnitude:

▶ The size n of the subject sample is a key contributing factor to the magnitude of the margin of error. An increase in number of participating subjects will lead to a decrease in the margin of error. However adding more subjects in an inter-rater reliability experiment will make it more expensive. Therefore a compromise must be found between the desired precision level for your estimate and the cost that you can afford for the experiment.

▶ A second important contributing factor is the size of our target population. Note that all variance expressions involve a multiplicative finite-population correction factor $1 - f = 1 - n/N$, which indicates that for a fixed sample size n, a smaller target population (i.e. smaller value for N) will lead to a smaller variance; and therefore to a smaller margin of error. Therefore for a limited budget, an inexpensive way to improve the accuracy of estimates is to limit the scope of the inter-rater reliability study by reducing the size of the target subject population.

▶ The last contributing factor is the magnitude of the "true" and unknown agreement coefficient. If the extent of agreement among raters is expected to be high, one may expect the margin of error to be small for the same sample size. This suggests that providing some training to the raters prior to the reliability experiment will improve the coefficient's precision in addition to increasing its magnitude.

Although very useful for computing the variances of inter-rater reliability coefficients when the number of raters is limited to 2, the variance equations presented in this section are not applicable to experiments involving 3 raters or more. This problem is addressed next.

5.3.1B ESTIMATED VARIANCES IN MULTIPLE-RATER RELIABILITY EXPERIMENTS

Gwet (2008a) proposed variance estimators for the multiple-rater version of AC$_1$, and Fleiss' Kappa in addition to proving their validity with a Monte-Carlo simulation experiment. The objective in this sub-section is to summarize these results, and to expand them in order to cover the weighted agreement coefficients, the missing ratings, as well as Conger's Kappa, and Krippendorff's alpha. In order to shorten the presentation of these results, we will show variance expressions only for the weighted versions of the coefficients. These expressions will cover unweighted coefficients as well by using identity weights.

Let n be the number of subjects rated by one rater or more, and n' the number of subjects rated by two raters or more. The percent agreement on a specific subject i is denoted by $p_{a|i}$ and is formulated as follows:

$$p_{a|i} = \sum_{k=1}^{q} \frac{r_{ik}(r_{ik}^* - 1)}{r_i(r_i - 1)}, \text{ if } r_i \geq 2, \text{ and } p_{a|i} = 0 \text{ otherwise.} \qquad (5.3.22)$$

You may want to refer to equation 5.2.4 for a definition of the different variables used in this equation.

▶ **The AC$_2$ Coefficient**

Let $f = n/N$ be the sampling fraction, and w_{kl} the set of weights to be used in the analysis. The AC$_2$ coefficient is defined by equation 4.18 of chapter 4, and its variance given by,

$$v(\widehat{\kappa}_{\mathrm{G}}) = \frac{1-f}{n}\frac{1}{n-1}\sum_{i=1}^{n}\left(\widehat{\kappa}_{\mathrm{G}|i}^{\star} - \widehat{\kappa}_{\mathrm{G}}\right)^2, \qquad (5.3.23)$$

where,

- $\widehat{\kappa}_{\mathrm{G}|i}^{\star} = \widehat{\kappa}_{\mathrm{G}|i} - 2(1-\widehat{\kappa}_{\mathrm{G}})\dfrac{p_{e|i} - p_e}{1 - p_e},$

- $\widehat{\kappa}_{\mathrm{G}|i} = \begin{cases} (n/n')(p_{a|i} - p_e)/(1-p_e), & \text{if } r_i \geq 2, \\ 0, & \text{otherwise,} \end{cases}$

- $p_{e|i} = \dfrac{T_w}{q(q-1)}\sum_{k=1}^{q}\dfrac{r_{ik}}{r_i}(1 - \pi_k).$

▶ **Fleiss' Kappa Coefficient $\widehat{\kappa}_{\mathrm{F}}$**

The variance of Fleiss' Kappa coefficient (see section 3.4 of chapter 3 for a definition of the weighted Fleiss' coefficient) is given by,

$$v(\widehat{\kappa}_{\mathrm{F}}) = \frac{1-f}{n}\frac{1}{n-1}\sum_{i=1}^{n}\left(\widehat{\kappa}_{\mathrm{F}|i}^{\star} - \widehat{\kappa}_{\mathrm{F}}\right)^2, \qquad (5.3.24)$$

where,

- $\widehat{\kappa}_{\mathrm{F}|i}^{\star} = \widehat{\kappa}_{\mathrm{F}|i} - 2(1-\kappa_{\mathrm{F}})\dfrac{p_{e|i} - p_e}{1 - p_e},$

  $\widehat{\kappa}_{\mathrm{F}|i} = \begin{cases} (n/n')(p_{a|i} - p_e)/(1-p_e), & \text{if } r_i \geq 2, \\ 0, & \text{otherwise,} \end{cases}$

- $p_{e|i} = \sum_{k=1}^{q}\overline{\pi}_k r_{ik}/r_i$, with $\overline{\pi}_k = (\overline{\pi}_{k+} + \overline{\pi}_{+k})/2,$

  $\overline{\pi}_{k+} = \sum_{l=1}^{q} w_{kl}\pi_l$, and $\overline{\pi}_{+l} = \sum_{k=1}^{q} w_{kl}\pi_k.$

The weight matrix is generally symmetric, in which case $\overline{\pi}_{k+} = \overline{\pi}_{+k}$.

▶ **Brennan-Prediger Coefficient $\widehat{\kappa}_{\mathrm{BP}}$**

The weighted Brennan-Prediger agreement coefficient (Brennan & Prediger, 1981) was defined in chapter 3 (see section 3.4). Its variance is defined as follows:

$$v(\widehat{\kappa}_q) = \frac{1-f}{n}\frac{1}{n-1}\sum_{i=1}^{n}\left(\widehat{\kappa}_{q|i} - \widehat{\kappa}_q\right)^2,$$

where,

$$\widehat{\kappa}_{q|i} = \begin{cases} (n/n')(p_{a|i} - p_e)/(1 - p_e), & \textit{if } r_i \geq 2, \\ 0, & \textit{otherwise,} \end{cases}$$

▶ Krippendorff's Alpha Coefficient

The weighted Krippendorff's alpha coefficient was defined in chapter 3 (see section 3.5.2). Its variance is defined as follows:

$$v(\widehat{\alpha}_{\mathrm{K}}) = \frac{1-f}{n} \frac{1}{n-1} \sum_{i=1}^{n} \left(\alpha_{\mathrm{K}|i}^{\star} - \alpha_{\mathrm{K}} \right)^2,$$

where, $\widehat{\alpha}_{\mathrm{K}|i}^{\star} = \widehat{\alpha}_{\mathrm{K}|i} - (1 - \alpha_{\mathrm{K}})(p_{e|i} - p_e)/(1 - p_e)$ and,

- $\widehat{\alpha}_{\mathrm{K}|i} = (p_{a\varepsilon_n|i} - p_e)/(1 - p_e)$,

- $p_{a\varepsilon_n|i} = (1 - \varepsilon_n)\left[p_{a|i} - p_a(r_i - \overline{r})/\overline{r} \right] + \varepsilon_n$, where $p_{a|i} = \sum_{k=1}^{q} \dfrac{r_{ik}(r_{ik}^{\star} - 1)}{\overline{r}(r_i - 1)}$,

$p_a = \dfrac{1}{n} \sum_{i=1}^{n} p_{a|i}$, $p_{e|i} = \sum_{k=1}^{q} \overline{\pi}_k \dfrac{r_{ik}}{\overline{r}} - (r_i - \overline{r})/\overline{r}$, $\overline{\pi}_k = (\overline{\pi}_{k+} + \overline{\pi}_{+k})/2$, and

$\overline{\pi}_{k+} = \sum_{l=1}^{q} w_{kl}\pi_l$, $\overline{\pi}_{+l} = \sum_{k=1}^{q} w_{kl}\pi_k$.

▶ Conger's Kappa Coefficient

The weighted Conger's Kappa coefficient (see Conger, 1980) was defined in chapter 3 (see section 3.4). Its variance is defined by,

$$v(\widehat{\kappa}_{\mathrm{C}}) = \frac{(1-f)}{n} \frac{1}{n-1} \sum_{i=1}^{n} \left(\kappa_{\mathrm{C}|i}^{\star} - \kappa_{\mathrm{C}} \right)^2,$$

where,

- $\widehat{\kappa}_{\mathrm{C}|i}^{\star} = \widehat{\kappa}_{\mathrm{C}|i} - 2(1 - \kappa_{\mathrm{C}})(p_{e|i} - p_e)/(1 - p_e)$,

- $\widehat{\kappa}_{\mathrm{C}|i} = \begin{cases} (n/n')(p_{a|i} - p_e)/(1 - p_e), & \textit{if } r_i \geq 2, \\ 0, & \textit{otherwise,} \end{cases}$

- $p_{e|i} = \dfrac{1}{r(r-1)} \sum_{g=1}^{r} \sum_{k=1}^{q} \overline{w}_{gk}^{(i)} \left(r\overline{p}_{+k} - p_{gk} \right)$.

- $\overline{w}_{gk}^{(i)} = \sum_{l=1}^{q} \delta_{gl}^{(i)} (w_{kl} + w_{lk})/2$, with $\delta_{gl}^{(i)}$ being 1 if rater g classifies subject i
  into category l, and 0 otherwise.

Computing the correct variances associated with the agreement coefficients discussed in the past few chapters involves a large number of calculations. This is especially true if your dataset contains missing ratings, and you use the weighted coefficients. Although these calculations can be done with a spreadsheet such as Excel, they are done more effectively with a computer program. The commercial user-friendly Excel VBA program AgreeStat (see `http://www.agreestat.com/agreestat.html`) implements all agreement coefficients presented in the past few chapters along with their associated variances. Alternatively, you may want to use the free R functions developed by the author, if you are an R user. These functions can be downloaded from the webpage `http://www.agreestat.com/r_functions.html`.

Example 5.2

To illustrate variance calculation in the context of multiple-rater reliability experiments, let us consider the Stickleback fish data of Table A.3 in appendix A. Table 5.5 shows the inter-rater reliability estimations and associated standard errors for the unweighted and the weighted analyzes. The weighted analysis is based on quadratic weights. Both analyzes include Conger's kappa, Gwet's AC_1, Fleiss' Kappa, Krippendorff's alpha, and BP coefficient. The percent agreement p_a is included in the analysis for comparison.

The standard error represents the square root of the variance, and quantifies the sampling error associated with the inter-rater reliability coefficient. The sampling error occurs when raters rate only a portion of the subject population, rather than rating that population in its entirety. The smaller the sampled portion of the population (i.e. the sampling fraction) the higher the sampling error. Other non-sampling errors such as clerical errors, or changes in experimental conditions are not quantified and should be minimized with a careful planning of the study.

Table 5.5: Agreement Coefficients and Associated Variances, and Standard Errors for the Stickleback Fish Data

Method	Unweighted Analysis		Weighted Analysis[a]	
	Coefficient	S.E[b]	Coefficient	S.E[b]
Conger's Kappa	0.4129	0.0778	0.7341	0.0668
Gwet's AC_1	0.4897	0.0694	0.7616	0.0403
Fleiss' Kappa	0.4103	0.0787	0.7338	0.0669
Krippendorff's Alpha	0.4154	0.0777	0.7361	0.0546
Brenann-Prediger	0.4756	0.0706	0.6825	0.0541
Percent Agreement	0.5805	0.0565	0.9206	0.0135

[a]The weighted analysis is based on Quadratic Weights
[b]S.E = Standard Error

It appears from Table 5.5 that the weighted coefficients based on quadratic weights are higher that their unweighted counterparts and have smaller standard errors. This is partly explained by the fact that weighted agreement coefficients include all full agreements as well as some disagreements in the form of partial agreements, and are therefore based on more data.

5.3.1C SOME FINITE-POPULATION SAMPLING TECHNIQUES

The purpose of this subsection is to give interested readers a glimpse into the calculation of expectations, and variances within the framework of finite population inference. Those who have not previously been exposed to finite population sampling techniques will gain further insight into the techniques leading to the variances discussed in the past few sections. However, this sub-section is not essential for understanding the topics discussed in subsequent sections, and can be skipped by readers with no interest in the nature of finite population sampling techniques.

We will first show that conditionally upon the rater sample, the sample-based overall percent agreement p_a is an unbiased estimator of the population parameter P_a (i.e. the expected value of p_a matches the subject population parameter it approximates[9]). We are choosing the overall percent agreement p_a as an example to illustrate the important statistical notion of unbiasedness. Consider all possible random samples of n subjects that could be selected out of the subject population containing a total of N. We indicated earlier that the number of such samples was the number of combinations of n subjects out of N, which is $C_N^n = N!/(n!(N-n)!$. List all these samples in any order and let $s_n^{(b)}$ be the bth sample on the list. The percent agreement based on that particular sample is given by[10] :

$$p_a\big(s_n^{(b)}\big) = \frac{1}{n} \sum_{i \in s_n^{(b)}} \sum_{k=1}^{q} \frac{r_{ik}(r_{ik}-1)}{r(r-1)},$$

$$= \frac{1}{n} \sum_{i=1}^{N} \sum_{k=1}^{q} \frac{r_{ik}(r_{ik}-1)}{r(r-1)} \epsilon_i^{(b)}, \quad \text{where } \epsilon_i^{(b)} = \begin{cases} 1 & if \ s_n^{(b)} \ni i \\ 0 & otherwise. \end{cases}$$

It follows that the expectation of p_a conditionally upon the rater sample is given by:

$$E(p_a|s_r^\star) = \sum_{b=1}^{C_N^n} p_a\big(s_n^{(b)}\big) P\big(s_n^{(b)}\big) = \frac{1}{n} \sum_{i=1}^{N} \sum_{k=1}^{q} \frac{r_{ik}(r_{ik}-1)}{r(r-1)} \left(\frac{1}{C_N^n} \sum_{b=1}^{C_N^n} \epsilon_i^{(b)} \right), \quad (5.3.25)$$

---

[9]The notion of unbiasedness tells us how far we can expect any given statistic to stray from the population parameter they approximate. Ideally, a statistic will be unbiased (or have a 0 bias), which indicates that its mean value equals the target parameter

[10]In order to keep the discussion at the basic level, we assume that there is no missing rating. That is, each of the r raters rate all n subjects under investigation.

where $P\left(s_n^{(b)}\right)$ is the probability of selecting the specific sample $s_n^{(b)}$. Note that the quantity in parentheses in equation (5.25a) is the ratio of the number of samples of size n containing subject i, to the total number of samples of size n. That ratio equals $C_{N-1}^{n-1}/C_N^n = n/N$. Consequently,

$$E(p_a|s_r^\star) = P_a = \frac{1}{N}\sum_{i=1}^{N}\sum_{k=1}^{q} \frac{r_{ik}(r_{ik}-1)}{r(r-1)}, \qquad (5.3.26)$$

which is the overall percent agreement calculated at the subject population level. To compute the variance, the different expectations involved will be calculated based on the same approach used here.

5.3.2 *Inference Conditionally Upon the Subject Sample*

There are models and standards for software process assessment and improvement such as the ISO/IEC 15504. In a typical inter-rater reliability study of an ISO/IEC 15504 assessment, independent assessors evaluate a number of software engineering and management practices (i.e. subjects) and are expected to show a high level of agreement. In such reliability experiments, the selection of assessors (i.e. raters) is the main source of variation affecting agreement since organizations will only be concerned with the subset of processes relevant to their business objectives as indicated by Park and Jung (2003). Consequently the set of processes will be considered fixed for inferential purposes, and the group of assessors seen as the sole source of random variation upon which statistical inference will be based.

Good statistical inference in this context will be done conditionally upon the specific set of attributes being evaluated (i.e. the subject sample). Therefore, all findings resulting from such an experiment will not be extrapolated to a set of software process attributes other than that used in the experiment. Let s_n denote the predetermined and fixed set of n process attributes retained for assessment, and $s_r^\star$ the group of r raters randomly selected from the target pool of R population raters. A total of B such samples[11] labeled as $s_r^{\star(1)}, \cdots, s_r^{\star(b)}, \cdots, s_r^{\star(B)}$ can possibly be selected, each of which with a probability $P\left(s_r^{\star(b)}\right)$ to be determined. Each specific rater sample $s_r^{\star(b)}$ will lead to a percent agreement $p_a\left(s_r^{\star(b)}\right)$, and to a percent chance agreement $p_e\left(s_r^{\star(b)}\right)$. These two probabilities can be used to obtain an agreement coefficient $\widehat{\kappa}\left(s_r^{\star(b)}\right)$. Therefore, using the same predetermined and fixed subject sample s_n, one can generate B agreement coefficients $\widehat{\kappa}\left(s_r^{\star(1)}\right), \cdots, \widehat{\kappa}\left(s_r^{\star(b)}\right), \cdots, \widehat{\kappa}\left(s_r^{\star(B)}\right)$.

---

[11]Note that $B = C_R^r = \binom{R}{r} = R!/[r!(R-r)!]$, the number of combinations of r out of R. MS Excel could be used to compute this number as " $=$ COMBIN(R, r)"

The "conditional" expected value of an agreement coefficient $\widehat{\kappa}$ given the subject sample s_n is by definition the weighted mean of all B agreement coefficients $\widehat{\kappa}\big(s_r^{\star(b)}\big)$ and is given by:

$$E\big(\widehat{\kappa}(s_r^\star)|s_n\big) = \sum_{b=1}^{\mathrm{B}} P\big(s_r^{\star(b)}\big)\widehat{\kappa}\big(s_r^{\star(b)}\big), \qquad (5.3.27)$$

and its variance given by:

$$V\big(\widehat{\kappa}(s_r^\star)|s_n\big) = \sum_{b=1}^{\mathrm{B}} P\big(s_r^{\star(b)}\big)\Big(\widehat{\kappa}\big(s_r^{\star(b)}\big) - E\big(\widehat{\kappa}(s_r^\star)|s_n\big)\Big)^2. \qquad (5.3.28)$$

Equations (5.3.27) and (5.3.28) are primarily used as definitional expressions, which are not convenient for computing expectations and variances.

To be more concrete, let us assume that the sampling of raters is based on the Simple Random Sampling (SRS) design where all samples $s_r^{\star(b)}$ have the same selection chance. That is, each of the B rater samples would be selected with the exact same probability $P\big(s_r^{\star(b)}\big) = 1/B$. Under these conditions, the variance of equation (5.3.28) can be approximated from a single rater sample $s_r^\star$ using the following "Jackknife" variance estimator:

$$v_{\mathrm{J}}\big(\widehat{\kappa}\big) = \frac{(1 - g_r)(r - 1)}{r} \sum_{g=1}^{r}\big(\widehat{\kappa}^{(-g)} - \widehat{\kappa}^{(\bullet)}\big)^2, \qquad (5.3.29)$$

where $g_r = r/R$ is the rater sampling fraction[12], $\widehat{\kappa}^{(-g)}$ is the extent of agreement among all raters except rater g, and $\widehat{\kappa}^{(\bullet)}$ is the average of all r values $\widehat{\kappa}^{(-g)}$. Equation (5.3.29) is applicable to any of the kappa-like agreement coefficients $\widehat{\kappa}$ discussed until now, and requires the availability of raw ratings as described in Table 5.1 with 3 raters or more. Conditional inference given a specific subject sample is not feasible when the number of raters in the sample is limited to 2. By removing one column at a time from the raw data table, and calculating the agreement coefficient based on the reduced table, one can generate all r agreement coefficients $\widehat{\kappa}^{(-g)}$ $(g = 1, \cdots, r)$ necessary to compute the "Jackknife" variance of equation 5.3.29. Kraemer (1979) previously mentioned the idea of using the jackknife methodology for estimating the variance of an agreement coefficient.

---

[12]When the size R of the rater population is unknown, then the rater sampling fraction must be set to 0. A zero rater sampling fraction may overestimate the variance if the rater population is small.

Example 5.3 ───

Let us consider Table 5.1 reliability data. We assume that the 10 subjects are the only ones of interest to the researcher, making the selection of raters the sole source of variation affecting the precision of the agreement coefficient. Column 2 of Table 5.6 shows the extent of agreement among raters based on the AC_1, Pi, Kappa, and BP coefficients, and on the full rater sample.

Table 5.6:
Conditional Variance of Agreement Coefficients given the Subject Sample

Coefficient	Full Sample	Replicate Sample				Jackknife Variance
		1	**2**	**3**	**4**	
$\widehat{\kappa}_G$	0.252	0.200	0.301	0.205	0.310	0.0080
$\widehat{\kappa}_F$	0.247	0.200	0.298	0.189	0.278	0.0067
$\widehat{\kappa}_C$	0.263	0.227	0.320	0.212	0.293	0.0061
$\widehat{\kappa}_{BP}$	0.250	0.200	0.300	0.200	0.300	0.0075

The sample of 4 raters could generate 4 replicate rater samples of size 3 each. Each replicate rater sample is obtained after removing one rater from the full sample. The Table 5.6 columns labeled as 1, 2, 3, and 4 contain the agreement coefficients based on these replicate samples. For example 0.301 is the AC_1 coefficient measuring the extent of agreement among raters 1, 3, and 4 (rater 2 being removed from the rater sample). For each of the agreement coefficients listed in the first column of Table 5.6, the jackknife variance is calculated in the last column, using corresponding replicate agreement coefficients and equation 5.3.29. Table 5.6 indicates that the Jackknife variance of the different coefficients ranges from 0.0061 for Kappa to 0.008 for AC_1.

───

More background on the Jackknife variance estimation can be found in Tukey (1958) who adapted to variance estimation, the Jackknife method that Quenouille (1949, 1956) initially introduced as a bias-reduction technique. As a variance estimation technique, the jackknife belongs to the more general class of replication methods that estimate the variance of a statistic by computing the same statistic several times using each time a different sub-sample (also known as "replicate sample") of the original sample and by averaging the squared differences of the replicate estimates to their mean. Other replication techniques not discussed in this book include the Balanced Repeated Replication (BRR) by McCarthy (1966) and the bootstrap by Efron (1979).

5.4   Unconditional Inference

Many inter-reliability studies are designed to produce findings that can be projected to a single population of interest. This population of interest is either the subject population or the rater population. However, there are situations common in the medical research field for example, where a classification system being tested is expected to be used by raters other than those who provided the ratings, and on subjects other than those who were rated. In this case, the precision of the inter-rater reliability coefficient must be evaluated with respect to both the target rater population as well as the target subject population. The recommended approach is to start with a clear description of the make-up of both the subject and rater populations. For example "all residents of a given city aged 35 to 65 who have once been hospitalized for a cardiovascular disease" could be a target subject population. As a second step, a sample of subjects should be randomly selected from the subject population, and a rater sample randomly selected from the rater population. Randomness here ensures that the selected samples will be representative of their respective target populations.

5.4.1   *Definition of Unconditional Variance*

Because the inter-rater reliability experiment involves two populations, expectations, variances, and standard errors must account for not one, but two sources of variation. One source of variation is due to the random selection of subjects, while the second source of variation is due to the sampling of raters. If $\widehat{\kappa}$ represents an inter-rater reliability coefficient computed from a sample s_n of n subjects, and a sample $s_r^\star$ of r raters, $\widehat{\kappa}$ will be a function of the two samples, and could be denoted as $\widehat{\kappa}(s_n, s_r^\star)$. Since there is a total of $D \times B$ possible combinations[13] of subject samples of size n, and rater samples of size r that can be selected from the two populations of inference, the expected value of $\widehat{\kappa}(s_n, s_r^\star)$ is defined as the average of all $\widehat{\kappa}(s_n, s_r^\star)$ coefficients. That is,

$$E\left(\widehat{\kappa}(s_n, s_r^\star)\right) = \sum_{d=1}^{D}\sum_{b=1}^{B} \widehat{\kappa}\left(s_n^{(d)}, s_r^{\star(b)}\right) P\left(s_n^{(d)}, s_r^{\star(b)}\right),$$

$$= \sum_{d=1}^{D}\sum_{b=1}^{B} \widehat{\kappa}\left(s_n^{(d)}, s_r^{\star(b)}\right) P\left(s_n^{(d)}\right) P\left(s_r^{\star(b)}\right), \qquad (5.4.1)$$

where $P\left(s_n^{(d)}, s_r^{\star(b)}\right)$ is the probability of selecting the specific subject and rater samples $s_n^{(d)}$ and $s_r^{\star(b)}$. A special case of interest often occurs in practice when each

---

[13]In this case $D = \mathrm{C}_{\mathrm{N}}^{n}$ is the number of combinations of n subjects taken out of N, and $B = \mathrm{C}_{\mathrm{R}}^{r}$ is the number of combinations of r raters taken out of a total of R.

of the D subject samples has the same probability of selection, and each of the B rater samples has the same selection probability. In this case, both subject and rater samples are referred to as simple random samples. Under the Simple Random Sampling (or SRS) design, the expectation in equation 5.24 becomes,

$$E\left(\widehat{\kappa}(s_n, s_r^\star)\right) = \frac{1}{D \cdot B} \sum_{d=1}^{D} \sum_{b=1}^{B} \widehat{\kappa}\left(s_n^{(d)}, s_r^{\star(b)}\right) \qquad (5.4.2)$$

The variance of an estimated agreement coefficient $\widehat{\kappa}(s_n, s_r^\star)$ is given by:

$$V\left(\widehat{\kappa}(s_n, s_r^\star)\right) = E\left\{\widehat{\kappa}(s_n, s_r^\star) - E\left(\widehat{\kappa}(s_n, s_r^\star)\right)\right\}^2, \qquad (5.4.3)$$

where $E\left(\widehat{\kappa}(s_n, s_r^\star)\right)$ is defined by equation 5.4.2. Note that equation 5.4.3 indicates that the variance of an inter-rater reliability is the average over all possible pairs of subject-rater samples of the squared differences of the agreement coefficients to their overall average.

The definitional equations 5.4.2, and 5.4.3 are good for understanding the notions of expectation and variance under finite population inference, but cannot be used to compute these statistical measures. The main obstacle is due to the very nature of reliability experiments that generally produce rating data from a single subject sample and a single rater sample, and not from all possible samples. In practice, this variance must be approximated as discussed by Gwet (2008*b*).

5.4.2 *Calculating the Unconditional Variance*

In this section, we will show how the unconditional variance of an agreement coefficient may be calculated based on ratings from a single sample of subjects, and a single sample of raters. These techniques were discussed in Gwet (2008*b*) for unweighted agreement coefficients, based on data which contains no missing ratings. The expression proposed by Gwet (2008*b*) for computing the unconditional variance of an agreement coefficient $\widehat{\kappa}$ is the sum of the variance $v_s(\widehat{\kappa})$ due to the sampling of subjects and the variance $v_r(\widehat{\kappa})$ due to the sampling of raters. That is,

$$v(\widehat{\kappa}) = v_s(\widehat{\kappa}) + v_r(\widehat{\kappa}). \qquad (5.4.4)$$

Gwet (2008*b*) proposed a close mathematical expression for evaluating $v_r(\widehat{\kappa})$ from the samples, and presented simulation results, which indicate that the rater variance component could account for a large percentage of total variance. It should therefore not be neglected if the reliability experiment aims at projecting the inter-rater reliability coefficient to a larger universe of raters as well as a larger universe of subjects.

What practitioners need, is a more general approach for calculating the unconditional variance associated with agreement coefficients, which can accommodate the presence of missing ratings as well as the use of weights. Such an approach is implemented by first calculating the subject-induced variance $v_s(\widehat{\kappa})$ using the appropriate expression from section 5.3.1, then by calculating the rater-induced variance $v_r(\widehat{\kappa})$ using the jackknife variance expression 5.3.29, and summing both variances as in equation 5.4.4. Some inter-rater reliability studies may involve many subjects, and generally involve only a few raters. Consequently, calculating the rater variance with the jackknife method will require minimal computational resources. As for the subject variance, using one of the close expressions of section 5.3.1 is recommended, since the jackknife method may take considerable computing time if the number of subjects exceeds several thousands. The next example illustrates the calculation of the subject variance, the rater variance, as well as the unconditional variance due to the combined subject and rater effects.

Example 5.4 ─────────────────────────────────────

To illustrate the calculation of the unconditional variance of an inter-rater reliability coefficient, we still consider the same Stickleback fish data of Example 5.2. Table 5.7 shows inter-rater reliability evaluated with 5 unweighted agreement coefficients, which are Conger's Kappa, Gwet's AC_1, Fleiss' Kappa, Krippendorff's alpha, and Brennan-Prediger coefficient. The percent agreement was added for comparison. The content of this Table includes the agreement coefficient's value, its standard error due to the selection of subjects (SE_s), its standard error due to the selection of raters (SE_r), and its standard error due to both the selection of subjects and raters (SE). It appears that the subject and rater variances (i.e. the square of the standard error) represent respectively overall approximately 85% and 15% of the total variance. Therefore, if you like to project your results to the larger population of raters, the rater variance must be taken into consideration.

Table 5.7: Unweighted Agreement Coefficients and Associated Conditional and Unconditional Standard Errors for the Stickleback Fish Data

Method	Coeff.	$SE_s(\widehat{\kappa})$	$SE_r(\widehat{\kappa})$	$SE(\widehat{\kappa})$
Conger's Kappa	0.4129	0.0778	0.0302	0.0834
Gwet's AC_1	0.4897	0.0694	0.0272	0.0745
Fleiss' Kappa	0.4103	0.0787	0.0323	0.0851
Krippendorff's α	0.4154	0.0777	0.0320	0.0840
Brenann-Prediger	0.4756	0.0706	0.0278	0.0759
Percent Agreement	0.5805	0.0565	0.0223	0.0607

Table 5.8 on the other hand, shows inter-rater reliability evaluated with 5 weighted agreement coefficients, using quadratic weights. This time the variance due the selection of raters represents between 20% and 50% of total variance. These proportions may vary substantially depending on the set of weights being used.

Table 5.8: Weighted Agreement Coefficients and Associated Conditional and Unconditional Standard Errors for the Stickleback Fish Data

Method	Coeff.	$SE_s(\hat{\kappa})$	$SE_r(\hat{\kappa})$	$SE(\hat{\kappa})$
Conger's Kappa	0.7341	0.0668	0.0340	0.0750
Gwet's AC_2	0.7616	0.0403	0.0373	0.0549
Fleiss' Kappa	0.7338	0.0669	0.0340	0.0751
Krippendorff's α	0.7361	0.0546	0.0336	0.0641
Brenann-Prediger	0.6825	0.0541	0.0538	0.0763
Percent Agreement	0.9206	0.0135	0.0134	0.0191

5.5 Sample Size Estimation

In this section, we discuss the important problem of sample size estimation. When designing an inter-rater reliability study, the researcher must generally resolve the problem of deciding how many subjects should be selected and how many raters should rate them. Very few practical guidelines are offered in the literature to our knowledge. Flack et al. (1988) have recommended a method for calculating the optimal number of subjects for Cohen's kappa coefficient when the number of raters is limited to two. Their approach requires the availability of past data and some assumptions regarding the raters' classification probabilities. Working on the simpler case of two raters and two categories, Cantor (1996) recommended another approach for calculating the optimal number of subjects for Cohen's kappa coefficient. The two approaches proposed by Cantor (1996) and Flack et al.(1988) are limited to the two-rater Cohen's kappa coefficient and are based on practical and clear-cut procedure.

I want to propose in this section a two-step procedure, which allows you to first calculate the optimal number of subjects required to achieve a certainly level of accuracy and if necessary a second step could be carried out to compute the optimal number of raters. Obtaining the optimal number of raters may be unnecessary if you have a fixed number of raters that must take part of the experiment. The proposed procedure is more of a convenient rule of thumb that should satisfy most researchers. I avoided recommending an elaborate statistical procedure that would be theoretically sound but practically confusing for practitioners.

Many chance-corrected agreement coefficients are based on two components, which are the percent agreement and the percent chance agreement. While the percent chance agreement often differs from one coefficient to another one, they generally share the same percent agreement. Since researchers often compute and report two agreement coefficients or more, I recommend that the sample of subjects as well as that of raters for multiple-rater studies be optimized on the percent agreement alone[14]. The optimal numbers of subjects and raters will ensure that the percent agreement is estimated with an error margin that does not exceed its prescribed value. Moreover, these optimal numbers will apply to all coefficients that share the same percent agreement.

5.5.1   *Optimal Number of Subjects*

The optimal number of subjects for a given inter-rater reliability coefficient is defined here as the number of subjects that minimizes the standard error associated with the percent agreement between two arbitrary raters. The variance of the percent agreement (denoted by p_a) between two raters is given by: $v = p_a(1 - p_a)/n$, where n is the number of subjects. It can be shown that this variance is always smaller than $1/(4 \times n)$. The 95% error margin associated with the percent agreement is $2\sqrt{v}$, and if you want it to remain below a desired value E then this goal will be accomplished by any number of subjects n that exceeds $1/E^2$ (i.e $n \geq 1/E^2$). Since the smaller the number of subjects the better, the optimal number of subjects is given by,

$$n = 1/E^2 \tag{5.5.1}$$

Note that the desired error margin can be considered reasonable only with respect to the magnitude of the percent agreement itself. If the percent of agreement is 0.6 for example, then an error margin of ± 0.2 (or $\pm 20\%$) may well be deemed reasonable. However, if the percent agreement is around 15% then an error margin of 0.2 would be horrendous. A desirable error margin would likely be smaller than 10%.

Table 5.9 shows the minimum number of subjects required to achieve the desired 95% error margin. It follows that, if you want the estimated percent agreement to fall within 5% of its "true" error-free value, you will need to collect data on 400 subjects. This may appear excessive at first sight, but the required number of subjects decreases fast as the desired error margin goes up. If you are willing to tolerate an error margin of 0.3 (or 30%), then you may achieve with only 11 subjects.

How to know what our desired error margin should be ? Two options are possible: (*a*) The first option is start with the number of subjects you can afford then find out what error margin should be prescribed. (*b*) The second option is to use the percent agreement p_a from a previous or a pilot study, then set the error margin value at

---

[14]Focussing on the percent agreement as opposed to the agreement coefficient itself is motivated by simplicity, and convenience (all coefficients would use the same optimal number of subjects). But it is also motivated by the fact that the component of the agreement coefficient variation that is due to the percent agreement dominates the other component due to the percent chance agreement, especially when the extent of agreement among raters is high.

approximately $0.20 \times p_a$ for example. If the percent agreement is much lower than 0.50, you may want to consider giving additional training to the raters before using them in full-scale experiment.

Table 5.9: Required Subject Sample Size by Desired Error Margin

Desired Error Margin	Required Subject Sample Size
5%	400
10%	100
15%	44
20%	25
25%	16
30%	11

5.5.2   *Optimal Number of Raters*

Another important issue that researchers often face when designing multiple-rater reliability studies, is about the number of raters that must participate n the experiment to ensure an adequate precision of the resulting agreement coefficients. Once again, I recommend selecting a number of raters that will yield a predetermined desired precision for the percent agreement among raters. The multiple-rater version of the percent agreement and its variance are discussed in chapters 3, and 5. For a given number of subjects, you can consider the variation of the percent agreement due solely to the sampling of raters. One can prove that the percent agreement variance is smaller than $4p_a^2/r^2$, where p_a and r are respectively the percent agreement, and the number of raters. Consequently, the ratio of the variance to the squared percent agreement is smaller than $4/r^2$. This proves that the coefficient of variation (cv) of the percent agreement (i.e. the ratio of the standard error to the percent agreement) is smaller than $2/r$. The required number of raters is determined as follows:

$$r = 2/cv, \tag{5.5.2}$$

where cv is the anticipated coefficient of variation.

Table 5.10 shows the required number of raters for various values of the coefficient of variation based on equation 5.5.2. It follows from this table that if you use 10 raters in a multiple-rater reliability experiment, you can expect the standard error to represent about 20% of the magnitude of the percent agreement. That is the percent agreement turns out to be 60% then you would expect the associated standard error not to exceed 12%, and a 95% error margin not to exceed $2 \times 12\% = 24\%$. These upper bounds are very conservative and should be expected to be at times substantially higher than the actual precision measures.

Table 5.10: Required Number of Raters by Desired Variation Coefficient

Desired Coefficient of Variation	Required Number Of Raters
5%	40
10%	20
15%	14
20%	10
25%	8
30%	7
40%	5
50%	4
70%	3
100%	2

5.6   Concluding Remarks

Chapter 5 presents a framework for statistical inference suitable for the analysis of inter-rater reliability data, and based on the randomization of the procedures for selecting subjects and raters. The main difference with alternative frameworks found in the inter-rater reliability literature is the absence of a theoretical statistical model. Statistical models commonly used in the literature are based on a hypothetical probability distribution associated with the ratings, and which serves as basis for calculating expectations and variances. A second difference appears in the way the randomization approach makes explicit the contribution of subjects and raters to the overall variation associated with the inter-rater reliability coefficients. Before the work of Gwet (2008b), the selection of raters was generally not treated as a source of variation affecting inter-rater reliability coefficients, except when the intraclass correlation coefficient was used for measuring the extent of agreement among raters.

In situations where the practitioner wants to extrapolate the findings to a larger universe of subjects, but not to any universe of raters larger than the group of participating raters, inference will be done conditionally on the rater sample made up of the specific raters who provided the ratings being analyzed. The validity of our analysis will then be limited to this particular group of raters. If the results of your analysis must be extrapolated to a larger universe of raters, but not to a universe of subjects larger than the group of participating subjects, inference is carried out conditionally upon the subject sample. Inference will be unconditional when the practitioner wants to extrapolate the findings to larger universes of raters and subjects simultaneously. Consequently, three types of inferences (two conditional and one unconditional) can be implemented with any of the chance-corrected inter-rater reliability coefficients studied in the past few chapters. After providing a formal definition of the inter-rater reliability variance for each of the three types of inferences, we also proposed variance estimation procedures that practitioners can use with actual ratings. We saw through some examples, that raters alone may account for as much as 50% of the total variance, and should therefore not be neglected when computing the variance unless conditional inference is deemed appropriate.

The expressions used for computing the variance of the various agreement coefficients are often complex, and cannot be conveniently used to determine the optimal number of subjects or of raters when designing inter-rater reliability studies. In this chapter, I proposed simple rules of thumb that can be used to overcome these difficulties. These simple procedures will generally lead to sample sizes that produce adequate precision levels for all agreement coefficients, even though they were initially designed to control the variance of the percent agreement.

Benchmarking Inter-Rater Reliability Coefficients

OBJECTIVE

In this chapter, I will discuss about several ways in which the extent of agreement among raters can be interpreted once it has been quantified with one of the agreement coefficients discussed in the past few chapters. Given the agreement coefficient's magnitude, should you conclude that the extent of agreement among raters is "Excellent", "Good", or "Poor?" To answer this question, I will review some benchmark scales proposed in the literature, will discuss their weaknesses, and will recommend an alternative benchmarking model that accounts for the precision with which the agreement coefficient has been estimated. I argue that the magnitude of the agreement coefficient alone is insufficient to qualify the extent of agreement among raters. It is because accurate numbers based on a well-designed experiment must lead to a stronger statement than inaccurate numbers based on a limited and ill-designed experiment.

CONTENTS

"Concrete measures can determine progress, but they do not really measure values."
  Peter Block : "The Answer to How Is Yes : Acting on What Matters"
  (Berrett-Koehler, 2002)

6.1   Overview

"Extent of agreement among raters" is often a vague notion in our imagination. The inter-rater reliability coefficient codifies it in a logical way, allowing researchers to have a common and concrete representation of an abstract concept. The many different logics used in this codification led to various forms of the agreement coefficient. However, for an inter-rater reliability coefficient to be useful, researchers must be able to interpret its magnitude. Although concrete agreement coefficients determine the extent to which raters agree among themselves, these measures do not tell researchers how valuable that information is. Should an agreement coefficient of 0.5 for example be considered good, fair, or bad? Should it be considered acceptable? What are the practical implications for implementing a classification system that is backed up with a 0.50 inter-rater reliability coefficient? These are some of the questions that are addressed in this chapter.

In the course of the development of inter-rater reliability coefficients, it appeared early that a rule of thumb was needed to help researchers relate the magnitude of the estimated inter-rater reliability coefficient to the notion of extent of agreement. Practitioners wanted a threshold for Kappa, beyond which the extent of agreement will be considered "good." The process of comparing estimated inter-rater reliability coefficients to a predetermined threshold before deciding whether the extent of agreement is good or bad is called *Benchmarking*, and the thresholds used to make the comparison are the *Benchmarks*.

Many scientific fields use standards of quality to distinguish the acceptable from the unacceptable. These standards are expected to vary from one field to another one. Regarding inter-rater reliability coefficients, the following two questions should be answered:

- What makes a good extent of agreement good?
- How high should the inter-rater reliability coefficient be for the extent of agreement as a construct to be considered good?

Accumulated experience in a particular discipline have generally provided the answer to these two questions as far as the use of Kappa is concerned. Landis and Koch (1977) provided one of the most widely-used benchmark scales among practitioners, and which will be discussed in section 6.2. Researchers having used the

Kappa statistic over a long period have found the proposed benchmark scale useful.

While the use of accumulated experience for benchmarking has undeniable merits, ignoring the influence that experimental conditions have on the magnitude of estimated agreement coefficients will lead to an incomplete interpretation of their significance. I demonstrate in the next few sections that a benchmarking model that does not account for the number of subjects and raters that participated in the reliability experiment, as well as the number of response categories could validate an agreement coefficient, which carries a large error margin. An agreement coefficient of 0.50 for example, is labeled as "moderate" according to all benchmark scales known in the literature. While this may be acceptable in a study involving 25 subjects, 3 raters and 4 response categories, I show in section 6.2 that an agreement coefficient of this magnitude is not even *statistically significant* if the study is based on 10 subjects, 2 raters and 2 response categories. The lack of statistical significance indicates that the "true" value of the coefficient (i.e. free of sampling errors) could well be as small as 0. In the absence of the "true" agreement coefficient, the error margin associated with the estimated agreement coefficient becomes informative ; because it provides the only description of the neighborhood where the truth is situated. If an error-free inter-rater reliability coefficient is 0, its value estimated from small samples of subjects or raters may appear as high as 0.5 or even higher due to sampling errors alone.

> *If an inter-rater reliability coefficient is not "Statistically significant," then any characterization of the agreement among raters other than "Poor" would be misleading. The sample-based estimated agreement coefficient which is not statistically significant does not provide strong enough evidence that the "true" magnitude of the agreement coefficient (i.e. free of sampling errors) is better than 0. Under this circumstance, the extent of agreement among raters, which is more dependent on the true agreement coefficient than on its estimated value is logically expected to be poor.*

I propose in this chapter, a new approach for interpreting the inter-rater reliability coefficient that uses existing benchmark scales as well as actual experimental parameters such as the number of subjects, raters, and response categories. Moreover, different benchmarking models are proposed for different agreement coefficients. The current approach to benchmarking is reviewed in section 6.2, while a description of the newly-proposed method is described in section 6.3.

6.2   Benchmarking the Agreement Coefficient

This section's objective is to review various benchmark scales proposed in the literature for interpreting the magnitude of the Kappa statistic, and to discuss some of their limitations. I will identify key factors affecting the meaning of the estimated inter-rater reliability, and will demonstrate the need to make them an integral part of any viable benchmarking method.

6.2.1   *Existing Benchmarks*

Benchmarking is essential for communicating the results of a reliability study to a wide audience, in addition to providing guidelines to help practitioners with the use of agreement statistics. Three benchmarking models proposed in the literature will be reviewed in this section. Although most of these models were developed to be used with the Kappa coefficient, they are often used in practice with other agreement coefficients as well.

Table 6.1 describes the benchmark scale that Landis and Koch (1977) proposed. It follows from this table that the extent of agreement can be qualified as "Poor", "Slight", "Fair", "Moderate", "Substantial", and "Almost Perfect" depending on the magnitude of Kappa. A Kappa value between 40% and 60% for example indicates a moderate agreement level, while ranges of values (60% − 80%), and (80% − 100%) indicate substantial and almost perfect agreement levels respectively. Although the authors acknowledge the subjective nature of their benchmarks, they recommended them as a useful guideline for practitioners. Other authors such as Everitt (1992) have supported this benchmark scale.

Table 6.1:
Landis and Koch Kappa's Benchmark Scale

Kappa Statistic	Strength of Agreement
< 0.0	Poor
0.0 to 0.20	Slight
0.21 to 0.40	Fair
0.41 to 0.60	Moderate
0.61 to 0.80	Substantial
0.81 to 1.00	Almost Perfect

Fleiss (1981) proposed another benchmark scale where the first three value ranges of the Landis-Koch benchmark are collapsed into a single range "0.40 or less" labeled as "Poor." Table 6.2 shows the 3 ranges of values that make up Fleiss' benchmarking scale. Kappa values in the 40% − 75% range for example represent an "Intermediate to Good" extent of agreement, while all Kappa values in the 75% − 100% range indicate an "Excellent" extent of agreement. This scale has the advantage of having a small number of categories while presenting the middle category as that of acceptable values, the low-end category as that of the unacceptable, and the high-end category as that of excellence.

Table 6.2: Fleiss' Kappa Benchmark Scale

Kappa Statistic	Strength of Agreement
< 0.40	Poor
0.40 to 0.75	Intermediate to Good
More than 0.75	Excellent

Altman (1991) proposed his benchmark scale summarized in Table 6.3, and which represents a modified version of the Landis-Koch's proposal. The only noticeable difference is the first two ranges of values of Landis-Koch's proposal that Altman collapsed into a single category labeled as "Poor." Landis-Koch's proposed benchmarking method was published several years before Alman's, and is still being used. Therefore, the argument for supporting the newer Altman's benchmarks remains unclear.

Table 6.3: Altman's Kappa Benchmark Scale

Kappa Statistic	Strength of Agreement
< 0.20	Poor
0.21 to 0.40	Fair
0.41 to 0.60	Moderate
0.61 to 0.80	Good
0.81 to 1.00	Very Good

Our objective in this chapter is not to recommend the use of a specific benchmark scale. Practitioners who want to use these scales could choose one that meets their analytical goals. For example, those who only want to know whether the extent of agreement is excellent or poor will want to use Fleiss' benchmarks, whereas researchers with a desire for a finer categorization may prefer either Landis-Koch or Altman proposals. The more critical issue we must address is that of the error margin associated with agreement coefficients. The magnitude of the error margin alone may lead to a spurious characterization of the agreement coefficient.

A larger number of subjects will generally lead to a more precise agreement coefficient, which is expected to be close to the true value it approximates. Therefore, a straight comparison of a precise coefficient with existing benchmarks will yield conclusions that will apply to the true parameter of interest as well. A small number of subjects on the other hand, reduces the precision of the inter-rater reliability coefficient, in addition to exposing that precision to further degradation due possibly to a small number of raters, or a small number of response categories. Comparing an agreement coefficient loaded with errors to a predetermined quality benchmark can only produce a questionable characterization of the extent of agreement among raters. Consequently, accounting for the number of subjects, raters, and response categories becomes critical when interpreting the magnitude of sample-based agreement coefficients. Section 6.2.2 aims at demonstrating that the number of subjects (n), raters (r), and categories (q) can substantially affect the agreement coefficient probability distribution[1], and therefore its error margin. This will prove that these factors must be taken into consideration when interpreting agreement coefficients.

6.2.2   *Agreement Coefficient's Sources of Variation*

To demonstrate how the number of subjects (n), raters (r), and categories (q) affect the agreement coefficient's distribution, a well-established statistical approach is to simulate an inter-rater reliability study with a computer, and to repeat the experiment many times in order to obtain the agreement coefficient's probability distribution. For this particular problem, I have used the Random Rating (RR) model where raters classify subjects into categories in a purely random manner. More specifically, I want to study how the quantities n, r, and q affect the 95th percentile[2] of an agreement coefficient. For this purpose, I used Kappa and Pi as examples of coefficients for illustration purposes.

Consider an agreement coefficient calculated with observed ratings, and which exceeds the RR-based 95th percentile (also called *Critical Value*) . If the observed ratings were randomly generated then this could be perceived as a rare event. Statistical reasoning generally recommends to reject any assumption that leads to a rare event, and in this case to consider the observed ratings as being non-random. Therefore, the observed ratings are unlikely to have been done randomly, and likely to convey a genuine agreement among raters. Now consider an agreement coefficient that is smaller than the critical value. If the observed ratings were randomly generated then this would be considered rather as a common (or normal) event. The common event is generally considered to be consistent with the assumption that led to it. Therefore, an agreement coefficient that is smaller than the critical value raises serious doubts about the very existence of an intrinsic agreement among raters. The

---

[1]For all practical purposes, the agreement coefficient distribution in this context essentially refers to what can be expected from an agreement coefficient in terms of magnitude and variation

[2]The 95th percentile is a threshold that an agreement coefficient can exceed only with a small chance below 5%.

purpose of this discussion was to help us understand the relationship between the calculated agreement coefficient and the reality it is supposed to quantify, and which is ultimately of interest to us.

For any particular set of values associated with n, r, and q, the RR-based 95th percentile is obtained by repeating the simulation of the Random Rating model a large number of times. Each iteration of the experiment yields one agreement coefficient. After several iterations, a series of values are generated providing the probability distribution of the agreement coefficient of interest. Repeating the Monte-Carlo[3] experiment for different values of n, q and r allows us to evaluate their impact on the inter-rater reliability distribution. The Monte-Carlo experiment is implemented as described in the following steps:

The Monte-Carlo Experiment

| 1 | *Assign specific values to n, r, and q. For example, one may decide to simulate a reliability study based on random rating, with $n = 8$ subjects, $r = 3$ raters, and $q = 5$.* |

| 2 | *Generate a table of ratings similar to Table 6.4, where the table entries are computer-generated random integers between 1 and 5.* |

| 3 | *Use Table 6.4 data to compute all agreement coefficients of interest and record them.* |

| 4 | *Steps 2 and 3 are repeated 100,000 times. However, the number of iterations will not exceed the number of rating tables that can possibly be created.* |

Table 6.4: Raw Ratings from a Monte-Carlo Experiment

Rater 1	Rater 2	Rater 3
5	5	4
2	3	1
3	3	3
5	5	5
4	3	5
5	5	4
1	1	2
3	2	2

This Monte-Carlo experiment was carried out several times with n taking the values $\{2, 5, 10, 15, 20, 25, 30, 35, 40, 45, 50, 55, 60\}$, q taking the values $\{2, 3, 4,$

---

[3]Randomness and its relationship with games of chance popular in the city of Monte-Carlo (Monaco) led Metropolis and Ulam (1949) to refer to this method as the Monte-Carlo method

5}, and r the values {2, 3, 4, 5, 10, 20}. The results obtained are depicted in Figures 6.2.1, 6.2.2, and 6.2.3.

Figure 6.2.1 shows the variation of the 95th percentile of Kappa for 2 raters only, as a function of the number of subjects (n) and the number of categories (q) under the RR model. It follows from this graph that if the number of subjects is 10 and the number of categories is 2, then the 95th percentile of Kappa will be greater than 0.5. This example shows that 2 raters scoring 10 subjects in a purely random manner, making no effort to categorize them in any logical way can still achieve a Kappa above 0.5 more than 5% of the times. Why is this possible? It is because any agreement coefficient based on only 10 subjects, 2 raters, and 2 categories is exposed to substantial error margin and cannot always have a value in the neighborhood of 0 where it is supposed to be under the RR model. The number of subjects in this case - limited to 10 - is too small for the concrete value of Kappa or any other agreement coefficient to be consistent with its conceptual definition and theoretical properties.

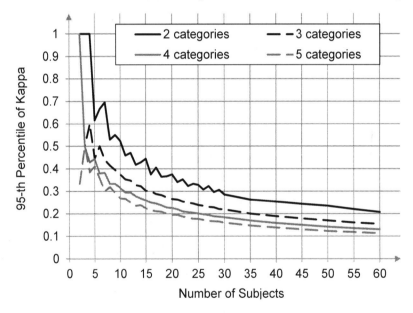

Figure 6.2.1: 95th Percentile of the kappa coefficient for 2 raters as a function of the number of subjects and number of categories

Figure 6.2.1 also shows that Kappa's critical value decreases as the number of subjects or the number of categories increases. As a result, more participating subjects or more categories in a reliability study make Kappa more accurate, and more consistent with its expected value. That the precision of Kappa is impacted by the number of categories may come as surprise to many. In fact the form of Kappa does not suggest any natural dependency upon the number of categories. Many authors (mainly kappa proponents) have criticized alternative agreement coefficients such as Brennan-Prediger, or Gwet's AC_1 on the ground that they depend on the number of categories[4] while Kappa does not. We now know that these criticisms are unfounded since Kappa too does depend on the number of categories.

As a matter of fact, most if not all chance-corrected agreement coefficients depend on the number of categories even though that dependency may be invisible to the naked eye as far as Kappa or Scott's Pi are concerned. If a particular category is not used by any rater during a inter-rater reliability experiment, it will certainly not affect the specific kappa coefficient obtained from the observed ratings. But it will still affect the sampling distribution of Kappa, since that category will eventually be used in subsequent experiments. When interpreting agreement coefficients, we must look beyond concrete numbers, and think in terms of their sampling distributions. These sampling distributions represent the only bridge between the numbers and the underlying realities they are supposed to quantify.

Based on what we have learned from Figure 6.2.1 can we claim that the observed relationship linking the critical value to the number of subjects, raters, and categories still holds for agreement coefficients other than Kappa? The answer to this question if yes. Figure 6.2.2 shows the 95th percentile of Scott's Pi statistic as a function of the number of subjects n and the number of categories q when the number of raters is limited to 2. You can still observe a decrease in the magnitude of the critical value when the number of subjects or the number of categories increases.

Figures 6.2.1 and 6.2.2 both depict a situation where the number of raters remains constant at 2 so that the critical value can be observed as the number of subjects and number of categories change. Figure 6.2.3 on the other hand shows the impact that the number of raters can have on an agreement coefficient's 95th percentile. Each curve refers to a specific number of raters, and displays the 95th percentile of Scott's Pi-statistic as a function of the number of subjects. An examination of these curves reveals that it is only when the number of raters or the number of subjects is large that the agreement gets sufficiently close to its expected value, which in this case is 0. Note that if the number of raters is 2 and the number of subjects 5 then the Pi coefficient may reach a level as high as 0.7 about 5% of the times. This is another reason why relying solely upon the concrete numbers without looking at the possible negative effects of statistical errors can be misleading.

---

[4]Note that the number of categories here refers to categories that are expected to be used. Categories not expected to be used by the raters should not count in the number of categories for the purpose of calculating Brennan-Prediger or Gwet's AC_1 coefficients.

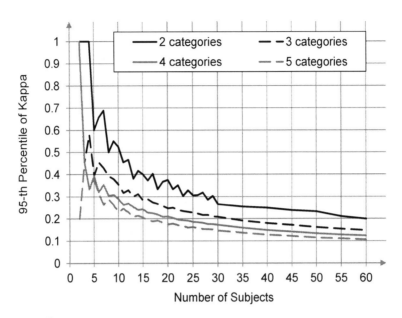

Figure 6.2.2: 95th Percentile of the π coefficient for 2 raters as a function of the number of subjects and number of raters

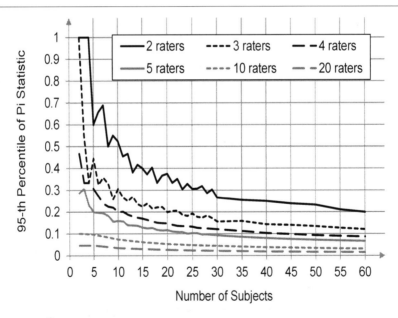

Figure 6.2.3: 95th Percentile of the π statistic for 2 categories as a function of the number of subjects and number of raters

Note that an inter-rater reliability coefficient of 0.30, even based on a small group of 5 subjects, is deemed as fair according to Landis-Koch, and Altman benchmark

scales. This would certainly be a reasonable assessment if such an agreement coefficient was obtained from ratings produced by 10 raters or more on the same 5
subjects. However qualifying an agreement coefficient of 0.3 as fair would be a highly
questionable characterization of the extent of agreement among 2 raters if the number of raters is limited to 5. In fact, Figure 6.2.3 shows that 2 raters rating 5 subjects
in a purely random manner could still achieve a Pi value around 0.60 about 5% of the
times. Consequently, under these circumstances an agreement coefficient of 0.30 does
not represent any intrinsic agreement between 2 raters, and should not be considered
fair.

In section 6.2.3, I will describe a new benchmarking model that consists of first
choosing a benchmark scale of your choice before computing the membership probabilities associated with each range of values. The range of values with the cumulative
membership probability deemed sufficiently large will determine the final characterization of the agreement coefficient.

6.3   The Proposed Benchmarking Method

As previously indicated, adequate benchmarking of an agreement coefficient must
take into consideration its precision, and the uncertainty surrounding its real value
caused by statistical errors. An agreement coefficient of 0.5 for example, whose error
margin is ± 0.05 tells us a far more powerful story about the real extent of agreement
among raters, than an agreement coefficient of the same value with and unduly high
error margin[5] of ± 0.3. As a matter of fact, we cannot draw a definitive conclusion
such as "our kappa value is good according to the Landis-Koch benchmark scale,"
using our calculated agreement coefficient alone. This would be as naive as visiting
a new city for the first time on a very sunny afternoon, then concluding that the sun
shines in that city all year long without even questioning what may have happened
in that city in the past and what could happen there next. The agreement coefficient
calculated from experimental data is a random number that changes with the subjects
and raters involved in the rating process. Therefore, its use for qualifying the extent
of agreement among raters must be probabilistic in nature. That is, we should make
a statement saying how confident we are that the extent of agreement among raters
is excellent. A good benchmarking will be statistical, not deterministic.

The calculated agreement coefficient is only a rough approximation of the ideal

---

[5]Note that an error margin of ± 0.05 associated with an estimated agreement coefficient of 0.5
suggests that the error-free parameter being approximated lies between 0.45 and 0.55 with high
certainty. If the error margin is ± 0.3 then the parameter will lie between 0.2 and 0.8 with high
certainty. This latter range of values is so wide that you wouldn't even know whether the true
parameter is high or low, making the estimated agrement coefficient of 0.5 useless.

error-free parameter we would obtain if all raters of interest to us were to rate all subjects of interest. The value of this ideal parameter is generally unknown, although it is the value that should normally be used for benchmarking purposes. One of the few reasonable options we have left is to evaluate the likelihood for this ideal parameter to belong to any given benchmark level (e.g. "Good," or "Moderate.").

6.3.1   *The Method*

The recommended benchmarking method is a three-step process:

(i) The first step consists of quantifying for any given agreement coefficient and benchmark scale of choice, the probability that the extent of agreement falls into each of the intervals defining the benchmark levels. For each interval, a membership probability will be calculated. I will show in the next sub-section how these likelihood probabilities are calculated.

(ii) As a second step, you would compute the cumulative probability for each interval starting from the top[6] and going down to the bottom. That is, the cumulative probability associated with the top interval is identical to the probability calculated in step (i) for that interval. For the second interval in descending order, the cumulative probability is the sum of probabilities calculated in step (i) for the two top intervals.

(iii) The final benchmark level is determined by the interval associated with the smallest cumulative probability that exceeds 95%. We will then be in a position to conclude with 95% certainty or more that the extent of agreement among raters is for example "Excellent." This approach allows for a fair comparison between different studies using the same agreement statistic even though they are based on different designs.

Let us first illustrate how our proposed benchmarking method works using a hypothetical inter-rater reliability experiment featuring two raters who have classified 100 psychiatric patients into one of 3 diagnosis categories named "Psychotic", "Neurotic", and "Organic." The outcome of this experiment is summarized in Table 6.5.

The analysis of Table 6.5 data with the AgreeStat software[7] has produced the results shown in Table 6.6. It appears that the different chance-corrected agreement coefficients vary from 0.675 to 0.868. A standard error, a 95% confidence interval, and a p-value are associated with each agreement coefficient. Since each coefficient is calculated based on one specific group of subjects, one would naturally expect

---

[6]The top interval is the one containing the highest values

[7]AgreeStat's website is the following: http://www.agreestat.com/agreestat.html

different groups of subjects to yield different coefficient values. The standard error is simply a number that tells you how far you can expect any given coefficient value to stray away for their average value. When this standard error is multiplied by 1.96, the product represents what is known as the 95% error margin associated with the estimated coefficient. If you subtract the error margin from the coefficient you will get the 95% lower confidence bound, while the 95% upper confidence bound is obtained by adding the error margin to the coefficient. The p-value associated with the kappa coefficient for example is 9.82×10^{-12}, which represents the ratio of 9.82 to 1 trillion, and should be considered as 0 for all practical purposes. Its value is tiny and represents a strong evidence that the observed kappa coefficient exceeds the value of 0 by a margin beyond any thing one would expect from statistical errors alone.

Table 6.5: Distribution of 100 psychiatric patients by rater and diagnostic group.

Rater A	Rater B			Total
	Psychotic	Neurotic	Organic	
Psychotic	75	1	4	80
Neurotic	5	4	1	10
Organic	0	0	10	10
Total	80	5	15	100

Table 6.6: Inter-rater reliability coefficients, and associated precision measures based on Table 6.5 data

Method	Coeff[a]	StdErr[b]	95% C.I.[c]	p-Value
Cohen's Kappa	0.676	0.088	0.502 to 0.850	9.82×10^{-12}
Gwet's AC$_1$	0.868	0.039	0.790 to 0.945	4.36×10^{-40}
Scott's Pi	0.675	0.089	0.499 to 0.851	1.55×10^{-11}
Krippendorff's Alpha	0.677	0.088	0.502 to 0.852	1.18×10^{-11}
Brenann-Prediger	0.835	0.047	0.742 to 0.928	1.33×10^{-32}
Percent Agreement	0.890	0.031	0.828 to 0.952	1.92×10^{-49}

[a]Coeff = Agreement Coefficient
[b]StdErr = Standard Error
[c]C.I. = Confidence Interval

Let us consider Altman's benchmark scale for illustration purposes. The discussions would be similar for the other benchmark scales. Table 6.7 shows for each agreement coefficient, the probability that its error-free parameter falls within each benchmark level range of values. This probability represents a p-value of some kind[8] associated with a benchmark level range of values. That is it quantifies the strength of the evidence in favor of the agreement coefficient membership in a particular benchmark interval. For example, based on the estimated kappa coefficient you can claim that the extent of agreement based on Kappa is "Very Good" with a very small probability of 0.079. However, it would be "Good" with a reasonably higher probability of 0.727. This probability decreases from that point on. It appears that only the AC_1 statistic produces an agreement coefficient that is "Very Good" with a probability as high as 0.959.

Table 6.7: Membership probabilities in Altman's benchmark ranges, by agreement coefficient

Benchmark Range	Description	Kappa	AC_1	Scott's Pi	Krippendorff	Brennan-Prediger
0.8 to 1.0	Very Good	0.079	0.959	0.080	0.081	0.772
0.6 to 0.8	Good	0.727	0.041	0.720	0.728	0.228
0.4 to 0.6	Moderate	0.193	0.000	0.199	0.190	0.000
0.2 to 0.4	Fair	0.001	0.000	0.001	0.001	0.000
less than 0.2	Poor	0.000	0.000	0.000	0.000	0.000

Table 6.8 shows the cumulative probabilities for the 5 agreement coefficients using the Altman's benchmark scale. Looking at the kappa coefficient for example, you can claim that the extent of agreement among raters based on Kappa is "very good" with a little certainty of 7.9%. You would not want to do that. But you can claim with an 81% certainty that the Kappa-based extent of agreement among raters is "Good" or better (i.e. "very good"). This is a far more reasonable certainty level that one can rely upon. You will be almost certain (i.e. with certainty level of 99.9%) with your statement when you claim that the Kappa-based agreement is "Moderate" or better. The interpretation of the other agreement coefficients is the same. Our recommended benchmarking procedure set the cut-off point for the cumulative probabilities at 95%. This "95% Rule" stipulates that the final benchmark level assigned to a particular agreement coefficient is the highest level on the scale, which is associated with a cumulative probability that exceeds 0.95. These final benchmark levels are identified in Table 6.8 with cumulative probabilities that are displayed in bold.

Table 6.9 shows the interpretation of 5 agreement coefficients according to the Landis-Foch, Fleiss, and Altman's benchmark scales. Using the Landis-Koch benchmark scale, the new benchmarking procedure demoted the extent of agreement among raters by one benchmark level for almost all agreement coefficients except AC_1. The

---

[8]The traditional p-value quantifies the extent to which the collected data supports our assumption that the parameter being estimated exceeds its hypothetical value.

situation is quite different with Fleiss' scale, where the intervals defining the benchmarks are so wide that the new procedure will rarely change the outcome obtained by the direct use of agreement coefficient estimates. The application of the new benchmarking procedure with the Altman's scale produced an outcome very similar to that obtained with Landis-Koch scale.

Table 6.8: Cumulative probabilities of membership in Altman's benchmark ranges, by agreement coefficient

Benchmark Range	Description	Kappa	AC$_1$	Scott's Pi	Krippendorff	Brennan-Prediger
0.8 to 1.0	Very Good	0.079	**0.959**	0.080	0.081	0.772
0.6 to 0.8	Good	0.806	1.000	0.800	0.809	**1.000**
0.4 to 0.6	Moderate	**0.999**	1.000	**0.999**	**0.999**	1.000
0.2 to 0.4	Fair	1.000	1.000	1.000	1.000	1.000
less than 0.2	Poor	1.000	1.000	1.000	1.000	1.000

Table 6.9: Benchmarking under the new method

Agreement Coefficient	Benchmark Scale		
	Landis-Koch	Fleiss	Altman
Cohen's Kappa	Moderate[a]	Intermediate to Good	Moderate[a]
Gwet's AC$_1$	Almost Perfect	Excellent	Very Good
Scott's Pi	Moderate[a]	Intermediate to Good	Moderate[a]
Krippendorff	Moderate[a]	Intermediate to Good	Moderate[a]
Brenann-Prediger	Substantial[a]	Excellent	Good[a]

[a]This new benchmark is one level below that of the classical approach

6.3.2   The Benchmark Probabilities and the Interpretation of the New Method

Let us first summarize the new benchmarking method, which is applied by implementing the following steps:

The Benchmarking Model

Estimation

1. Choose an agreement statistic of interest (e.g. AC$_1$, Kappa, Krippendorff, Brennan-Prediger,···), weighted or unweighted.

2. Compute the agreement coefficient (COEFF) selected in step 1 using the observed ratings.

Benchmark Probabilities

3   Chose a benchmark scale to be used (Landis-Koch, Fleiss, or Altman).

4   Compute the standard error (SE) associated with the agreement coefficient chosen.

5   For each interval (a, b) defining a benchmark level, compute the Interval Membership Probability (IMP). It is the probability that a standard Normal variate Z falls within the interval $[(\text{COEFF} - b)/\text{SE}, (\text{COEFF} - a)/\text{SE}]$.

That is,

$$\text{IMP} = P\left(\frac{\text{COEFF} - b}{\text{SE}} \le Z \le \frac{\text{COEFF} - a}{\text{SE}}\right). \qquad (6.3.1)$$

See further down how this probability can be calculated using MS Excel.

Cumulative Probabilities

6   Compute the cumulative benchmark probabilities starting from the highest benchmark level and moving down towards the lowest level.

Final Agreement Level

7   The final agreement corresponds to the highest benchmark level associated with the smallest cumulative probability that exceeds 0.95.

The benchmark probabilities of equation 6.3.1 can be computed using Microsoft Excel in a rather straightforward manner. For a given benchmark interval (a, b), proceed as follows:

- For Excel Windows 2010 or a more recent Windows version, and Excel Mac 2011 or a more recent Mac version, use the following formula:

  =NORM.S.DIST((COEFF-a)/SE,TRUE) - NORM.S.DIST((COEFF-b)/SE,TRUE)

- For Excel Windows 2007 or an older Windows version use the formula:

  =NORMSDIST((COEFF-a)/SE) - NORMSDIST((COEFF-b)/SE) .

- When dealing with an open interval such as $< a$, the associated benchmark probability would be calculated as follows:

  =NORM.S.DIST((COEFF-a)/SE,TRUE) for Excel Windows 2010 or a later version, and Excel Mac 2011 or a later version. For older versions of Excel use the formula =NORMSDIST((COEFF-a)/SE) .

Suppose that $\widehat{\kappa}_G$ is the estimated AC_1 agreement coefficient, κ_G its (error-free) estimand, and $\sigma\left(\widehat{\kappa}_G\right)$ its standard error. It has been demonstrated (see Gwet(2008b)) that the ratio $(\widehat{\kappa}_G - \kappa_G)/\sigma\left(\widehat{\kappa}_G\right)$ follows the standard Normal distribution. Consequently, if for example the probability for the standard Normal variate Z to exceed

$(\widehat{\kappa}_{G} - a)/\sigma(\widehat{\kappa}_{G})$ for any given number a, is very small then this must be seen as a strong evidence that the estimand κ_{G} is likely to be below a. This is the approach used to evaluate the benchmark probabilities.

I like to argue why using the probabilistic approach for benchmarking makes perfect sense, and to explain the statistical implications of using it. In the previous example, the AC_1 coefficient was estimated at 0.868 (c.f. Table 6.6) with a 95% confidence interval of (0.790 *to* 0.945). Looking at the Altman's Benchmark Scale of Table 6.3 for example, it appears that the 95% confidence interval overlaps the 2 ranges of values defining the "Good" and "Very Good" benchmarks. Therefore I can claim with 95% certainty that the extent of agreement based on AC_1 is either "Good" or "Very Good." Now, one can observe that it is the tiny segment (0.79 *to* 0.80) of the confidence interval that belongs to "Good" range of values, while the other much bigger segment (0.80 *to* 0.945) is contained into the "Very Good" range of values. Since (0.790, 0.945) is the 95% confidence interval, we know with 2.5% certainty that the true agreement coefficient may still exceed 0.945. The AC_1-based agreement coefficient has been considered "Very Good" because of this 2.5% certainty of being above 0.945, and the fact that the 95% confidence interval is included almost entirely into the upper segment of the Altman's scale.

Let us now consider Cohen's Kappa coefficient. It has an estimated value is 0.676 and a 95% confidence interval of (0.502 *to* 0.850). The confidence interval overlaps the top 3 benchmark categories on the Altman's scale. This indicates that the Kappa-based inter-rater reliability is either moderate, good, or very good. This is a weak claim that we can make with 95% certainty. It is pretty much like claiming in the month January with 95% certainty that your grade at the next exam will be D, C, B, or A. One will hardly rely upon such a weak statement, which tends to indicate that you are not really a good student after all. It is therefore more reasonable to label you as a D, or a C student. The Good range of values (0.6 to 0.8) is entirely contained inside the 95% confidence interval, and has without surprise the highest benchmark probability of 0.727. This probability may not look sufficiently large because large segments of the confidence interval are still located outside of the "Good" range of values. Therefore, it is only by combining the top three range of values that we can secure a cumulative probability that exceeds 0.95.

Throughout this chapter, I have recommended the use of the 95% confidence interval for benchmarking purposes. However, you may chose a lower confidence level such as 90% or even 85%. This will likely lead to a better qualification of the extent of agreement among raters. The price to be paid is a higher risk of errors associated with your conclusions.

6.4   Concluding Remarks

The primary objective of this chapter was to present an alternative benchmarking model for interpreting the extent of agreement among raters based on the magnitude of the calculated agreement coefficient. The approach currently advocated in the inter-rater reliability literature is based upon a straight comparison between the calculated agreement coefficient and a number of benchmarks proposed by various authors. Using a Monte-Carlo experiment, I demonstrated that this classical approach tends to provide an overly optimistic characterization of the extent of agreement among raters, ignoring the adverse effects that a small number of subjects or raters can have on the agreement coefficient precision. The Monte-Carlo experiment has proved that the classical benchmarking model would characterize the extent of agreement among raters as "Excellent" even when the ratings are obtained through a purely random process. A situation where no intrinsic agreement is expected to occur among raters. This problem is created by estimated agreement coefficients that are sometimes artificially inflated by errors due to the sampling of subjects, or that of raters. The experiment has also demonstrated that a small number of categories will increase the magnitude of theses errors.

In order to provide a fair comparison between agreement coefficients obtained from different studies based on different designs, I have recommended a new benchmarking process that is probabilistic. That is each benchmark range of values is assigned a membership probability. This probability represents the likelihood that the estimand of a particular agreement coefficient falls into the benchmark range of values. After computing these benchmark probabilities, one option would be to simply present them and leave it up to others to decide whether they want to characterize the extent of agreement as very good, intermediate or poor. They will still be able to use the benchmark probabilities to justify their decisions. Instead, I have decided to recommend a rule for characterizing the extent of agreement, which is to select the highest benchmark level that is associated with the smallest cumulative probability that exceeds 95%. The 95% cut-off point is a standard of acceptability in statistical science. Practitioners may decrease or increase that cut-off point if deemed necessary.

I believe that the choice of benchmark scale is less important than the way it is used for characterizing the extent of agreement among raters. Having said that, I do believe that Fleiss' benchmark scale presented in Table 6.2 is bad. It is because of the unduly large width of its benchmark intervals. For example the Intermediate-to-Good range of values goes from 0.4 to 0.75, and is too broad to be very helpful in practice. Moreover, the two words "Intermediate" and "Good" have meanings that are too different for them to be lumped into a single category. Intermediate generally means it could get much better, while good is always considered satisfactory. If and inter-rater reliability of 0.75 may be deemed acceptable, very few people will admit an inter-rater reliability of 0.4 as being acceptable. However the Landis-Koch and Altman's benchmark scales are both acceptable.

Unlike the classical benchmarking model that is applied uniformly to all agreement coefficients, the newly-proposed model is tailored to each agreement coefficient. The standard error of the estimated agreement coefficient plays a pivotal role in this new process. The standard error quantifies the quality of the study design, will reward well-designed studies with higher benchmark probabilities, while penalizing poorly designed studies. It prevents poorly-designed inter-rater reliability studies from producing an "Excellent" extent of agreement among raters based solely on an imprecise estimated agreement coefficient.

PART III

INTRACLASS CORRELATION COEFFICIENTS

## CHAPTER 7

Intraclass Correlation: A Measure of Raters' Agreement

OBJECTIVE

This chapter presents a general overview of the use of Intraclass Correlation Coefficients for quantifying the extent of agreement among raters when the ratings are in the form of quantitative measurements. A high-level description of the underlying statistical models is provided as well as a discussion on the limitations associated with their use. After reading this chapter the practitioner will be able to decide which model is appropriate for the study that was conducted, and will know the related challenges that must be overcome. This chapter also describes the Bland-Altman plot, a popular graphical method for analyzing agreement between two raters. The reader will find an introduction to sample size calculations in this chapter, and a more detailed treatment of the sample size problem in subsequent chapters. Figure 7.4.1 represents a flowchart showing how to find the correct intraclass correlation coefficients based on the way the ratings were gathered and the type of analysis to be done.

CONTENTS

7.1 Introduction

In the past few chapters of parts I and II, I presented many techniques for quantifying the extent of agreement among raters. Although some of these techniques were extended to interval and ratio data, the primary focus has been on nominal and ordinal data. This chapter as well as the other chapters of part III, are devoted to the study of inter-rater reliability for quantitative outcomes whose possible values are defined by a continuum, as opposed to being a predetermined set of specific values.

Why do we need to care about intraclass correlation when weighted versions of the chance-corrected measures can be used to handle quantitative outcomes? It is because the notion of "perfect" agreement associated with two raters assigning the exact same score to the same subject, does not translate well to quantitative measurements. Consider for example two electronic devices used to measure the knee joint laxity on 15 human subjects. Even if both devices are equally reliable, you would not expect them to produce the exact same quantitative measurement on the same subjects, since these values belong to a continuum. Likewise, two very competent raters that measure the height or the weight of the same human subject will likely produce slightly different numbers regardless of their proficiency level in the use of the measuring instrument. With agreement no longer referring to an exact match, the notions of chance agreement and percent agreement evaporate.

The solution to this problem is to use the portion of variation in the data that is due to subjects, and to compare it to the other portion of that variation due to raters. If the rater-induced variation exceeds that of the subject by a wide margin then the raters are said to have low inter-rater reliability. Otherwise, the raters are said to have high inter-rater reliability. But this approach will work only if the reliability experiment is designed in such a way that the different variation components can be separated. You will see in the next few sections how this task can be accomplished. Several approaches can be used to design an inter-rater reliability study, depending on the goal aimed at for the study. In the next section, I will describe a few designs commonly used in the context of inter-rater reliability analysis.

7.2 Statistical Models

Consider the reliability data shown in Table 7.1. That data represents scores that 4 raters assigned to 6 subjects, and could be interpreted in various ways depending on how it was collected. Here are 4 possible study designs (or data models) that could have produced Table 1 data:

▶ **Model 1A**: *Each subject is rated by a different group of raters*

According to this model, each row of Table 7.1 is not necessarily associated with the same set of 4 raters. Although the 4 raters are consistently labeled as 1, 2, 3, and 4, they could represent different individuals, or different measuring instruments. One may average this data row-wise to study the subject effect, but will not be able to average column-wise to obtain the rater effect. It is why this is often known as a one-factor (or one-way) model, the single factor here being the subject.

The main implication of this model is that one rater may not have the opportunity to score more than one subject. Consequently, this model makes it impossible to evaluate *Intra-rater Reliability*, which is a measure of the rater's self-consistency. However, the raters under this model still score the same subjects, making it possible to compute *Inter-rater reliability*.

The main advantage for using this model is that the raters could be located in different geographic areas, and rate local subjects. There is no need to move subjects around to allow different groups of raters to rate the same subjects. This model may also be suitable in situations where subjects are hard to recruit and the availability of the same group of raters cannot be guaranteed when a subject is able to participate in the experiment.

Table 7.1: Scores assigned by 4 raters to 6 subjects[a]

Subject	Rater				Average
	1	2	3	4	
1	9	2	5	8	6
2	6	1	3	2	3
3	8	4	6	8	6.5
4	7	1	2	6	4
5	10	5	6	9	7.5
6	6	2	4	7	4.75
Average	7.67	2.5	4.33	6.67	5.29

[a]This data is taken from Shrout & Fleiss (1979), although I replaced the terms Target and Judge with Subject and Rater respectively, and added row and column marginal averages.

▶ **Model 1B**: *Each rater rates a different group of subjects*

If Table 7.1 data were collected according to this design, then the 6 subjects may differ from rater to rater. That is, each rater scored his own set of subjects, even though I may have decided to consistently labeled them as 1, 2, 3, 4, 5, and 6. One may evaluate the rater effect by averaging Table 7.1's columns. Any row-wise averaging would be meaningless as such an operation would involve different subjects as well as different raters. Therefore, the only factor that can be studied is the rater factor, and this model will later be referred to as a one-factor or one-way model.

The main implication of this model is that it allows for the evaluation of intra-rater reliability, and not that of inter-rater reliability. Evaluating inter-rater reliability always requires different raters to score the same subjects.

▶ **Model 2**: *The Random Factorial Design*

According to this model, each subject is scored by the same group of raters. Both the subjects and the raters are random samples selected from the respective populations they represent, hence the naming "random" design. Moreover, the column and row marginal averages are meaningful, and the effects of subject and rater factors can be evaluated. It is because both factors (rater and subject) can be studied that this design is known as a "factorial design". The experimental design that produces Table 7.1 data is called a two-way factorial design.

▶ **Model 3**: *The Mixed Factorial Design*

According to this design, each subject is scored by the same group of raters, and is also in this regard a factorial design. Unlike Model 2, here only the group of subjects represents a random sample selected from a larger subject population, while the group of raters does not represent a random sample. Because the group of raters that participate in the reliability experiment is not randomly selected from a larger rater population, these raters only represent themselves. The resulting inter-rater reliability coefficient can therefore not be applied to raters beyond those in the experiment. Therefore, the subject effect is random, while the rater effect is fixed. This combination of random and fixed effects gave this design the name "Mixed Factorial Design." When the number of factors considered is limited to two as is the case for Table 7.1, it is renamed the "Two-Way Mixed Factorial Design."

Each of these models requires a different method for calculating the intraclass correlation coefficient. Shrout & Fleiss (1979) discussed models 1A (although it was referred to as model 1), 2, and 3. The same models were also discussed by McGraw and Wong (1996), who presented methods for computing the intraclass correlation for each of them. However, these authors did not deal with the important problem of missing ratings, which is very common in inter-rater reliability experiments. The next few chapters of Part III of this book discuss the missing-rating issue extensively.

7.3   The Bland-Altman Plot

An mainly graphical method often used as an alternative to the intraclass correlation for analyzing inter-rater reliability data was proposed by Bland and Altman (1986). It combines a graphical approach and a quantitative analysis of the magnitude of the rating differences. This method can only analyze two raters at a time, and has become popular over time among researchers, although many of its users are often unaware of its limitations. In this section, I will present an overview of this method, and will discuss its merits as well as its limitations.

Suppose that we want to study the extent of agreement between the two raters labeled as 3 and 4 using Table 7.1's ratings. The Bland-Altman method is implemented as follows:

- The first step consists of creating a scatterplot that depicts the differences in ratings between raters 4 and 3 as a function of their averages. Table 7.2 shows the ratings being analyzed as well as the two series of averages and differences used to create the scatterplot of Figure 7.3.1.

- The next step is to display on the scatterplot created in the previous step, the two "limits of agreement". The dotted line at the bottom is the lower limit of agreement and the one at the top represents the upper limit of agreement. The lower limit of agreement is -1.169 while the upper limit of agreement is 5.836. This indicates that you can expect the difference between raters 4 and 3 to be as high as 3.763 and as low as 0.904. Depending on the application at hand, such a gap may be acceptable or may be too wide. Ultimately, this gap will help the researcher decide whether the extent of agreement between the two raters 4 and 3 is acceptable or not. If $\overline{d}$ is the average difference and s the standard deviation of the differences, then the lower limit of agreement is $\overline{d} - 2s/n$ and the upper limit of agreement $\overline{d} + 2s/n$.

The two steps described above summarize what is known as the Bland-Altman method. It is intuitive and fairly straightforward to apply. Bland and Altman (1986) indicated that their plot can help study the relationship between the rating pairwise differences and the associated pairwise means, which by the way are used as surrogates for the true rating associated with the subject. The study of this relationship is one way of verifying whether the differences are independent or not. These differences must be approximately independent for the interpretation of the lower and upper limits of agreement to be valid. If these differences have for example a tendency to decrease as the averages increase, or if this relationship shows any other specific trend, this may an indication of a lack of independence. Transforming the initial ratings using the logarithm function for example may be the remedy for obtaining the independence needed.

Some researchers believe that the Bland-Altman method is the only realistic way of dealing with inter-rater agreement. That is no true. We will see in the next few chapters why the intraclass correlation is not only appropriate, but is often the better approach.

Table 7.2: Scores assigned by Raters 3 & 4 to 6 subjects

Subject	Rater #3	Rater #4	Mean Rating	Difference[a]
1	5	8	6.5	3
2	3	2	2.5	-1
3	6	8	7	2
4	2	6	4	4
5	6	9	7.5	3
6	4	7	5.5	3

[a]Difference = (Rater 4) - (Rater 3)

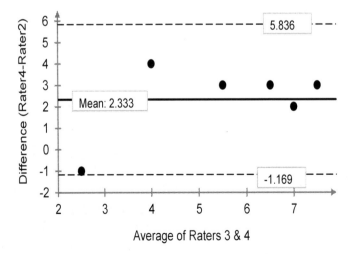

Figure 7.3.1: Rating Differences as a function of rating means

ISSUES WITH THE BLAND-ALTMAN METHOD

Part of the popularity of the Bland-Altman method stems from its graphical nature. You can look at the graph and see right in front of you the differences between the ratings obtained from the two raters you are analyzing. A simple visual exploration may even allow you to form an opinion about the extent to which they agree. Using the two limits of agreement helps you figure out how large the difference should be before it can be considered too large. Here are a few assumptions the Bland-Altman method is based upon, and which are often not satisfied:

- Bland and Altman (1986, p. 4) indicates that the "... *differences are likely to follow a Normal distribution because we have removed a lot of the variation between subjects and are left with the measurement error.*" The real problem with this assumption is that it is untrue if there is a subject-rater interaction. This is often the case when the rating is affected by the magnitude of the "true" score associated with the subjects. The subject-rater interaction does not preclude the differences from following the Normal distribution. However, the differences will be correlated and their actual standard deviation would be higher than the estimate s recommended by Bland and Altman(1986).

  If the standard deviation of the differences is underestimated then the Bland-Altman method may produce a false sense of agreement. When subjects and raters interact, inter-rater reliability is better analyzed with the intraclass correlation that relies on a formal modeling of the interaction effect.

- Another benefit of the Bland-Altman plot lies in the analysis of the the relationship between the differences and the average ratings. This relationship is important primarily because it allows you to see whether raters and subjects interact provided the average is a good surrogate for the subject's true score. The problem here is that the average is known to be close to the true value only if there is little variation in the ratings. That is if the raters are known to be in agreement, an assumption we cannot make since that very agreement is precisely what we are studying.

- The Bland-Altman method is meant for pairwise analyses only. It may not allow you to obtain a global picture of the extent of agreement among multiple raters. When the number of raters is moderately large such as 8, the number of pairwise analyses becomes as large as 28, which can be problematic.

I would recommend using the Bland-Altman plot mainly as an exploratory technique. It allows the researcher to have a first glimpse into the inter-rater reliability results. Ultimately, an intraclass correlation based on the appropriate statistical model should be calculated.

7.4 Sample Size Calculations

When designing an inter-rater (or intra-rater) reliability study, the researcher first needs to determine how many subjects and how many raters must be part of the experiment. Sometimes, there is also a need to determine the number of trials also known as the number of replicates if replication is desired. Note that replication is about a rater taking more than one measurement from the same subject. Each of the next three chapters has a section on sample size calculation. These sections provide detailed procedures showing how the number of raters, the number of subjects and the number of trials can be determined depending on which data model is chosen.

Traditionally power calculation as done in statistics is based on the test of hypothesis involving population means, and consists of finding the optimal sample size that yields the desired power[1] for the statistical test. This procedure generally requires the researcher to specify the effect size (or the detectable difference)[2], the statistical significance (also known as α or alpha), and the desired power. The approach proposed here for the ICC is slightly different. It requires the researcher to specify the desired confidence interval length (this is equivalent to specifying the effect size), the confidence level associated with the confidence interval (this often takes the values 90%, 95%, or 99%), and the anticipated ICC value. The anticipated ICC value may be known from prior studies or from a pilot experiment. If such a value is unknown then I will recommend a conservative approach based on the anticipated ICC value that will yield the largest confidence interval length.

Our investigation has revealed that you need about 5 raters to optimize your inter-rater reliability coefficient for a given total number of ratings. The total number of ratings is the product of the number of raters by the number of subjects (assuming one trial per rater and per subject). Therefore, if your experiment is going to generate 140 ratings for example, then it would be more efficient to have 5 raters and 28 subjects instead of having 10 raters and 14 subjects. A design is said to be more efficient in this context when it yields the smaller confidence interval length. Consequently increasing the number of subjects is more rewarding than increasing the number of raters beyond 5. However, if recruiting raters is cheaper than recruiting subjects then you may have to increase the number of raters beyond 5 and reduce the number of subjects.

In practice, it often happens that the researcher has to use a specific model, due

---

[1]The power of a statistical test represents the probability for that test to reject the "null" hypothesis when it is false. This "null" hypothesis could be the equality of two population means, or the equality of a population mean to a hypothetical value.

[2]The detectable difference is the smallest difference between the two population means under comparison, which will cause the null hypothesis to be rejected.

to various practical constraints. If you have the opportunity to chose the model you want, the question becomes which one to chose and how to chose it. The answer depends on whether you want to optimize the inter-rater reliability calculation, the intra-rater reliability calculation or both. Let us start with the inter-rater reliability optimization first.

For the purpose of optimizing the inter-rater reliability assessment, I recommend the use of models 2 or 3 if possible. Model 3, if appropriate, is expected to yield more accurate intra-rater reliability coefficients than model 2 for the same number of raters, and subjects. However, the discussions in subsequent chapters may give you the impression that using models 1A or 2 will produce similar results. This is not accurate. Model 1A allows you to use a different group of raters for each subject. While this may be convenient when the same group of raters cannot be present to rate the same subjects, the inter-rater reliability calculation comes with a price tag. The use of different groups of raters is expected to increase the variation in ratings due to the rater effect, which in turn will reduce the magnitude of the inter-rater reliability coefficient. Model 1A does not allow for an in-depth analysis of the impact of having different groups of raters, since it does not specify the mechanism underlying the selection of these raters for each subject. The choice between models 2 and 3 depends on whether the raters used in the experiment are the only ones you are interested in (model 3), or whether they are part of a larger universe of raters you like to infer to (model 2). Under models 2 and 3, each rater is expected to rate all subjects, making it easier for you to decide how many raters, subjects, and possibly trials will produce the ratings you need. This is one of the key advantages of these two models.

For the purpose of optimizing the intra-rater reliability, I still recommend the use of models 2 or 3 if possible. You may nevertheless use the simple model 1B with a single subject being rated multiple times by each of the participating raters. However, using model 1B makes the intra-rater reliability very dependent upon the one subject being rated. An alternative approach would be to use model 1A with one rater rating each subject multiple times. Again this approach will make the intra-rater reliability very dependent on the specific rater used in the experiment. This may or may not be what you want. The approach I recommend is the use of models 2 or 3, with model 2 (if appropriate) expected to produce more accurate intra-rater reliability coefficient for the same number of raters than model 3. For a fixed number of ratings per rater, you need no more than 4, 5, or 6 trials to obtain the most accurate intra-rater reliability coefficient under models 2 and 3. That is if a rater must produce 40 ratings, it would be more effective to use 8 subjects and 5 trials rather than 20 subjects and 2 trials. All these issues and many more are discussed in-depth in the next three chapters.

Figure 7.4.1 represents a decision tree showing which equations or subsections in the subsequent chapters should be used to compute the correct agreement coefficient and associated p-values and confidence intervals, depending on the model dictated by your study design. The numbering of these equations (or subsections) is descriptive, and the first digit refers to the chapter number, the second digit to the section within the chapter, and the third number to a specific equation or subsection.

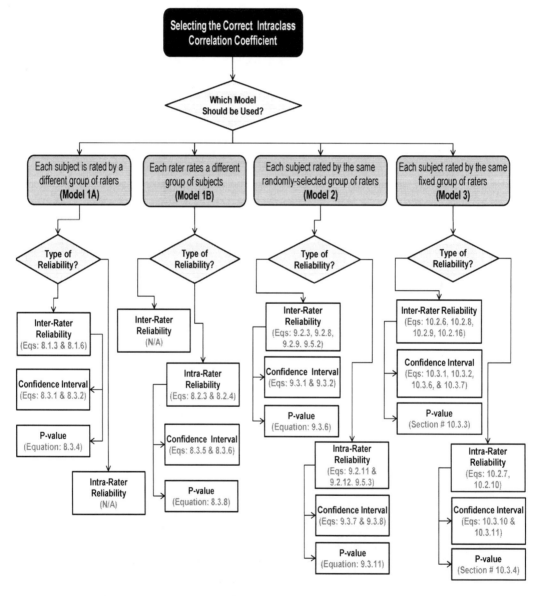

Figure 7.4.1: Choosing the Correct Intraclass Correlation

CHAPTER ⎣8⎦

Intraclass Correlations in One-Factor Studies

OBJECTIVE

The objective of this chapter is to present methods and techniques for calculating the intraclass correlation coefficient and associated precision measures in single-factor reliability studies based on model 1A or model 1B. I consider situations where the quantitative measurement is studied as a function of either the rater effect or the subject effect, but not both. Intraclass correlation is first defined as an abstract construct before the computation procedures are described. Methods for obtaining confidence intervals and p-values will be presented as well. I also discuss some approaches for calculating the optimal number of subjects and raters needed while planning an inter-rater reliability experiment.

CONTENTS

8.1   Intraclass Correlation under Model 1A

Let us consider a reliability experiment where r raters must each take m measurements (or replicate measurements or trial measurements) from n subjects. However, each subject could be rated by a different group of r raters. One could say with respect to Table 8.1 that $n = 6$, $r = 4$, and $m = 1$, since there are 6 subjects, 4 raters, and 1 replicate (i.e. there is a single measurement taken by the raters on each subject). Let y_{ijk} be the abstract representation of the quantitative score assigned to subject i by rater j on the kth trial. The rater may change from subject to subject as stipulated in model 1A. The mathematical translation of this model is as follows:

$$y_{ijk} = \mu + s_i + e_{ijk}, \tag{8.1.1}$$

where μ is the expected score, s_i is subject i's effect, and e_{ijk} the error effect. Both effects are assumed to be random, independent[1] and to follow the Normal distribution with mean 0, and variances σ_s^2, and σ_e^2 respectively.

8.1.1   *Defining Inter-Rater Reliability*

The *Intraclass Correlation Coefficient* (ICC) needed to measure inter-rater reliability is by definition the correlation coefficient between the two quantitative scores y_{ijk} and $y_{ij'k}$ associated with the same subject i, and the same replicate number k, but with two raters j and j'. It follows from equation 8.1.1 that this particular correlation coefficient (denoted by ρ) is given by,

$$\rho = \frac{\sigma_s^2}{\sigma_s^2 + \sigma_e^2}. \tag{8.1.2}$$

Equation 8.1.2 provides the theoretical definition of ICC as the ratio of the subject variance to the total variance (i.e. the sum of subject and error variances) based on model 8.1.1. This ratio shows that the ICC will be high when the subject variance exceeds the error variance by a wide margin. This quantity indeed represents the extent of agreement among the r raters. To see this, you must first realize that the error variance σ_e^2 is actually the variance of two factors blended together, which are the rater factor and the error factor. However, the design represented by model 1A makes it impossible to separate them[2]. Therefore, a small error variance under model

---

[1] Independence is taken here in a statistical sense. That is the knowledge of the magnitude of one effect tells nothing about the magnitude of the other effect

[2] You would separate the rater and error variances only if each rater scores a whole set of subjects, which is not the case under model 1A

1A, actually means that both the error and rater variances have to be small. It is that small (and unknown) rater variance that ensures a small variation in the rater's scores and a high inter-rater reliability.

8.1.2   *Calculating Inter-Rater Reliability*

Shrout and Fleiss (1979) as well as McGraw and Wong (1996) presented ways to actually compute the intraclass correlation from raw data. Their methods are based on the use on various means of squares, and assume that your dataset is complete (i.e. does not contain missing values). This could be problematic in practice as missing values are common in many applications. However, the use of the means of squares is particularly useful for planning purposes, and will help determine the required sample sizes, and number of replicates prior to conducting the actual study (see section 8.3.3). This section focuses on computation methods needed to analyze data already collected, and that may contain missing values.

The approach that I present here is a simplified version of the methods described by Searle (1997, page 474). Let m_{ij} be the number of measurements (or replicates) associated with subject i and rater j. In the case of Table 8.1, $m_{ij} = 1$ for all subjects and all raters. If rater j does not score subject i then $m_{ij} = 0$, indicating that these ratings are missing. Let M be the total number measurements collected for the whole study (i.e. M is the summation of all m_{ij} values). For Table 8.1, $M = 6 \times 4 = 24$. Here are a few quantities that we are going to need:

- $m_{i\cdot}$ = number of measurements associated with subject i. In Table 8.1 there are 4 values associated with each subject since none is missing. That is $m_{1\cdot} = m_{2\cdot} = \cdots = m_{6\cdot} = 4$.

- $m_{\cdot j}$ = number of measurements associated with rater j. In Table 8.1, there are 6 values associated with each rater since none is missing. That is, $m_{\cdot 1} = m_{\cdot 2} = m_{\cdot 3} = m_{\cdot 4} = 6$.

- $y_{i\cdot\cdot}^2$ is the squared value of subject i's total score, and T_{2s} the sum of squares of all subject total scores (i.e. the sum of $y_{i\cdot\cdot}^2$ values).

- Let T_y be the total score (i.e. the summation of all y_{ijk} values), and T_{2y} the total sum of squares (i.e. the summation of all squared scores y_{ijk}^2).

In practice, the ICC of equation 8.1.2 can only be approximated using experimental data. This is done by calculating the two variance components from the raw experimental data. While the theoretical subject variance is σ_s^2, its calculated value is denoted by $\widehat{\sigma}_s^2$ (read sigma hat s square). Likewise, the calculated error variance is denoted by $\widehat{\sigma}_e^2$. The calculated intraclass correlation coefficient associated with model

1A is denoted by $\text{ICC}(1A,1)^3$ and given by,

$$\boxed{\text{ICC}(1A,1) = \frac{\widehat{\sigma}_s^2}{\widehat{\sigma}_s^2 + \widehat{\sigma}_e^2},} \qquad (8.1.3)$$

where,

$$\widehat{\sigma}_e^2 = (T_{2y} - T_{2s})/(M - n), \qquad (8.1.4)$$

$$\widehat{\sigma}_s^2 = \frac{T_{2s} - T_y^2/M - (n-1)\widehat{\sigma}_e^2}{M - k_0}, \qquad (8.1.5)$$

and k_0 is the expected number of measurements per subject and is calculated by summing all factors $m_{ij}^2/m_{.j}$ over all n subjects and all raters. If there is no missing rating then $k_0 = rm$.

Example 8.1 _____

To illustrate the calculation of ICC(1A,1), let us consider the data of Table 8.1 and assume that it was collected following the 1A design. Tables 8.1 and 8.2 show the different steps for calculating the intraclass correlation coefficients. Table 8.2 aims at showing the calculation of $k_0 = 4$, obtained by summing the last column. Columns 6, 7, 9, and 10 of Table 8.1 show the numbers $T_y = 127$, $M = 24$, $T_{2s} = 728.25$, and $T_{2y} = 841$. It follows from equations 8.1.4 and 8.1.5 that,

$$\widehat{\sigma}_e^2 = (841 - 728.25)/(24 - 6) = 6.264,$$
$$\widehat{\sigma}_s^2 = (728.25 - 127^2/24 - (6 - 1) \times 6.264)/(24 - 4) = 1.2444.$$

After plugging these variance components into equation 8.1.3, one obtains the intraclass correlation, $\text{ICC}(1A, 1) = 1.2444/(1.2444 + 6.264) = 0.1657$.
Interested readers may download the Excel spreadsheet,

        www.agreestat.com/book4/chapter8examples.xlsx

which shows the step-by-step calculation of this ICC.

The approach used in Example 8.1 for computing $\text{ICC}(1A, 1)$ yields the exact same answer as the standard approach based on means of squares advocated by Shrout and Fleiss (1979), or McGraw and Wong (1996). Their standard approach however, can only work when there is no missing rating, and is given by,

$$\text{ICC}(1A, 1) = \frac{\text{MSS} - \text{MSE}}{\text{MSS} + (rm - 1)\text{MSE}}, \qquad (8.1.6)$$

---

[3] "1A" in this notation indicates that ICC is based on model 1A, and the number 1 on the right side of the comma sign indicates that each rating used in the analysis represents 1 measurement, as opposed to being an average of several measurements. Some authors (e.g. Shrout & Fleiss, 1979) discussed the situation where the rating being analyzed is an average of k measurements. However, it is unclear how useful this scenario is in practice.

where MSS is the mean of squares for subjects, and MSE the mean of squares for errors. These means of squares are calculated as follows:

- MSS is calculated by summing all squared differences $(\overline{y}_{i..} - \overline{y})^2$ over all n subjects, and by multiplying the summation by $rm/(n-1)$. Note that $\overline{y}_{i..}$ represents the average of all measurements associated with subject i, while $\overline{y}$ is the overall average.

- MSE is calculated by summing all squared differences $(y_{ijk} - \overline{y}_{i..})^2$ over all n subjects, and by dividing the summation by $n(rm-1)$.

Table 8.1: Ratings of 6 Subjects from 4 Raters, and Calculation of ICC(1A,1) based on equation 8.1.3

| Subject (i) | Rater (j) | | | | $y_{i..}$ | $m_{i..}$ | $y_{i..}^2$ | $y_{i..}^2/m_{i.}$ | $y_{2i..}$ [a] |
	1	2	3	4					
1	9	2	5	8	24	4	576	144	174
2	6	1	3	2	12	4	144	36	50
3	8	4	6	8	26	4	676	169	180
4	7	1	2	6	16	4	256	64	90
5	10	5	6	9	30	4	900	225	242
6	6	2	4	7	19	4	361	90.25	105
$y_{.j.}$	46	15	26	40	127	24		728.25	841
$m_{.j}$	6	6	6	6					

[a]Note that $y_{2i..}$ in the last column represents the row-wise summation of the squared raw values.

Table 8.2: Calculating k_0 using the values $m_{ij}^2/m_{.j}$

| Subject (i) | Rater (j) | | | | |
	1	2	3	4	Total
1	0.16667	0.16667	0.16667	0.16667	0.66667
2	0.16667	0.16667	0.16667	0.16667	0.66667
3	0.16667	0.16667	0.16667	0.16667	0.66667
4	0.16667	0.16667	0.16667	0.16667	0.66667
5	0.16667	0.16667	0.16667	0.16667	0.66667
6	0.16667	0.16667	0.16667	0.16667	0.66667
					$k_0 = 4$

8.1.3   *Defining Intra-Rater Reliability*

A question one may ask is whether an intraclass correlation coefficient defined under model 1A can adequately measure intra-rater reliability[4]. In general, the answer would be no. However, there is an exception that would allow experimental data generated under Model 1A to be used for calculating intra-rater reliability. This exception is an experiment with replication, involving two trials or more that are carried out on each subject. Such an experiment allows equation 8.1.2 to be interpreted as an intra-rater reliability coefficient as well. The intraclass correlation coefficient is then defined as the correlation coefficient between two replicate measurements y_{ijk} and $y_{ijk'}$. This coefficient is also known as the test-retest reliability coefficient.

Under model 1A, the notions of rater and replication are confounded. That is, two ratings associated with the same subject are treated the same way whether they were generated by two raters or by the same rater on two occasions. That explains why there a unique ICC of equation 8.1.2 that represents both the inter-rater and the intra-rater reliability coefficient. Although this general reliability measure can serve several purposes, it also possesses several drawbacks. For example, if equation 8.1.2 is used as an intra-rater reliability coefficient and yields a low value, then you may never know whether this is due to low reproducibility or to a high rater effect. To resolve this problem, some researchers design intra-rater reliability experiments with a single rater and a number of replicate measurements per subject. This approach will work fine except that it is based on a single rater, which means that the use of a different rater will potentially change the intra-rater coefficient substantially. This will not be a problem if the different raters are already known to have high inter-rater reliability.

8.1.4   *Recommendations*

The use model 1A is highly recommended if the reliability experiment is designed in such a way that each subject is rated by multiple raters, and the researcher cannot guarantee that the same group of raters will be available to rate more than on subject. If that is the case, I recommend that only inter-rater reliability be calculated. Equation 8.1.2 is not a good measure of intra-rater reliability.

If the main study objective is intra-rater reliability, I would recommend the use of model 1B of section 8.2. Model 1B requires the use of two raters or more, and yields a valid intra-rater coefficient.

---

[4]Intra-rater reliability represents the extent of self-consistency of the raters.

8.2   Intraclass Correlation under Model 1B

Under model 1B, each rater may rate a different group of subjects. Although there could be some overlap between the different groups of subjects, this is not a requirement under model 1B. This model is different from model 1A where each subject could be rated by a different group of raters. One reason why model 1B has not been mentioned often in the literature is that the ICC it can produce is inappropriate for calculating inter-rater reliability[5]. However, it is perfectly appropriate for evaluating intra-rater reliability. Therefore, model 1B is to be ignored if your primary focus is the calculation of inter-rater reliability.

The general mathematical formulation of the rating y_{ijk} associated with subject i, rater j, and replicate (or trial) k is as follows:

$$y_{ijk} = \mu + r_j + e_{ijk}, \tag{8.2.1}$$

where μ is the expected score, r_j the random effect due to rater j, and e_{ijk} the random error term representing any residual effect not attributed to the rater[6]. Both variables r_j and e_{ijk} are assumed to follow Normal distributions with a common mean 0 and the variances σ_r^2 and σ_e^2 respectively. Equation 8.2.1 is nothing else than an abstract representation of the rating that I use to lay down the mathematical foundation for calculating the intraclass correlation coefficient under model 1B.

8.2.1   *Defining Intra-Rater Reliability*

The ICC that quantifies intra-rater reliability under model 1B is by definition the correlation coefficient between the ratings y_{ijk} and $y_{ijk'}$ associated with two trials k and k', for the same subject i and the same rater j. Note that under model 1B, the subject and measurement (or error) effects are confounded. That is, only their combined effect can be evaluated. Consequently, having different subjects and one measurement per subject, or one subject and repeated measurements will not affect the way intra-rater reliability is calculated.

It follows from equation 8.2.1 that this particular correlation coefficient is given by:

$$\gamma = \frac{\sigma_r^2}{\sigma_r^2 + \sigma_e^2}, \tag{8.2.2}$$

---

[5]Calculating inter-rater reliability requires different raters to rate the same subjects (a condition that is necessary to have the subject effect under control), which is not required under model 1B

[6]Note that this residual effect could be due to the subject as well as to the any unspecified experimental error.

which is the relative magnitude of the rater variance with respect to the total variance of the measurements. γ can take values between 0 and 1, where 0 represents the weakest intra-rater reliability, and 1 the highest. Equation 8.2.2 indeed represents a good measure of self-consistency for raters. To see this, note that γ takes a high value when the rater variance σ_r^2 exceeds the error variance σ_e^2 by a wide margin (i.e. σ_r^2 is high and σ_e^2 is small). Since the subject and measurement effects are confounded under model 1B as previously indicated, a small σ_e^2 value is also an indication of small (unknown) subject and small measurement variances. This is a sign that the repeated measurements are in agreement.

Some researchers know intra-rater reliability as a measure of the extent of agreement among repeated measurements taken by the same rater on one subject. In reality, it is unwise to design an intra-rater reliability study based on a single rater and a single subject. If such a study yields high intra-rater reliability, you will not know whether that level of agreement will hold if you use a different rater and a different subject. To ensure the validity of the intra-rater reliability coefficient across a large group of raters and subjects, you may want to base your study on a sample of raters and a sample of subjects.

Using multiple subjects in an intra-rater reliability study to ensure its validity across a sizable sample of subjects carries some risks that must be mitigated. The design based on model 1B will be efficient only if the experimenter uses a homogeneous roster of subjects that is assigned to each rater, in order to minimize the experimental error. Otherwise, the measure of intra-rater reliability may be small even though the raters can reproduce their ratings very well. Model 1B has the advantage of being simple, and does not require the raters to be located in the same place, nor to rate the same subjects. Each rater may even rate a single subject on a few occasions. Each trial can then be analyzed as a separate subject. If a homogeneous roster of subjects is unavailable to the experimenter, then a better option would be to use an alternative design such as those discussed in subsequent chapters.

8.2.2   *Calculating Intra-Rater Reliability*

To compute the intraclass correlation coefficient of equation 8.2.2 from actual data, one option is the use the mean of squares for raters (MSR) and the mean of squares for errors (MSE) as suggested by McGraw and Wong (1996) or Shrout and Fleiss (1979). This approach is widely used by researchers across various fields of research. Its main disadvantage is that it works well when the following two conditions are met: (1) the experimental design is balanced (i.e. each rater must produce the same number of ratings), and (2) all ratings must be reported (i.e. there is no missing rating). These two conditions are rarely met in practice. The implication of this is that researchers must often throw data away so that a complete table can be analyzed. Luckily for us, there are some alternative methods that are presented in this section, and which can be used for unbalanced designs and with missing data.

An alternative method that can handle missing values and unbalanced designs is an adaptation of what Searle (1997, page 474) has proposed. What we gain in flexibility is obtained at the cost of more complexity. I will first present the first full-sample approach before discussing the more general method.

The calculated value of γ is denoted by ICC(1B,1), where 1B refers to the statistical model used, and digit 1 after the comma sign indicates that each rating is associated with a single subject and a single trial, and does not represent an average of several measurements. The notation ICC(1B,1) is well established today in the literature on inter-rater reliability assessment.

SPECIAL APPROACH FOR BALANCED DATA

When your experimental data do not contain missing ratings, you may compute ICC(1B,1) using the mean of squares for raters MSR and the mean of squares for errors MSE as follows,

$$\text{ICC(1B,1)} = \frac{\text{MSR} - \text{MSE}}{\text{MSR} + (nm-1)\text{MSE}}. \tag{8.2.3}$$

These means of squares are defined as follows:

- ▶ MSR is obtained by summing the squared differences $(\overline{y}_{.j.} - \overline{y})^2$, and by multiplying the summation by $nm/(r-1)$. Note that $\overline{y}_{.j.}$ represents the average of all measurements associated with rater j.

- ▶ MSE is obtained by summing the squared differences $(y_{ijk} - \overline{y}_{.j.})^2$, and by dividing the summation by $r(nm-1)$.

The general approach to be presented next, can handle both complete and incomplete datasets. However, both approaches yield the exact same results when the data is complete.

GENERAL APPROACH FOR UNBALANCED DATA

Using unbalanced data, the ICC of equation 8.2.2 is estimated by first calculating the two variance components σ_r^2 and σ_e^2. The calculated rater variance is denoted by $\widehat{\sigma}_r^2$ (read sigma hat r square). Likewise, the calculated error variance is denoted by $\widehat{\sigma}_e^2$. These two quantities lead to the calculated intraclass correlation coefficient given by,

$$\boxed{\text{ICC(1B, 1)} = \frac{\widehat{\sigma}_r^2}{\widehat{\sigma}_r^2 + \widehat{\sigma}_e^2},} \tag{8.2.4}$$

where,

$$\hat{\sigma}_e^2 = (T_{2y} - T_{2r})/(M - r), \tag{8.2.5}$$

$$\hat{\sigma}_r^2 = \frac{T_{2r} - T_y^2/M - (r-1)\hat{\sigma}_e^2}{M - k_1}, \tag{8.2.6}$$

and k_1 is calculated by summing all factors $m_{ij}^2/m_{i\cdot}$ over all subjects i and all raters[7] j. The other terms in equations 8.2.5 and 8.2.6 are defined as follows:

▶ $m_{i\cdot}$ and $m_{\cdot j}$ represent the number of ratings associated with subject i and rater j respectively, while M is the total number of all ratings generated by the experiment.

▶ T_y is the summation of all ratings (y_{ijk}), while T_{2y} is the summation of all squared ratings (y_{ijk}^2).

▶ T_{2r} is the summation of all factors $y_{\cdot j\cdot}^2/m_{\cdot j}$, where $y_{\cdot j\cdot}$ is the summation of all ratings associated with rater j.

Note that for balanced data, the estimated error variance becomes equivalent to the mean of squares for errors MSE (i.e. $\hat{\sigma}_e^2 = $ MSE), and the estimated rater variance can be rewritten as $\hat{\sigma}_r^2 = (\text{MSR} - \text{MSE})/(nm)$, where MSR is the mean of squares for raters. The two expressions 8.2.3 and 8.2.4 will yield the same answer for balanced data.

The following example illustrates the calculation of the intra-rater reliability coefficient ICC(1B,1) using Table 8.3 data. Although this data is balanced, the calculation of ICC(1B,1) is done using both the general approach for unbalanced data and the special approach for balanced data.

Example 8.2 _____

Let us consider the reliability data shown in Table 8.3. Assume that the 6 subjects represent 1 subject rated 6 times, and that different raters may have rated a different subject. This design is consistent with model 1B discussed in this section.

If follows from equation 8.2.5 that calculating the error variance component $\hat{\sigma}_e^2$ requires the knowledge of T_{2y}, T_{2r}, M and r. We have $M = 24$, which is the total number of non-missing measurements, and $r = 4$ the number of raters. Table 8.3 also shows the steps for calculating $T_{2r} = 769.5$ from the raw y_{ijk} data, while Table 8.4 shows the calculation of $T_{2y} = 841$ from the squared scores y_{ijk}^2. Therefore,

$$\hat{\sigma}_e^2 = (841 - 769.5)/(24 - 4) = 3.575$$

_____

[7]Note that when each subject is scored no more than once (i.e. $m_{ij} = 0$ or $m_{ij} = 1$), then k_1 always equals the number of subjects n. If the same number m of ratings are produced for each subject, then $k_1 = nm$, which is the total number of ratings produced by each rater for all subjects.

It follows from equation 8.2.6 that T_y and k_1 are the two additional elements needed to compute the rater variance components. Table 8.3 shows the steps for calculating $T_y = 127$, and $k_1 = 6$. Therefore,

$$\widehat{\sigma}_r^2 = (769.50 - 127^2/24 - (4-1) \times 3.575)/(24-6) = 4.8185.$$

Consequently, ICC(1B,1) $= 4.8185/(4.8185 + 3.575) = 0.574$. Interested readers may download the Excel spreadsheet,

<code>www.agreestat.com/book4/chapter8examples.xlsx</code>,

and look at the particular worksheet labeled as "Example 8.2" which shows the step-by-step calculation of ICC(1B,1).

Table 8.3: Statistics based on y_{ijk}'s

Subject	Rater (j)				Total
(i)	1	2	3	4	
1	9	2	5	8	
2	6	1	3	2	
3	8	4	6	8	
4	7	1	2	6	
5	10	5	6	9	
6	6	2	4	7	
$y_{\cdot j \cdot}$	46	15	26	40	127
$y_{\cdot j \cdot}^2$	2116	225	676	1600	
$m_{\cdot j}$	6	6	6	6	
$y_{\cdot j \cdot}^2/m_{\cdot j}$	352.67	37.5	112.67	266.67	769.5

Table 8.4: Statistics based on y_{ijk}^2's

Subject	Rater (j)				Total
(i)	1	2	3	4	
1	81	4	25	64	174
2	36	1	9	4	50
3	64	16	36	64	180
4	49	1	4	36	90
5	100	25	36	81	242
6	36	4	16	49	105
Total	366	51	126	298	841

Since the data being analyzed in this example is balanced, identical results can be obtained using the mean of squares for errors (MSE), and the mean of squares for raters (MSR) as shown in equation 8.2.3. The mean rating is $\bar{y} = 5.292$. Therefore,

$$
\begin{aligned}
\text{MSR} &= \left[(7.667 - 5.292)^2 + (2.500 - 5.292)^2 + (4.333 - 5.292)^2 + \right. \\
&\quad \left. + (6.667 - 5.292)^2 \right] \times 6 \times 1/(4-1), \\
&= (5.6406 + 7.7934 + 0.9184 + 1.8906) \times 6/3 = 32.4861.
\end{aligned}
$$

As for the MSE, it is calculated as follows:

$$
\begin{aligned}
\text{MSE} &= (1.7778 + 2.7778 + 0.1111 + 0.4444 + 5.4444 + 2.7778 + \\
&\quad + 0.25 + 2.25 + 2.25 + 2.25 + 6.25 + 0.25 + \\
&\quad + 0.4444 + 1.7778 + 2.7778 + 5.4444 + 2.7778 + 0.1111 + \\
&\quad + 1.7778 + 21.7778 + 1.7778 + 0.4444 + 5.4444 + 0.1111)/(4*(6-1)) = 3.575.
\end{aligned}
$$

Consequently, ICC(1B,1) $= (32.4861 - 3.575)/(32.4861 + (6-1) * 3.575) = 0.574$.

8.3   Statistical Inference about ICC under Models 1A and 1B

In the past few sections, I presented methods for calculating intraclass correlation from experimental data, under one of the two statistical models 1A and 1B. The ICC so obtained is intimately tied to the specific subjects and raters that participated in the reliability experiment. Oftentimes, these participating subjects and raters only represent small samples selected from larger subject and rater populations, which constitute the primary interest of the researcher. Including entire populations in a reliability experiment would be a costly task that few researchers can afford. This is why studies are usually based on smaller samples to reduce the cost of conducting them. Although the ICC associated with the entire subject and rater populations is the "true" ICC, it is actually their calculated versions that we have to work with. The question now is how to use experimental data and the calculated ICC in order to make a statement about the magnitude of the "true" intraclass correlation coefficient[8] .

There are two ways that a researcher can appreciate the magnitude of the true ICC. One is the Confidence Interval (CI), and the other is the test of hypothesis. The confidence interval is a range of values that you would calculate using the ratings produced during the experiment. What is peculiar about that range of values is that it is expected to contain the true ICC with a predetermined probability known as the Confidence Level[9]. A narrow confidence interval gives us a reasonably good idea about the magnitude of the true ICC. The test of hypothesis on the other hand, consists of calculating the *p*-value, which measures the extent to which the data supports a conjecture about the magnitude of the true ICC value.

The methods discussed in this section assumed the rating dataset being used to be complete. That is, your original dataset contains missing ratings, you will need to remove those before performing the confidence interval and *p*-value calculations. The precision associated with these calculations will be good if the number of missing values is limited, but will deteriorate as the number of missing ratings increases.

---

[8]This process of using collected facts to draw conclusions about the larger universe is called "inference." When this process involves any randomization in the selection of subjects and/or raters, then it is referred to as "Statistical Inference." Throughout this book, I will use statistical inference as the only method of inference. Note that other authors use to the randomization of the rating process described by a theoretical statistical model to perform statistical inference. This alternative approach is not considered in this book.

[9]Our calculated ICC is obtained using data from a single sample of the rater population, and a single sample of the subject population. Different samples are expected to yield different ICC values and therefore different confidence intervals. The confidence level is set by you the researcher and is the relative number of times you want the constructed confidence intervals to include the "true" intraclass correlation.

8.3.1 *Confidence Interval for ρ under Model 1A*

The "true" ICC under model 1A is defined by equation 8.1.2. The confidence interval associated with it represents all the values between a lower confidence bound (LCB), and an upper confidence bound (UCB) defined in such a way that they will enclose the true ICC value ρ with a probability that matches the predetermined confidence level[10]. The LCB and UCB are defined as follows,

$$\text{LCB} = \frac{F_{\text{L}} - 1}{F_{\text{L}} + (M/n - 1)}, \text{ with } F_{\text{L}} = F_{obs}/C_{\text{L}}, \tag{8.3.1}$$

$$\text{UCB} = \frac{F_{\text{U}} - 1}{F_{\text{U}} + (M/n - 1)}, \text{ with } F_{\text{U}} = F_{obs} \times C_{\text{U}}, \tag{8.3.2}$$

where M is the total number of reported ratings, F_{obs}, C_{L}, and C_{U} are defined as follows,

▶ $F_{obs} = \text{MSS/MSE}$, where MSS and MSE are respectively the Mean of Squares for Subjects and for Errors, calculated as follows:

    (a) For MSE, sum all squared differences $(y_{ijk} - \overline{y}_{i\cdot\cdot})^2$ from observations to the subject-level mean, then divide by $M - n$ *(this term is referred to as the "number of degrees of freedom" associated with the MSE).*

    (b) For MSS, sum all factors $m_{i\cdot}(\overline{y}_{i\cdot\cdot} - \overline{y})^2$ where $m_{i\cdot}$ is the number of reported ratings associated with subject i, then divide the summation by $n-1$ *(Note that $n-1$ is known as the "number of degrees of freedom" associated with MSS).*

▶ The two quantities C_{L} and C_{U} must be obtained from a statistical table, computed with a statistical software, or with MS Excel. C_{L} represents the $100 \cdot (1 - \alpha/2)^{th}$ percentile (with $\alpha = 1 - $ *(Confidence Level)*) of the F distribution with $n-1$ and $M-n$ degrees of freedom respectively. The second quantity C_{U} represents the $100 \cdot (1 - \alpha/2)^{th}$ percentiles of the F distribution with the $M - n$ and $n - 1$ degrees of freedom respectively.

Although all statistical packages offer functions for computing these quantities, our preferred method for calculating them, in terms of practicality and convenience is MS Excel. We will illustrate this approach in the next example.

---

[10]The confidence level is generally a high probability ; the typical values being 90%, 95%, or 99%. Increasing this value generally results in a wider and less useful confidence interval. Decreasing it will result in a narrower interval, which gives a more accurate location of the "true" ICC. But you will have less trust (or confidence) in this narrow interval's ability to actually contain the "true" ICC. Therefore, a compromise must always be found between a reasonable confidence level and an acceptable interval width.

Example 8.3

In Example 8.1, we analyzed Table 8.1 data under the assumption that it was collected according to the specifications of model 1A. The calculated intraclass correlation coefficient was $\text{ICC}(1A, 1) = 0.1657$. We now want to calculate the associated confidence interval at the 95% confidence level.

The first step is to compute the MSS and the MSE. It follows from Table 8.5 that $\text{MSS} = 11.24167$, and was calculated as described above. We first calculated the row marginal averages $\overline{y}_{i..}$, and the squared differences $(\overline{y}_{i..} - \overline{y})^2$, before summing them and multiplying the sum by $rm/(n-1)$ (note that $m_{i.} = rm$ for each subject i). Interested readers may want to look at the "Example 8.3" worksheet in the Excel workbook,

$$\texttt{www.agreestat.com/book4/chapter8examples.xlsx,}$$

for more details regarding these calculations. Table 8.6, on the other hand shows that $\text{MSE} = 6.26389$. This calculation is based on the squared differences $(y_{ijk} - \overline{y}_{i..})^2$.

Table 8.5: Calculating the Mean Square for Subjects (MSS)

Subject	Rater (j)					
(i)	1	2	3	4	$\overline{y}_{i..}$	$(\overline{y}_{i..} - \overline{y})^2$
1	9	2	5	8	6.00	0.50174
2	6	1	3	2	3.00	5.25174
3	8	4	6	8	6.50	1.46007
4	7	1	2	6	4.00	1.66840
5	10	5	6	9	7.50	4.87674
6	6	2	4	7	4.75	0.29340
					$\overline{y} = 5.29$	$\text{MSS} = 11.24167$

Table 8.6: Calculating the Mean Square Error (MSE)

Subject		$(y_{ijk} - \overline{y}_{i..})^2$ factors by rater (j)			
(i)	$\overline{y}_{i..}$	1	2	3	4
1	6	9	16	1	4
2	3	9	4	0	1
3	6.5	2.25	6.25	0.25	2.25
4	4	9	9	4	4
5	7.5	6.25	6.25	2.25	2.25
6	4.75	1.5625	7.5625	0.5625	5.0625
					$\text{MSE} = 6.26389$

The confidence level of 95% leads to $\alpha = 1 - 0.95 = 0.05$. Therefore the factors C_{L}

and C_{υ} of equations 8.3.1 and 8.3.2 both represent the 97.5% percentiles (Note that $97.5\% = 100 \times (1 - \alpha/2)\% = 100 \times (1 - 0.05/2)\%$) of the F distributions with 5 and 18 degrees of freedom for C_{L}, and 18 and 5 degrees of freedom for C_{υ}. If you are using Windows Excel 2007 or an earlier version (or Mac Excel 2008 or an earlier version), then you could conveniently calculate the first factor as C_{L} =FINV(0.05/2,5,18) to obtain $C_{\mathrm{L}} = 3.38197$. With Windows Excel 2010 (or Mac Excel 2011) or a more recent version (at the time of this writing, Windows Excel 2010 is the most recent version), you may also calculate C_{L} as =F.INV(1-0.05/2,5,18) and obtain the same result. Likewise $C_{\upsilon} = 6.36188$, and this is obtained with Windows Excel 2007 and Mac Excel 2008 as "=FINV(0.05/2,18,5)," or with the more recent Windows Excel 2010 and Mac Excel 2011 as "=F.INV(1-0.05/2,18,5)."

Therefore, $F_{obs} = \mathrm{MSS}/\mathrm{MSE} = 1.79468$. Since $F_{\mathrm{L}} = 1.79468/3.38197 = 0.53066$, and $F_{\upsilon} = 1.79468 \times 6.36188 = 11.41753$, the confidence limits are calculated as follows (note that $rm = M/n$ since the data is balanced):

$$\mathrm{LCB} = (F_{\mathrm{L}} - 1)/\big[F_{\mathrm{L}} + (M/n - 1)\big] = (0.53066 - 1)/(0.53066 + (4 - 1)) = -0.13293,$$
$$\mathrm{UCB} = (F_{\upsilon} - 1)/\big[F_{\upsilon} + (M/n - 1)\big] = (11.41753 - 1)/(11.41753 + (4 - 1)) = 0.72256.$$

However, the intraclass correlation coefficient is by definition a positive number. Therefore, we should consider (LCB, UCB) = $(0, 0.72256)$ as the 95% confidence interval for ρ.

8.3.2   *p-Value for ρ under Model 1A*

In this section, I assume that the researcher wants to evaluate the extent to which the ratings are consistent with the hypothesis that the true inter-rater reliability ρ exceeds a predetermined value ρ_0 that may represent a standard of acceptability in the profession. The p-value performs an indirect comparison of the two quantities ρ and ρ_0. The process starts with a summary measure of the ratings that is a decreasing function of ρ, and whose sampling distribution is known. The p-value evaluates how often this summary measure exceeds its observed value based on actual ratings and the hypothesized value ρ_0. A small p-value provides a strong indication that the true ICC value ρ exceeds ρ_0.

Let F and F_{obs} be defined as follows,

$$F = \frac{\mathrm{MSS}}{\mathrm{MSE}\big(1 + M\rho/[n(1 - \rho)]\big)}, \text{ and } F_{obs} = \frac{\mathrm{MSS}}{\mathrm{MSE}\big(1 + M\rho_0/[n(1 - \rho_0)]\big)}, \quad (8.3.3)$$

where M is the number of reported ratings, while MSS and MSE are the Means of Squares for Subjects and for Errors, calculated as shown in section 8.3.1. Note that the ratio M/n in equation 8.3.3 represents the average number of ratings per subject, which reduces to rm for balanced data. F is known to follow the F-distribution with

$n - 1$ and $M - n$ degrees of freedom for any value of ρ. While MSS and MSE are abstract quantities when used with the F statistic, it is their respective calculated values that are used with F_{obs} after experimental data had be gathered.

The p-value is defined as the probability for the random variable F to exceed F_{obs}. That is,

$$p-value = P(F \geq F_{obs}). \tag{8.3.4}$$

The rule of thumb regarding the use of the p-value in practice is to support the hypothesis that $\rho > \rho_0$ whenever the p-value is smaller than 0.05. If you are already familiar with standard statistical packages (R, SPSS, SAS, $\cdots$), you may use them to compute the probability in equation 8.3.4. Otherwise, my advice is to use MS Excel[11] as follows:

$= \text{F.DIST.RT}(F_{obs}, n - 1, M - n)$ *(for Excel 2010/2011 or more recent),*

$= \text{FDIST}(F_{obs}, n - 1, M - n)$ *(for Excel 2007/2008 or an earlier version)*

Example 8.4 _____

To illustrate the calculation of the p-value, consider Table 8.1 ratings once again. In Example 8.1 we calculated the intraclass correlation $ICC(1A, 1) = 0.1657$. In Example 8.3, we calculated the two means of squares MSS $= 11.24167$ and MSE $= 6.26389$, which we can use along with equations 8.3.3 and 8.3.4 to get the p-value.

Table 8.7 shows the p-value for various values of ρ_0. It appears that even for a value of ρ_0 as small as 0, the p-value exceeds the threshold of 0.05 by a wide margin. Consequently, the reliability data of Table 8.1 does not even support the hypothesis that $\rho > 0$. In statistical jargon, one would say that the estimate $ICC(1A, 1) = 0.1657$ is not statistically significant.

Table 8.7: p-Values associated with $ICC(1A, 1)$ for Various ρ_0 Values

ρ_0	F_{obs}	p-Value[a]
0	1.7947	0.1648
0.05	1.4826	0.2443
0.1	1.2425	0.3306
0.15	1.0521	0.4184
0.2	0.8973	0.5038
0.25	0.7691	0.5841

[a]For more details regarding these calculations, you may want to look at the "Example 8.4" worksheet in the Excel workbook www.agreestat.com/book4/chapter8examples.xlsx.

---

[11]From now on, I will use the slash symbol "/" to separate the Windows and Mac versions of Excel. For example Excel 2007/2008 refers to the Windows Excel 2007 or Mac Excel 2008.

8.3.3   Sample Size Calculations under Model 1A

When designing an inter-rater reliability study, the researcher must decide how many raters and how many subjects to recruit. The general approach I recommend here applies to model 1A only and is similar to the method proposed by Giraudeau & Mary (2011). This technique consists of finding the optimal number of observations (i.e. the total number of measurements taken on all subjects) that minimizes the length of the ICC's confidence interval. Additional information on previous efforts in this area is provided by Doros and Lew (2010).

As previously mentioned, under model 1A the rater and replicate (or error) effects are confounded. That is, they are indistinguishable and only their combined effect can be evaluated. Consequently, when designing a study under model 1A, you only need to predict two numbers:

- The optimal number of measurements per subject. Let m designate that number.

- The optimal number of subjects. Let n be that number.

Once the optimal number of measurements per subject m is calculated, then the researcher will have to decide whether that number will represent the number of raters (for inter-rater reliability assessment) or the number of replicates (for intra-rater reliability assessment) or any combination of raters and replicates. However, under model 1A there is no benefit in using raters and replicates simultaneously. These effects are confounded and only their combined impact can be evaluated. Instead, one will use raters only to evaluate inter-rater reliability, and replicates only for intra-rater reliability. For example, if $m = 10$ then one would use 10 raters and 1 measurement per rater, or 1 rater and 10 replicate measurements. Using 5 raters and 2 replicates per rater for example will weaken both the inter-rater and the intra-rater reliability.

Figure 8.3.1 depicts the expected length of the 95% confidence interval as a function of the "true" value of the ICC, under the assumption that the total number of measurements from all subjects is 20 (i.e. $n \times m = 20$). The two continuous curves represent cases where the number of subjects is 4 for the black curve and 5 for the gray one. The two dotted lines on the other hand, represent experiments based on 10 and 2 subjects. The actual value of the ICC is generally unknown, and will have to be hypothesized by the researcher at the design stage. To be more concrete, you need to know whether the raters you are investigating have high agreement or low agreement in order to develop an effective design. The purpose of the study is to measure agreement; yet we need some information about that same agreement in order to devise an effective design. What, if you do not have any preliminary information regarding the extent of agreement among the raters under investigation?

The solution could be to conduct a pilot study with a small number of observations (i.e. approximately 10 observations), and use the crude estimate of the ICC obtained to finalize a more refined sample size calculation.

It appears from Figure 8.3.1 that the expected confidence interval length decreases as the ICC increases. That is, if the anticipated ICC is high, then the number of observations required to obtain a narrow confidence interval (i.e. a more accurate estimation) will generally be small. In other words, the study of raters known to have high agreement is cheaper than the study of raters known to have low agreement. This is logical. If raters have high agreement, ratings collected by a few raters on a few subjects will tell the whole story. Other raters who did not participate in the study, but who agree with the participants will not add any more information to the extent of agreement. But if a group of raters are known to have low agreement, then ratings collected by a few of them will reveal very little about the extent of agreement among all raters in that heterogeneous group. A sizeable number of raters and subjects must be recruited in order to obtain an effective study.

Figures 8.3.2 through 8.3.6 depict the relationship between the 95% confidence interval length and the "True" ICC for various values of the total number of measurements. Figure 8.3.2 for example is based 40 measurements, and the different curves on that figure represent different distributions of the 40 measurements between the number of subjects and the number raters. All 6 figures 8.3.1 to 8.3.6 show that for any given ICC value, having 4 or 5 raters (or 4 or 5 measurements per subject for intr-rater reliability studies) appears to minimize the confidence interval length. Readers interested to know how these graphs are created, are invited to read the last few paragraphs at the end of this section.

How to determine the sample size ?

One possible approach that I recommend for determining the optimal sample size is the following three-step process:
- Start with an anticipated value for the intraclass correlation. The situation where you have no prior information at all about the possible magnitude of the intraclass correlation is addressed in the next subsection.
- Set your desired confidence interval length to be approximately $0.8 \times$ ICC, where ICC is the predicted extent of agreement among raters of the previous step[12].
- Review the different graphs and the expected 95% confidence interval length that is associated with the anticipated ICC value. One curve should lead to

---

[12]This rule of thumb is derived from the classical confidence intervals for means. The length of a 95% confidence interval length is 4 times the standard deviation (STD). If the coefficient of variation (i.e. the ratio of the STD to the actual mean) is required to be 0.2 or less then the confidence interval length will have to be 0.8 times the true mean or less ($0.8 = 0.2 \times 4$)

a confidence interval length that is sufficiently close to our desired value of $0.8 \times$ ICC. The number of observations associated with that curve will be the optimal sample size. If no curve is found matching our desired confidence interval length, one should use the closest value available.

Suppose that you anticipate the ICC to be around 0.6, a value on which the sample size determination will be based. Since $0.8 \times 0.6 = 0.48$, you are then looking for a sample size that will yield a 95% confidence interval length that does not exceed 0.48. Figure 8.3.1 (based on 20 observations) indicates that for ICC=0.6, both curves show a confidence interval length that exceeds 0.7. Consequently, you will need more than 20 observations. In Figure 8.3.2, all curves yield an interval length that exceeds 0.5 for ICC=0.6. In Figure 8.3.3 however, it appears that for ICC=0.6 a few curves yield a confidence interval length close to 0.45. Now we know that we will need approximately 60 measurements overall.

Now that you will need 60 measurements, the question becomes how should you distribute them across subjects and raters? Figure 8.3.3 also shows that using 20 subjects and 3 raters will produce the smallest confidence interval length for $ICC = 0.6$. However, a second viable option would be to use 15 subjects and 4 raters. Figures 8.3.4, 8.3.5, and 8.3.6 indicate that one may obtain much shorter intervals by increasing the number of measurements. In most cases, using approximately 3 or 4 raters is sufficient to minimize the confidence interval length.

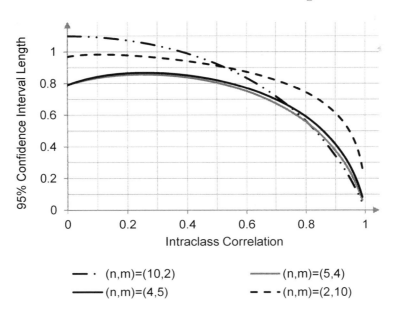

Figure 8.3.1: Expected width of the 95% confidence interval as a function of ICC for $n \times m = 20$ measurements.

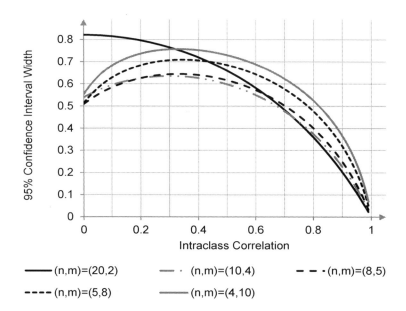

Figure 8.3.2: Expected width of the 95% confidence interval as a function of ICC for $n \times m = 40$ measurements.

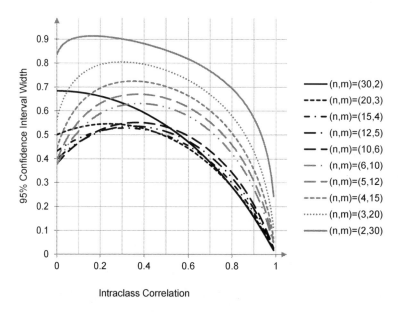

Figure 8.3.3: Expected width of the 95% confidence interval as a function of ICC for $n \times m = 60$ measurements.

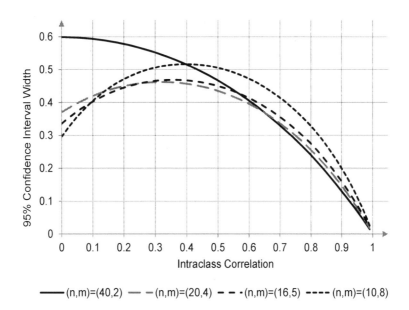

Figure 8.3.4: Expected width of the 95% confidence interval as a function of ICC for $n \times m = 80$ measurements.

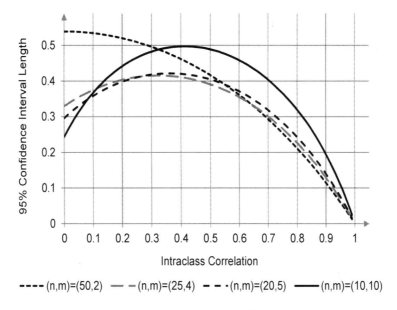

Figure 8.3.5: Expected width of the 95% confidence interval as a function of ICC for $n \times m = 100$ measurements.

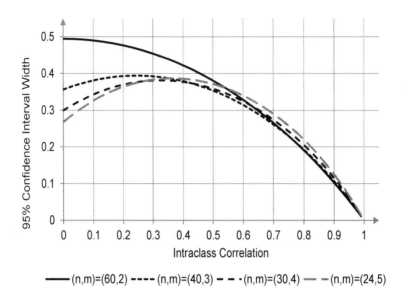

Figure 8.3.6: Expected width of the 95% confidence interval as a function of ICC for $n \times m = 120$ measurements.

Dealing with Unknown ICC

When designing an inter-rater reliability study, some researchers will not have a reasonable starting ICC value to optimize their design on, and may not want to do a pilot study to obtain that value as previously suggested in this section. What I recommend in that situation is to assume that $ICC = 0.5$. This assumption produces a conservative approach likely to require a sample size that exceeds what any other ICC value would lead to. It is the price to be paid for not having any prior knowledge of your rater and subject populations when designing your study.

Finding the optimal number of subjects and raters (or replicates) can be accomplished in a two-step process based on Figures 8.3.7 and 8.3.8. Figure 8.3.7 is used to determine the optimal number of measurements, while Figure 8.3.8 is used to determine the corresponding number of subjects and raters.

Figure 8.3.7 depicts the desired confidence interval length (vertical axis) as a function of the total number of measurements the experiment produces (horizontal axis) when $ICC = 0.5$. You first set your desired confidence interval length, then you use one of the 5 curves to determine the corresponding total number of measurements required to achieved that length. The 5 curves on this chart are associated with different confidence levels. How to determine the desired confidence interval length ? With a hypothesized ICC value of 0.5, I recommend a target confidence interval length that does not exceed 0.4 (obtained according the 0.8-rule of thumb discussed earlier in this section, that recommends an optimal interval length of $0.8 \times ICC = 0.8 \times 0.5$). It follows from Figure 8.3.7 that an interval length of 0.4 requires 40 measurements at the 80% confidence level, or 90 measurements at the 95% confidence level.

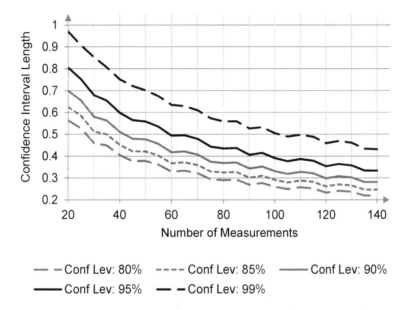

Figure 8.3.7: Expected Confidence Interval Width as Function of the Optimal Number of Measurements when ICC=0.5.

It is very tempting to opt for a lower confidence level such as 80%, which always requires a smaller number of measurements compared to higher confidence levels. However, a design based on lower confidence levels will yield desired narrow confidence intervals that carry a higher risk of not including the "true" ICC (i.e. not telling us a credible story about the real magnitude of the ICC). For all practical purposes, the confidence level should be interpreted as follows: if a study based on an 80% confidence level is conducted 100 times producing 100 confidence intervals, only 80 of them are expected to include the true value of the ICC.

Figure 8.3.8 displays the optimal number of subjects and raters as functions of the total number of measurements obtained from Figure 8.3.7. Once the total number of measurements is obtained from Figure 8.3.7, it is used in Figure 8.3.8 to determine the optimal number of subjects and raters. Note that each value for total number of measurements is associated with a unique pair of number of subjects and raters in Figure 8.3.8, which yields the smallest confidence interval length of Figure 8.3.7.

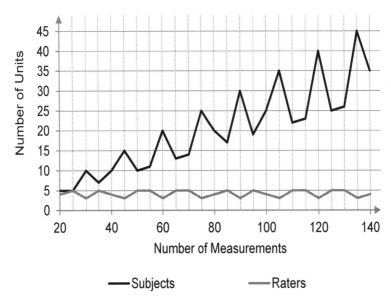

Figure 8.3.8: Optimal Number of Subjects and Raters as Function of the Optimal Number of Measurements

8.3.4   *Confidence Interval for γ under Model 1B*

The "true" ICC (named γ) under model 1B is defined by equation 8.2.2, and its value is calculated from observed ratings using equation 8.2.4. The confidence interval associated with γ (the true ICC) represents all the values between a lower confidence bound (LCB), and an upper confidence bound (UCB) defined in such a way that they will enclose the true ICC value of γ with a probability that matches the predetermined confidence level. The LCB and UCB are defined as follows,

$$\text{LCB} = \frac{F_{\text{L}} - 1}{F_{\text{L}} + (M/r - 1)}, \text{ with } F_{\text{L}} = F_{obs}/C_{\text{L}}, \tag{8.3.5}$$

$$\text{UCB} = \frac{F_{\text{U}} - 1}{F_{\text{U}} + (M/r - 1)}, \text{ with } F_{\text{U}} = F_{obs} \times C_{\text{U}}, \tag{8.3.6}$$

where M is the total number of reported ratings and r the number of raters. Let $\alpha = 1 - \textit{(Confidence Interval)}$, and C_{L}, and C_{U} defined as follows:

- C_{L} is the $100 \cdot (1 - \alpha/2)^{th}$ percentile of the F-distribution with $r - 1$ and $M - r$ degrees of freedom.

- C_{U} is the $100 \cdot (1 - \alpha/2)^{th}$ percentile of the F-distribution with $M - r$ and $r - 1$ degrees of freedom.

To compute these two percentiles using MS EXCEL, proceed as follows:

EXCEL 2007/2008 or older $\text{=FINV}(\alpha/2, r-1, M-r)$, *for* C_{L},

$\text{=FINV}(\alpha/2, M-r, r-1)$, *for* C_{U},

EXCEL 2010/2011 or newer $\text{=F.INV}(1-\alpha/2, r-1, M-r)$, *for* C_{L},

$\text{=F.INV}(1-\alpha/2, M-r, r-1)$, *for* C_{U}.

F_{obs} on the other hand, would be calculated as follows:

$F_{obs} = \text{MSR}/\text{MSE}$, with MSR and MSE being respectively the Mean of Squares for Raters, and the Mean of Squares for Errors.

(a) MSE is a ratio, which is obtained by first summing all squared differences $(y_{ijk}-\overline{y}_{\cdot j\cdot})^2$ from the observations to the rater-level mean, then by dividing that summation by $M-r$ *(this later term is known as the "number of degrees of freedom" associated with the MSE).*

(b) MSR is obtained by dividing the summation of all factors $m_{\cdot j}(\overline{y}_{\cdot j\cdot} - \overline{y})^2$ by $r-1$, with $m_{\cdot j}$ being the number of reported ratings associated with rater j. *Note that $r-1$ is also known as the "number of degrees of freedom" associated with MSR, and $\overline{y}_{\cdot j\cdot}$ is the average of all measurements associated with rater j.*

The following example illustrates the process for calculating the confidence interval associated with model 1B's intraclass correlation coefficient.

Example 8.5 _____

Using Table 8.1 data with model 1B in Example 8.2, we calculated the intraclass correlation coefficient to be $\text{ICC}(1B, 1) = 0.574$. We now want to calculate the associated confidence interval at the 95% confidence level.

The first step is to compute the MSR and the MSE. It follows from Table 8.8 that MSR = 32.4861, which is calculated from the squared differences $(\overline{y}_{\cdot j\cdot} - \overline{y})^2$ as explained above. We first calculated the column marginal averages $\overline{y}_{\cdot j\cdot}$, and the squared differences $(\overline{y}_{\cdot j\cdot} - \overline{y})^2$, before summing them and multiplying the summation by $nm/(r-1)$. Interested readers may want to look at the "Example 8.5" worksheet in the Excel workbook,

www.agreestat.com/book4/chapter8examples.xlsx,

for more details regarding these calculations. Table 8.9, on the other hand shows that MSE = 3.575. This calculation is based on the squared differences $(y_{ijk} - \overline{y}_{\cdot j\cdot})^2$ as explained earlier.

Table 8.8: Calculating the Mean of Squares for Raters (MSR) from Input Data

Subject	Rater (j)				
(i)	1	2	3	4	
1	9	2	5	8	
2	6	1	3	2	
3	8	4	6	8	
4	7	1	2	6	
5	10	5	6	9	
6	6	2	4	7	
$\overline{y}_{\cdot j\cdot}$	7.6667	2.5	4.3333	6.6667	$\overline{y} = 5.2917$
$(\overline{y}_{\cdot j\cdot} - \overline{y})^2$	5.6406	7.7934	0.9184	1.8906	MSR = 32.4861

The confidence level of 95% leads to $\alpha = 1 - 0.95 = 0.05$. Therefore the factors C_{L} and C_{U} of equations 8.3.5 and 8.3.6 represent the 97.5^{th} percentiles (Note that $97.5 = 100 \times (1 - \alpha/2) = 100 \times (1 - 0.05/2)$) of the F distributions with 3 and 20 degrees of freedom for C_{L}, and 20 and 3 degrees of freedom for C_{U}. Note that $3 = r - 1$ and $20 = r(nm - 1)$.

If you are using Excel 2010, 2007 or an earlier version, then you could conveniently calculate C_{L} as =FINV(0.05/2,3,20) to obtain $C_{\mathrm{L}} = 3.8587$. With Excel 2010/2011 or a more recent version, you have an additional option for calculating C_{L} as =F.INV(1-0.05/2,3,20), which yields the same result. Likewise $C_{\mathrm{U}} = 14.16738$, and it is obtained with the Excel 2007 function =FINV(0.05/2,20,3), or with the more recent Excel 2010 function =F.INV(1-0.05/2,20,3).

Table 8.9: Calculating the Mean Square Error (MSE)

Subject	$(y_{ijk} - \overline{y}_{\cdot j\cdot})^2$ factors by rater (j)			
(i)	1	2	3	4
1	1.7778	0.25	0.4444	1.7778
2	2.7778	2.25	1.7778	21.7778
3	0.1111	2.25	2.7778	1.7778
4	0.4444	2.25	5.4444	0.4444
5	5.4444	6.25	2.7778	5.4444
6	2.7778	0.25	0.1111	0.1111
			MSE = 3.575	

Therefore, $F_{obs} = \mathrm{MSR/MSE} = 9.08702$. Furthermore, $F_{\mathrm{L}} = 9.08702/3.85870 = 2.35495$, and $F_{\mathrm{U}} = 9.08702 \times 14.16738 = 128.73934$. The confidence limits are calculated as follows:

$$\mathrm{LCB} = (F_{\mathrm{L}} - 1)/[F_{\mathrm{L}} + (nm - 1)],$$
$$= (2.35495 - 1)/(2.35495 + (6 \times 1 - 1)) = 0.18422.$$

$$\text{UCB} = (F_\text{ι} - 1)/\big[F_\text{ι} + (nm - 1)\big],$$
$$= (31.71537 - 1)/(31.71537 + (6 \times 1 - 1)) = 0.95514.$$

Thus, $(\text{LCB}, \text{UCB}) = (0.184, 0.955)$ is the 95% confidence interval for γ.

8.3.5   *p-Value for γ under Model 1B*

In this section, I assume that the researcher wants to evaluate the extent to which the ratings are consistent with the hypothesis that γ exceeds a predetermined value γ_0 that may represent a standard of acceptability in the profession. Section 8.3.2 describes how the p-value is used to achieve this goal.

Let F_{obs} be defined as follows,

$$F_{obs} = \frac{\text{MSR}}{\text{MSE}\big(1 + M\gamma_0/[r(1 - \gamma_0)]\big)}, \qquad (8.3.7)$$

where MSR and MSE are the mean of squares for raters and the mean of squares for errors respectively. The definitions and calculation procedures related to these means of squares were presented in section 8.3.4. If you replace γ_0 with γ in equation 8.3.7, and you consider the means of squares as abstract statistics, you will obtain a statistic named F that follows the F-distribution with $r - 1$ and $M - r$ degrees of freedom. The p-value is defined as the probability that F exceeds its observed value F_{obs}. That is,

$$p\text{-}Value = P\big(F \geq F_{obs}\big), \qquad (8.3.8)$$

Those familiar with standard statistical packages may use them to compute the probability in equation 8.3.8. For the rest, I advise the use of MS Excel as follows:

$= \text{F.DIST.RT}(F_{obs}, r - 1, M - r)$ *(for Excel 2010/2011 or more recent),*

$= \text{FDIST}(F_{obs}, r - 1, M - r)$ *(for Excel 2007/2008 or earlier version)*

Example 8.6 _____

Using Table 8.1 data, we calculated the ICC under model 1B in Example 8.2 as $ICC(1B, 1) = 0.574$. The associated 95% confidence interval $(0.184, 0.955)$ was obtained in Example 8.5. That is, 0.574 is our best estimation of the magnitude of the intraclass correlation under model 1B. Moreover we can claim with 95% certainty that the true value of the intraclass correlation is between 0.184 and 0.955. This confidence interval is wide, and does not provide very useful information regarding the magnitude of γ. This may be an indication that the number of subjects who participated in the experiment was too small.

In this example we want to know whether the ratings of Table 8.1 are consistent with the research hypothesis that $\gamma > \gamma_0$, using the p-value. Table 8.10 shows the p-value[13] for various levels of γ_0. It appears that the p-value is below the threshold 0.05 for all values γ_0 equal to or smaller than 0.3, and is above 0.05 for γ_0 that exceeds 0.3. Therefore, we may conclude that the true value of the intraclass correlation likely exceeds 0.3.

Table 8.10: p-Value Calculation using Table 8.1 Data

γ_0	F_{obs}	$p\text{-}value$
0.1	6.2910	0.0035
0.2	4.5435	0.0139
0.3	3.3479	0.0396
0.4	2.4783	0.0908
0.5	1.8174	0.1765
0.6	1.2981	0.3025

8.3.6   Sample Size Calculations under Model 1B

Under Model 1B, the subject and error effects are confounded as previously mentioned, and only the rater effect is identifiable. When designing an intra-rater reliability study under this model, you will have to determine the rater and subject sample size requirements, as was done for model 1A. While the rater sample size requirements will be met only by recruiting the prescribed number of raters, the subject sample size requirements could be met by recruiting some subjects and by replicating some measurements on the same subjects.

The method for calculating the required rater and subject sample sizes is almost identical to the one described for model 1A. The only difference is the reverse roles the rater and the subject play under these two models. The required number of subjects under model 1A equals the required number of raters under model 1B. Likewise, the required number of raters/replicates under model 1A equals the required number of subjects/replicates under model 1B. If sample size calculations under model 1B reveal for example that you need 10 subjects, then you may decide to fulfill that requirement by recruiting 5 subjects and taking 2 measurements per subject. How many subjects to recruit will depend on how representative you want your subject sample to be.

---

[13]For more details regarding these calculations, you may look at the "Example 8.6" worksheet in the Excel workbook www.agreestat.com/book4/chapter8examples.xlsx.

How are figures 8.3.1 to 8.3.6 obtained?

All the graphs displayed in figures 8.3.1 to 8.3.6 are obtained through a Monte-Carlo simulation. If ρ is the true value of the ICC, equation 8.3.3 shows that the ratio $F_s = \text{MSS}/\text{MSE}$ can be expressed as $F_s = F \times (1 + rm\rho/(1-\rho))$ where F is a random variable that follows the F-distribution with $n-1$ and $n(rm-1)$ degrees of freedom. To generate each curve of figure 8.3.1 for example, I proceeded as follows:

(1) I started by setting a value to n (the number of subjects) and another value to rm (the product of the number of raters by the number of replicates, which I labeled on the graph as m for simplicity) representing the total number of measurements per subject.

(2) Next, I assigned an ICC value to ρ.

(3) I then generate 100,000 random variates from the F-distribution with $n-1$ and $n(rm-1)$ degrees of freedom. These random variates allowed me to compute 100,000 F_s values as defined above.

(4) The F_s values were used as suggested in equations 8.3.1 and 8.3.2 to derive 100,000 confidence intervals and associated lengths. The average of these 100,000 interval lengths and the hypothesized value ρ produce one point on the curve.

(5) This process is repeated for each of 100 ρ values 0, 0.1, 0.2, until 0.99. For the sake of efficiency, I would generally create the confidence intervals associated with all 100 ρ values for each random variate generated. This allows me to obtain all 100 averages at once, generating thereby the 100 points needed to create the curve.

8.4 Concluding Remarks

In this chapter, I have presented two simple models the researcher can use to design an inter-rater or an intra-rater reliability study. These two models were designated as model 1A and model 1B. Model 1A describes the situation where each subject is rated by a different group of raters[14], while model 1B describes a situation when each rater rates a different group of subjects[15]. We learned that model 1A could be used to investigate both the inter-rater reliability and the intra-rater reliability, unlike model 1B that may be considered only for investigating intra-rater reliability.

Because each subject can be rated by a different group of raters under model 1A, its use presents the following advantages:

---

[14]There may be some overlap between the different groups of raters
[15]There may be some overlap between the different groups of subjects

- The subjects can be located in different places, and be rated by local raters.

- Even if the subjects are all located in the same place, the rating process itself can be spread over the course of a relatively long period of time without having to worry wether the same group of raters will always be available in its entirety. The subjects can always be rated by the group of raters that happens to be available.

However, the use of model 1A has some disadvantages that the researcher should be aware of. Although the measure of inter-rater reliability under model 1A is valid, its estimation using actual ratings will have a potentially high variance if each rater produces very few ratings. That is, under this model you will want to have some overlap between the different groups of raters to give each rater the opportunity to rate multiple subjects. The calculation of the intra-rater reliability coefficient under model 1A requires the use of a single rater. This will make it more sensitive to the particular rater used to generate the ratings.

Because each rater can rate a different group of subjects under model 1B, its use presents the following advantages:

- The raters can be located in different places and will have the opportunity to rate subjects recruited locally.

- Even if the raters are all located in the same place, the rating process itself can be spread over the course of a relatively long period of time without having to worry about the same group of subjects being available to each rater. Some subjects that may be unavailable to one rater can well be replaced with new ones, without the validity of model 1B being affected.

The use of model 1B has some disadvantages that should be mentioned. Evaluating inter-rater reliability under model 1B is an impossible task. It is because, different raters are not required to rate the same subjects making it impossible to assess the extent of agreement among them. As for the intra-rater reliability coefficient, it can be calculated under model 1B although the researcher will need to use a single subject, which will be rated multiple times by each rater. However the single subject being rated could be different for each rater. This will make the intra-rater reliability coefficient very sensitive to the particular subject the ratings are based upon.

If the disadvantages associated with each of the two models presented here are unacceptable to the researcher, then more elaborate models discussed in subsequent chapters must be considered. The new models explored in these chapters will describe more restrictive experimental designs, but will produce more accurate reliability coefficients.

CHAPTER 9

Intraclass Correlations under the Random Factorial Design

OBJECTIVE

The objective of this chapter is to present methods for calculating various intraclass correlation coefficients and associated precision measures, in reliability studies where the rater and subject factors are fully crossed. Each rater is expected to rate all participating subjects, but may take more measurements on some subjects and less on others. The rater and subject samples are both assumed to have been randomly selected from larger rater and subject populations, which represent the primarily interest of the researcher. I define two types of intraclass correlation coefficients: (i) the intraclass correlation coefficient for quantifying inter-rater reliability, and (ii) the intraclass correlation coefficient for quantifying intra-rater reliability. For both types of intraclass correlation, methods for obtaining confidence intervals, p-values, and optimal sample sizes (i.e. required number of subjects and raters during the design of experiments) will be presented as well.

CONTENTS

9.1   The Issues

The Intraclass Correlation Coefficient (ICC) that is associated with Model 1A, is the ratio of the subject variance to the sum of the subject and error variances. What was termed error variance in the previous chapter is in reality the variance of a combination of three effects, which are the rater effect, a possible rater-subject interaction effect[1], and the experimental error effect. Because these three effects are blended together, they are interdependent, and their combined variance is expected to be higher than if the experiment was designed to keep them independent[2]. Therefore, the researcher can improve the magnitude of the ICC substantially by designing the experiment so as to keep all the factors at play independent from one another. This is accomplished by getting each rater to score all subjects. Such a design is known as the factorial design and is the subject of this chapter.

The ICC associated with Model 1B on the other hand, quantifies the intra-rater reliability and was defined in the previous chapter as the ratio of the rater variance to the sum of the rater and error variances. Once again, the error variance in the context of model 1B is actually the variance of the combined effect due to the subject, the rater-subject interaction and the experimental error. The experimental design that underlies model 1B (i.e. each rater scores a different group of subjects) has blended these three effects into one. Consequently, the variance of the combined effect will often be high, reducing thereby the magnitude of the ICC. If an experiment is designed so that the rater, rater-subject interaction, and error effects are independent from one another, then the variance due to their interdependency will be eliminated leading to a higher ICC for the same amount of data collected. This is the factorial design mentioned in the previous paragraph.

There are different types of factorial designs that may achieve different objectives. We will now review some of them.

Types of Factorial Designs

The factorial design, is an experimental design where each rater is expected to rate all subjects participating in the experiment. The main advantage of this design is that all the factors involved in the experiment are kept independent from one another. That is, you can fix a specific rater and study the subject effect; just as you may

---

[1]The rater-subject interaction can be seen as the portion of the rater effect that may be attributed to the specific subject being rated.

[2]Note that if a and b are 2 dependent effects, then their combined variance will be $var(a + b) = var(a) + var(b) + 2cov(a,b)$, where $cov(a,b)$ is the covariance between a and b. If the effects are independent, the covariance term will vanish, the joint variance will decrease (assuming a positive covariance, which is usually the case in agreement studies).

fix a specific subject so as to study the rater effect. If two measurements or more are taken from one subject by the same rater, then one may study the rater-subject interaction effect independently from the experimental error.

Rater-subject interaction is bad for both inter-rater and intra-rater reliability, but is sometimes unavoidable. It induces more variation in the data, in addition to the portion of total variation that is due to raters and subjects. This extra variation will further reduce the magnitude of the ICC. Figure 9.1.1 depicts the reliability data of Table 8.1 of chapter 8. Without interaction, all 4 curves associated with the raters would be reasonably parallel, which is the case for raters 1, 2, and 3. Rater 4 however, appears to assign scores to subjects with a gap with other raters that changes from subject to subject. This is an indication of the existence of rater-subject interaction. Rater 4 alone is likely to bring the ICC down in a significant way.

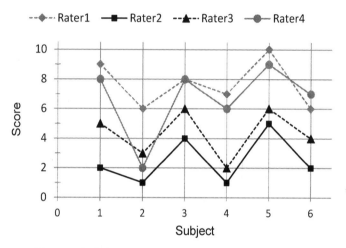

Figure 9.1.1: Ratings of 6 subjects by rater

Two types of factorial designs involving the subject and rater factors are the random and mixed factorial designs. The random factorial design is a design where the rater and the subject effects are random, while the mixed factorial design is one where the rater effect is fixed and the subject effect random.

In the random factorial design, the raters participating in the experiment are selected randomly from a larger universe of raters, and the participating subjects are selected randomly from a larger universe of subjects. The subjects and raters in their respective universes are actually those the researcher wants to investigate in the first place. The samples representing subgroups of these universes are used to minimize the costs of conducting experiments. It is the desire to draw meaningful conclusions about entire universes from their smaller representative samples that creates the need to use statistical methods.

In the mixed factorial design on the other hand, only participating subjects are selected randomly from a larger subject universe. The participating raters are not tied to any other group of raters. They represent themselves, and are the only ones being investigated by the researcher. The study findings will only apply to these raters, and cannot be generalized to raters who did not participate in the experiment. For example, consider a reliability experiment whose purpose is to evaluate the consistency level between two measuring devices used in rheumatology clinical examinations. The researcher in this case, will want the study findings to be limited to the two specific measuring devices being investigated, and not be generalized to other devices that may not be similar to those used in the experiment. Experiments based on mixed factorial designs will often yield a higher ICC than those based on the random factorial designs, because no variation is generated by the rater effect when the design is mixed.

In this chapter, I will focus on the statistical methods used for analyzing experimental data based on the random factorial design. Methods needed for analyzing mixed factorial designs will be discussed in the next chapter.

9.2   The Intraclass Correlation Coefficients

The random factorial design involves a single group of raters as well as a single group of subjects, all of which are rated by each rater. That is the rater and subject factors are fully crossed. Table 9.1 shows lung functions data of 15 children representing their peak expiratory flow rates. Four measurements were taken on each subject by 4 raters. The raters here could represent 4 individuals operating the same measuring device, or one individual using the same measuring device on 4 different occasions. The data produced in these two scenarios can be analyzed with the same methods discussed in this section, although the results may be interpreted differently depending on the context.

Table 9.1 data were generated by a single group of 4 raters, each of whom rated all members of the same group of 15 subjects. We assume that the 4 raters are representative of a larger pool of raters they were selected from. Likewise, the 15 children are assumed to represent the larger population of children of interest they were randomly selected from.

The resulting scores are described mathematically as follows:

$$y_{ijk} = \mu + s_i + r_j + (sr)_{ij} + e_{ijk}, \tag{9.2.1}$$

where y_{ijk} is the score assigned to subject i by rater j on the kth trial[3]. The remaining terms of model 9.2.1 are defined as follows:

---

[3]Many reliability experiments only involves one trial (the first one)

▶ μ is the expected value of the y-score for all subjects and raters.

▶ s_i is the random subject effect, assumed to follow the Normal distribution with 0 mean, and a variance σ_s^2.

▶ r_j is the random rater effect, assumed to follow the Normal distribution with mean 0, and variance σ_r^2.

▶ $(sr)_{ij}$ is the random subject-rater interaction effect, assumed to follow the Normal distribution with mean 0, and variance σ_{sr}^2.

▶ e_{ijk} is the random error effect, assumed to follow the Normal distribution with mean 0, and variance σ_e^2.

▶ The subject, rater, and interaction effects are considered to be mutually independent. That is, the magnitude of one does not affect that of another effect.

Table 9.1: 15 children lung function measurements representing the peak expiratory flow rates (PEFR)[a]

Subject	Rater (j)			
(i)	1	2	3	4
1	190	220	200	200
2	220	200	240	230
3	260	260	240	280
4	210	300	280	265
5	270	265	280	270
6	280	280	270	275
7	260	280	280	300
8	275	275	275	305
9	280	290	300	290
10	320	290	300	290
11	300	300	310	300
12	270	250	330	370
13	320	330	330	330
14	335	320	335	375
15	350	320	340	365

[a]Source: Bland MJ, Altman DG. Statistics Notes: Measurement error. British Medical Journal 1996;312:1654 (extract)

It is essential for researchers to have a good understanding of the practical implications of some of these assumptions. Let us assume that the reliability experiment being analyzed involves n subjects, r raters, and m replicates (or trials). The fact that all rater effects (i.e. the r_j factors for raters $j = 1, \cdots, r$) share the same mean and the same variance σ_r^2 indicates that all these raters have a similar understanding of the rating processes with their differences being random. If one rater systematically assigns high ratings to subjects, while a second rater assigns very low ratings to the same subjects, then the analysis of these ratings with model 9.1 may not be conclusive. This model will make the error term absorb most of the unexplained variation in ratings, which will result in low inter-rater and intra-rater reliability coefficients. Consequently, the ratings being analyzed must come from raters with a common understanding of the rating processes, which can be acquired with basic training.

Model 9.2.1 (also referred to as Model 2 in the inter-rater reliability literature - see Shrout & Fleiss, 1979) stipulates that under the random factorial design, the different effects are additive, independent, and follow the Normal distribution. Unlike model 1A and 1B of the previous chapter, Model 9.2.1 allows for the calculation of both the inter-rater, and intra-rater reliability coefficients. I will review each of these coefficients in the next few sub-sections.

9.2.1   *Inter-Rater Reliability Coefficient*

An inter-rater reliability based on model 9.2.1 is by definition the correlation coefficient between the scores y_{ijk} and $y_{ij'k}$ associated with two raters j and j', the same subject i, and the same trial number k. It follows from equation 9.2.1 that the inter-rater reliability (denoted by ρ) is defined[4] as,

$$\rho = \frac{\sigma_s^2}{\sigma_s^2 + \sigma_r^2 + \sigma_{sr}^2 + \sigma_e^2} \tag{9.2.2}$$

The question to be asked at this stage is whether equation 9.2.2 actually measures the extent of agreement among the r raters that participated in the experiment. A carefully examination of expression 9.2.2 suggests that ρ varies from 0 to 1, and takes a high value closer to 1 only when the subject variance σ_s^2 exceeds the combined variance $\sigma_r^2 + \sigma_{sr}^2 + \sigma_e^2$ by a wide margin. This will happen when the sum $\sigma_r^2 + \sigma_{sr}^2 + \sigma_e^2$ is small, which in turn indicates that the rater variance σ_r^2 is small. And a small rater variance σ_r^2 is a clear indication of high agreement among raters.

If a large value of ρ is a strong indication of good inter-rater agreement, can we say that a good inter-rater agreement will also result in a high value for ρ? The answer is unfortunately *"not necessarily."* In reality, a good inter-rater agreement will result in a high value for ρ only if the experiment is sufficiently well designed so

---

[4]Note that $\rho = \mathsf{Corr}(y_{ijk}, y_{ij'k}) = \mathsf{Cov}(y_{ijk}, y_{ij'k}) / \left[\sqrt{\mathsf{Var}(y_{ijk})} \sqrt{\mathsf{Var}(y_{ij'k})} \right]$

as to keep the experimental error to the minimum. Again, it follows from equation 9.2.2 that a large error variance σ_e^2 will bring the whole ICC expression down even if the rater variance is small. Consequently,

> *if the ICC yields a high value, you can be certain that the extent of agreement among raters is good. However, if the ICC value is low, it is not necessarily an indication of poor agreement. It could be an indication of a poorly-designed experiment, and you may need to conduct additional analyzes.*

The experimental error may become unduly large, if your experiment is conducted in such a way that there are many uncontrolled factors that affect the magnitude of the scores other than the subject and the rater. These uncontrolled factors could be the location of the subject, major changes in experimental conditions such as the temperature, the measuring equipment or others. If the primary study objective is to obtain the ICC then the experimenter will want to design the experiment so that the subject and the rater are the most influential factors on the score magnitude. Adding more factors (controlled or uncontrolled) will negatively affect the ICC.

Calculating Inter-Rater Reliability

To compute the intraclass correlation coefficient from actual data, I again propose, a method that can handle missing scores, and which is an adaptation of what Searle (1997, page 474) has recommended. This method is more general than that proposed by Shrout & Fleiss (1979), which cannot handle missing values. But both approaches match perfectly well when the data do not contain missing values.

The ICC of equation 9.2.2 is estimated from raw experimental data by calculating the 4 variance components σ_s^2, σ_r^2, σ_{rs}^2, and σ_e^2. The calculated subject, rater, rater-subject interaction, and error variances are respectively denoted by $\widehat{\sigma}_s^2$, $\widehat{\sigma}_r^2$, $\widehat{\sigma}_{rs}^2$, and $\widehat{\sigma}_e^2$. The calculated intraclass correlation coefficient is denoted by ICC(2,1)[5] and given by:

$$\text{ICC}(2,1) = \frac{\widehat{\sigma}_s^2}{\widehat{\sigma}_s^2 + \widehat{\sigma}_r^2 + \widehat{\sigma}_{rs}^2 + \widehat{\sigma}_e^2}. \tag{9.2.3}$$

When there is no missing ratings, these variance components are conveniently calculated using a number of means of squares as shown in Shrout & Fleiss (1979), or McGraw & Wong (1996). The Shrout-Fleiss and McGraw-Wong procedures are discussed later in this section. The computation procedures presented here are less

---

[5]The notation ICC(2,1) is widely used in the inter-rater reliability literature. ICC stands for Intraclass Correlation Coefficient, while "2" refers to model 2, and "1" indicates that each rating represents a single raw measurement, and not an average of several measurements.

straightforward since they must account for missing values. The variance components are calculated as follows:

$$\widehat{\sigma}_e^2 = (T_{2y} - T_{2sr})/(M - \lambda_0), \tag{9.2.4}$$

$$\widehat{\sigma}_{sr}^2 = \Big[(M - k_1')\delta_r + (k_3 - k_2')\delta_s$$
$$- \Big(T_{2s} - T_y'^2 - (n-1)\widehat{\sigma}_e^2\Big)\Big]\Big/(M - k_1' - k_2' + k_5'), \tag{9.2.5}$$

$$\widehat{\sigma}_r^2 = \delta_s - \widehat{\sigma}_{sr}^2, \tag{9.2.6}$$

$$\widehat{\sigma}_s^2 = \delta_r - \widehat{\sigma}_{sr}^2, \tag{9.2.7}$$

where,

- T_{2y} is the summation of all squared values y_{ijk}^2.

- T_{2sr} is the summation of all factors $y_{ij.}^2/m_{ij}$, with $y_{ij.}$ being the total score value over all replicates associated with subject i and rater j, and m_{ij} the number of measurements taken on subject i by rater j.

- M is the total number of measurements produced by the experiment, while λ_0 is the number subject-rater combinations for which one measurement or more were produced (i.e. the number of (i, j)-cells for which $m_{ij} \geq 1$).

- $k_1' = k_1/M$, where k_1 is the summation of all $m_{i.}^2$ with $m_{i.}$ being the number of measurements taken on subject i.

- $\delta_r = \big[T_{2sr} - T_{2r} - (\lambda_0 - r)\widehat{\sigma}_e^2\big]/(M - k_4)$, where T_{2r} is obtained by summing all the terms $y_{.j.}^2/m_{.j}$, with $y_{.j.}$ being the total score value associated with rater j. Moreover k_4 is calculated by summing all the terms $m_{ij}^2/m_{.j}$, with $m_{.j}$ being the number of measurements taken by rater j on all subjects.

- $\delta_s = \big[T_{2sr} - T_{2s} - (\lambda_0 - n)\widehat{\sigma}_e^2\big]/(M - k_3)$, where T_{2s} is obtained by summing all the terms $y_{i..}^2/m_{i.}$, with $y_{i..}$ being the total score value associated with subject i. Moreover, k_3 is calculated by summing all the terms $m_{ij}^2/m_{i..}$.

- $k_2' = k_2/M$, where k_2 is calculated by summing the terms $m_{.j}^2$ over all raters.

- $T_y'^2 = T_y^2/M$, where T_y is the summation of all scores y_{ijk}, and $k_5' = k_5/M$ with k_5 calculated by summing the terms m_{ij}^2.

The calculation of the inter-rater reliability is described here for the factorial model with interaction effect. Such a model requires repeated measurements to be taken on the same subject. This is not always feasible, particularly if taking one measurement is very demanding on subjects. In this case, the researcher may prefer the use of a simpler model based on a single rating per subject and per rater, and in which the error and interaction effects are blended together. The calculation of the inter-rater reliability coefficient under this simpler model is discussed in section 9.5.1.

The following example illustrates how the intraclass correlation coefficient ICC(2,1) is calculated under model 9.2.1 data.

Example 9.1 _____

For the purpose of this example, I have made two modifications to Table 9.1 to obtain Table 9.2 that will be analyzed. First, the number of children is reduced to 8, and two or three measurements were taken on some of the children. Second, the number of ratings per subject may vary from one rater to another creating some missing ratings as shown in Table 9.2.

Table 9.2: Eight children lung function measurements representing the peak expiratory flow rates (PEFR)

| Subject | Rater (j) | | | | | Standard | Mean |
(i)	1	2	3	4	Mean Score	Deviation	Difference
1	190	220	200	200			
1	220	200	240	230	212.50	17.53	6.67
2	260	260	240	280			
2	210	300	280	265	261.88	27.51	15.42
3	270	265	280	270			
3	280	280	270	275			
3	260		280	300	275.45	10.60	6.53
4	275	275	275		275.00	0.00	0.00
5	280	290	300	290			
5	320	290	300	290	295.00	11.95	-3.33
6	300	300	310	300			
6	270	250	330	370	303.75	36.23	32.50
7	320	330	330	330			
7		320	335	375	334.29	18.80	17.50
8	350	320	340	365	343.75	18.87	10.83

Table 9.2 also contains some subject-level statistics such as the subject mean score, the subject standard deviation, and the the mean score difference[6] Figure 9.2.1 shows the graph of the subject mean score difference (c.f. column 8 of Table 9.2) against the subject mean score (c.f. column 6 of Table 9.2), and provides a visual assessment of the extent of agreement among the four raters. This graph can be seen as a version of what is known in the literature as the Bland-Altman plot (see Bland & Altman

_____

[6]The mean score difference is calculated separately for each subject by averaging all six pairwise differences associated with the six pairs of raters that can be formed out of the group of four raters. The way the two raters in a given pair are ordered when taking the difference is irrelevant. But the ordering adopted must remain the same for all subjects.

(1986)). It follows from this graph that the 4 raters agree reasonably well with a possible exception of an outlier associated with a mean score of 303.75 and a mean score difference of 32.5.

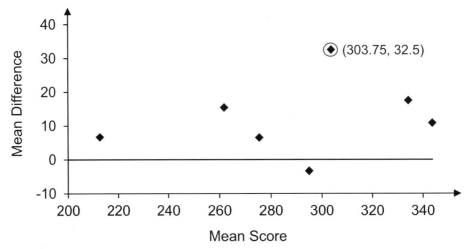

Figure 9.2.1: Agreement plot showing the mean score difference against the mean score based on Table 9.9 data.

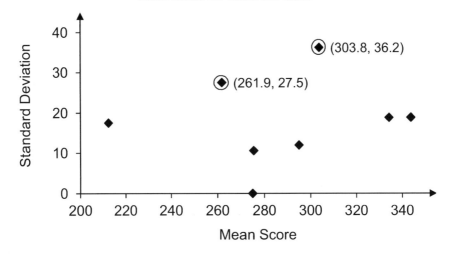

Figure 9.2.2: Repeatability plot showing the standard deviation against the mean score based on Table 9.9 data

Figure 9.2.2 on the other hand, depicts the subject standard deviation[7] as a function of their overall mean score. It offers another look at the rater agreement as the score magnitude changes, and is know in the literature as the repeatability plot. (See Bland & Altman - 1996 -). This plot is often used for repeated measures, and can identify more outliers that the first plot would not. Both figures 9.2 and 9.3 tell about the same

---

[7]This standard deviation is that of all scores associated with one subject.

story showing an overall good agreement with the exception of 1 or 2 outliers.

The intraclass correlation coefficient ICC(2,1) of equation 9.2.3 is given by,

$$\mathrm{ICC}(2,1) = \frac{1,627.395}{1,627.395 + 82.507 + 0 + 460.897},$$
$$= 0.7497,$$

where $\widehat{\sigma}_s = 1,627.395$, $\widehat{\sigma}_r = 82.507$, and $\widehat{\sigma}_e = 460.897$. As for the interaction variance component $\widehat{\sigma}_{rt}$, it was initially estimated to be a negative value -97.55, which was later replaced by 0 since the variance cannot be negative. The negative value obtained here is likely due to insufficient data for an accurate estimation of the interaction effect.

To see the details of these calculations, interested readers may look at the "Example 9.1" worksheet in the Excel spreadsheet,

<code>www.agreestat.com/book4/chapter9examples.xlsx</code>,

which shows the step-by-step calculations of ICC(2,1) for this example, from the input data of Table 9.2 to the final result of 0.7497.

Some Simplifications with Complete Rating Data

When your rating data is complete, that is the measurements expected from all raters have been recorded, then the intraclass correlation ICC(2, 1) of equation 9.3 can take its usual and better known form given by,

$$\mathrm{ICC}(2,1) = \frac{\mathrm{MSS} - \mathrm{MSI}}{\mathrm{MSS} + r(\mathrm{MSR} - \mathrm{MSI})/n + (r-1)\mathrm{MSI} + r(m-1)\mathrm{MSE}}, \qquad (9.2.8)$$

where MSS, MSR, MSI, and MSE are defined as follows:

▶ MSS is the mean of squares for subjects, which is calculated by summing the squared differences $(\overline{y}_{i..} - \overline{y})^2$, and by multiplying the summation by $rm/(n-1)$. Note that $\overline{y}_{i..}$ is the average of all ratings associated with subject i, while $\overline{y}$ is the overall average.

▶ MSR is the mean of squares for raters, calculated by summing the squared differences $(\overline{y}_{.j.} - \overline{y})^2$, and by multiplying the summation by $nm/(r-1)$. The term $\overline{y}_{.j.}$ represents the average of all ratings associated with rater j.

▶ MSI is the mean of squares for the rater-subject interaction, calculated by summing the squared differences $(\overline{y}_{ij.} - \overline{y}_{i..} - \overline{y}_{.j.} + \overline{y})^2$, and by multiplying the summation by $m/[(r-1)(n-1)]$. The term $\overline{y}_{ij.}$ represents the average of all ratings associated with subject i and rater j.

▶ MSE is the mean of squares for errors, calculated by summing the squared differences $(y_{ijk} - \overline{y}_{ij.})^2$ and by dividing the summation by $rn(m-1)$.

If your data is based on a single replication experimental design (i.e. only one measurement is taken on each subject), then the variances due to the error and the rater-subject interaction can no longer be calculated separately. In this case, only MSI must be calculated as described above, and be renamed as MSE. Equation 9.2.8 will then become,

$$\text{ICC}(2,1) = \frac{\text{MSS} - \text{MSE}}{\text{MSS} + r(\text{MSR} - \text{MSE})/n + (r-1)\text{MSE}}. \tag{9.2.9}$$

9.2.2   Intra-Rater Reliability Coefficient

The factorial design can be used for studying both the inter-rater and the intra-rater reliability. As previously discussed, intra-rater reliability is a measure of self-consistency for the raters. It represents the raters' ability to reproduce the same measurements on similar subjects. Therefore the intra-rater reliability study aims at investigating the reproducibility of the measurements. This task can be performed only if the same raters produce two ratings or more for the same subjects. That is, the notion of replication involving repeated trials plays a pivotal role in the study of intra-rater reliability.

The intra-rater reliability based on model 9.2.1, is by definition the correlation coefficient between the scores y_{ijk} and $y_{ijk'}$ associated with the two trials k and k', associated with the same subject i, and the same rater j. It follows from equation 9.2.1 that the intra-rater reliability (denoted by γ) is defined[8] as,

$$\gamma = \frac{\sigma_r^2 + \sigma_s^2 + \sigma_{sr}^2}{\sigma_r^2 + \sigma_s^2 + \sigma_{sr}^2 + \sigma_e^2}. \tag{9.2.10}$$

Does equation 9.2.10 actually measure raters' self-consistency? To answer this question, you should first note that γ would normally vary from 0 to 1, where 0 indicates no intra-rater reliability, and 1 a perfect intra-rater reliability. A high value for γ is an indication that the variance due to the error factor (σ_e^2) is relatively small compared to the total variance due to the rater, subject, and subject-rater interaction effects. Since the error variance is due to the combined effect of replication and experimental error, we can conclude that the variability due to replication is necessarily small. Therefore the ratings are highly reproducible. If γ is small (i.e. close to 0) then we can conclude that the combined effect of replication and experimental error is large. This may be due to a large variation in the repeated measurements (i.e.

---

[8]Note that $\gamma = \text{Corr}(y_{ijk}, y_{ijk'}) = \text{Cov}(y_{ijk}, y_{ijk'})/\left[\sqrt{\text{Var}(y_{ijk})}\sqrt{\text{Var}(y_{ijk'})}\right]$. The assumption of independence of the factors can be used here to obtain equation 9.11

poor reproducibility) or a large experimental error or both. We don't know. What we know is that the experiment aimed at demonstrating high reproducibility was inconclusive.

Calculating Intra-Rater Reliability

To compute the intraclass correlation coefficient of equation 9.2.10 from actual data, I propose once again a method that can handle missing values adapted from Searle (1997, page 474). The method proposed by Shrout & Fleiss (1979), and which is based on several means of squares, cannot handle missing values. This special approach for balanced data, and the general approach for unbalanced data yield the same ICC when the data is balanced. For illustration purposes only, I will first present the special approach for balanced data.

SPECIAL METHOD FOR BALANCED DATA

If your data is balanced then the intra-rater reliability coefficient can be calculated as follows:

$$\text{ICC}_a(2,1) = \frac{r\text{MSR} + n\text{MSS} + (rn - r - n)\text{MSI} - rn\text{MSE}}{r\text{MSR} + n\text{MSS} + (rn - r - n)\text{MSI} + rn(m-1)\text{MSE}}, \qquad (9.2.11)$$

where r is the number of raters, n the number of subjects, m the number of trials (or replicates), MSR the mean of squares for raters, MSS the mean of squares for subjects, MSI the mean of squares for the subject-rater interaction, and MSE the mean of squares for errors. These different means of squares are calculated as shown in section 9.2.1.

There is no need to know what this expression would be if there is only one measurement per rater and per subject. It is because the purpose of this section is to quantify reproducibility, which can be accomplished only in the context of replication involving two trials or more per subject.

GENERAL METHOD FOR UNBALANCED DATA

The ICC of equation 9.11 is calculated from raw experimental data by replacing the 4 variance components σ_s^2, σ_r^2, σ_{sr}^2, and σ_e^2 with their calculated values. The calculated subject, rater, interaction and error variances are respectively denoted by $\widehat{\sigma}_s^2$, $\widehat{\sigma}_r^2$, $\widehat{\sigma}_{sr}^2$ and $\widehat{\sigma}_e^2$. Therefore the calculated intraclass correlation coefficient for intra-rater reliability assessment is given by,

$$\text{ICC}_a(2,1) = \frac{\widehat{\sigma}_r^2 + \widehat{\sigma}_s^2 + \widehat{\sigma}_{sr}^2}{\widehat{\sigma}_r^2 + \widehat{\sigma}_s^2 + \widehat{\sigma}_{sr}^2 + \widehat{\sigma}_e^2}, \qquad (9.2.12)$$

where the variance components are calculated as shown in equations 9.2.4, 9.2.5, 9.2.6, and 9.2.7. Using Table 9.2 data and the variance components calculated in example 9.1, you can calculate the intra-rater reliability as,

$$\text{ICC}_a(2,1) = \frac{1,627.395 + 82.507 + 0}{1,627.395 + 82.507 + 460.897}, \tag{9.2.13}$$

$$= 0.788.$$

It appears that the intra-rater reliability is reasonably high in this case. This is due to the fact that the error variance is small compared to the other variance components.

9.3   Statistical Inference About the ICC

The primary objective of this section is the present methods that allow you to quantify the precision of the intraclass correlation coefficient calculated with equations 9.2.3, and 9.2.12. You will be able to make a statement regarding the magnitude of the true[9] intraclass correlation coefficient using your experimental data. The process used to accomplish this task is known as statistical inference. The two inferential approaches I will discuss are the confidence interval and the p-value. As mentioned in the previous chapter, the confidence interval represents the range of values expected to contain the true ICC with a pre-specified (high) probability called the *Confidence Level*. The p-value on the other hand, measures the extent to which the data supports a conjecture about the magnitude of the ICC.

The methods discussed in this section make use of various means of squares since they were developed within the classical framework of the analysis of variance for balanced data. However, these methods are adapted here to accommodate the missing ratings. Their statistical properties stated here will be satisfied if the number of missing ratings remains reasonably small.

9.3.1   *Statistical Inference about ρ*

In this section, we want to know how well ICC(2,1) approximates the theoretical inter-rater reliability ρ of equation 9.2.2. This task is accomplished by presenting two precision measures: the confidence interval, and the p-value. The confidence interval provides a range of values that expected to include the true value ρ with a high confidence level. The p-value on the other hand quantifies the likelihood that the true value of ρ exceeds a predetermined hypothetical value that the researcher is interested in.

---

[9]Recall that equations 9.2.3, or 9.2.12 can only give you an approximated value for the intraclass correlation based on the specific experimental data you have collected. The "true" ICC would require far more information about the entire population of subjects, than you can possibly collect.

The Confidence Interval

Let ρ be the inter-rater reliability of interest as defined by equation 9.2.2. I assume the objective to be the construction of a confidence interval around ρ at a specified confidence level (e.g. 90%, 95% or 99%). Let $\alpha = 1 - $ *(Confidence Level)*. The confidence interval represents all values between a lower confidence bound (LCB) and an upper confidence bound (UCB), defined as follows:

$$\text{LCB} = \frac{n(\text{MSS} - F_1 \cdot \text{MSI})}{n\text{MSS} + F_1 \left[r\text{MSR} + (rn - r - n)\text{MSI} + (M - rn)\text{MSE} \right]}, \tag{9.3.1}$$

$$\text{UCB} = \frac{n(F_2 \cdot \text{MSS} - \text{MSI})}{nF_2 \cdot \text{MSS} + r\text{MSR} + (rn - r - n)\text{MSI} + (M - rn)\text{MSE}}. \tag{9.3.2}$$

These two confidence bounds involves many terms that I will now define.

- MSS is the Mean of Squares for Subjects, and is calculated by summing the squared differences $m_{i\cdot}(\overline{y}_{i\cdot\cdot} - \overline{y})^2$ over all n subjects, and by dividing the summation by $(n - 1)$. The quantities $\overline{y}_{i\cdot\cdot}$ and $\overline{y}$ represent respectively the average of all non-missing ratings associated with subject i, and the average of all non-missing ratings.

- MSR is the Mean of Squares for Raters, and is calculated by summing $m_{\cdot j}(\overline{y}_{\cdot j\cdot} - \overline{y})^2$ over all r subjects, and dividing this summation by $(r - 1)$. Note that $\overline{y}_{\cdot j\cdot}$ represents the average of all non-missing ratings associated with rater j.

- MSI is the Mean of Squares for Interaction (i.e. the subject-rater interaction), and is calculated by summing $m_{ij}(\overline{y}_{ij\cdot} - \overline{y}_{i\cdot\cdot} - \overline{y}_{\cdot j\cdot} + \overline{y})^2$ over all n subjects, and r raters, with the summation being divided by $(r - 1)(n - 1)$. The average $\overline{y}_{ij\cdot}$ is that of all scores associated with subject i and rater j.

- MSE is the Mean of Squares for Errors, and is calculated by summing $(y_{ijk} - \overline{y}_{ij\cdot})^2$ over all rater, subjects, and replicates, and by dividing the summation by $(M - rn)$. This quantity will be 0 for single-trial experiments.

Any average associated with an empty cell should be set to 0. That is, if rater j does not rate subject i then the average $\overline{y}_{ij\cdot}$ will be 0. In addition to calculating the means of squares, you will need to calculate the two factors F_1 and F_2, which depend on the F probability distribution. Let a, b, and c be defined as follows:

$$a = \frac{r\rho}{n(1 - \rho)}, \quad b = 1 + \frac{r(n - 1)}{n}\frac{\rho}{1 - \rho}, \quad c = (M/n - r)\frac{\rho}{1 - \rho}, \tag{9.3.3}$$

and v given by,

$$v = \frac{(a\text{MSR} + b\text{MSI} + c\text{MSE})^2}{\dfrac{(a\text{MSR})^2}{r-1} + \dfrac{(b\text{MSI})^2}{(r-1)(n-1)} + \dfrac{(c\text{MSE})^2}{M - rn}} \tag{9.3.4}$$

The two factors F_1 and F_2, are defined as follows:

▶ F_1 is the $100(1-\alpha/2)^{th}$ percentile of the F distribution with $n-1$ and v degrees of freedom.

▶ F_2 is the $100(1-\alpha/2)^{th}$ percentile of the F distribution with v and $n-1$ degrees of freedom.

Researchers familiar with anyone of the major statistical packages (e.g. SAS, SPSS, STATA, and others) can calculate F_1 and F_2 using them. For those not familiar with any major statistical software, the most convenient way to obtain these factors is to use Excel. For example with Windows Excel 2010 or Mac Excel 2011, you can obtain these two factors as follows (assume that the confidence level is 95%, which implies that $\alpha = 1 - 0.95 = 0.05$):

$$= \text{F.INV}(1 - 0.05/2, n - 1, v) \quad \textit{(for } F_1\textit{)},$$

$$= \text{F.INV}(1 - 0.05/2, v, n - 1) \quad \textit{(for } F_2\textit{)},$$

v being a term that you will need to compute first using equation 9.3.3. Note that the function F.INV was introduced with Excel 2010 for Windows and Excel 2011 for Mac. If you are using an earlier version of Excel (e.g. Excel 2007/2008 or an older version)[10], then you will need to use the function FINV as follows:

$$= \text{FINV}(0.05/2, n - 1, v) \quad \textit{(for } F_1\textit{)},$$

$$= \text{FINV}(0.05/2, v, n - 1) \quad \textit{(for } F_2\textit{)}.$$

For readers who may want to understand the statistical theory underlying the confidence interval construction, I suggest to consider the statistic F defined as,

$$F = \frac{\text{MSS}}{a\text{MSR} + b\text{MSI} + c\text{MSE}}. \tag{9.3.5}$$

This statistic follows the F distribution with the degrees of freedom $n - 1$ and v, where v is given by equation 9.3.4. This result follows from the fact that $E(\text{MSS}) = aE(\text{MSR}) + bE(\text{MSI}) + cE(\text{MSE})$ and from Satterthwaite's approximation to the Chi-square distribution (see Satterthwaite (1946)). The F distribution may be derived from this Chi-square distribution, according to some standard results in mathematical statistics that are beyond the scope of this book.

---

[10] The notation "Excel 2007/2008" refers to Windows Excel 2010 or Mac Excel 2008, and is used throughout this book for simplicity sake.

> *If your experiment is based on a one-replicate factorial de-*
> *sign (i.e. a single measurement is taken on each subject*
> *($m = 1$)), then in equations 9.3.3, and 9.3.4, you will have*
> *$c = 0$ and $MSE = 0$.*

Example 9.2 _____

Let us consider once again, the reliability data of Table 9.2 (previously analyzed in example 9.1), where 4 raters scored 8 subjects participating in a multiple-trial reliability experiment. The inter-rater reliability calculated in example 9.1 is $ICC(2,1) = 0.7497$. The purpose of this example is to illustrate the construction of a 95% confidence interval for the "true" and unknown intraclass correlation ρ.

◊ The first step is to compute the means of squares MSS, MSR, MSI, and MSE. The three means of squares we are interested in are given by,

$$MSE = 479.33, \ MSS = 11,701.52, \ MSI = 319.17341, \text{ and } MSR = 1523.306.$$

If you want to see all the steps involved in the computation of these means of squares, you may download the Excel spreadsheet,

www.agreestat.com/book4/chapter9examples.xlsx

and look at the "Example 9.2" worksheet where all three means of squares are highlighted in yellow.

◊ The second step consists of computing a, b, c, and v of equations 9.3.3, and 9.3.4. Again, it follows from the calculations shown in the Excel workbook chapter9examples.xlsx, that $a = 1.49741$, $b = 11.48185$, $c = 9.358798$, and v given by,

$$v = \frac{(1.497 \times 11,701.52 + 11.481 \times 319.173 + 9.359 \times 479.333)^2}{\dfrac{(1.497 \times 11,701.52)^2}{4-1} + \dfrac{(11.481 \times 319.173)^2}{(4-1)(8-1)} + \dfrac{(9.359 \times 479.333)^2}{57 - 8 \times 4}} = 34.233.$$

◊ To calculate the F_1 and F_2 quantities of equations 9.3.1 and 9.3.2, I used the F.INV function available in Excel 2010/2011 as follows (the highlighted part is what goes into Excel):

$$F_1 = 2.688 \quad \boxed{\text{=F.INV(1-(1-0.95)/2,8-1,34.233)}}$$

$$F_2 = 4.337 \quad \boxed{\text{=F.INV(1-(1-0.95)/2,34.233,8-1)}} .$$

◊ Finally, the lower and upper confidence bounds can be calculated using equations 9.3.1, and 9.3.2. Therefore, LCB = 0.5444, and UCB = 0.937, which represent the boundaries of the 95% confidence interval associated with ρ.

Hypothesis Testing: The p-Value

After estimating the intraclass correlation ρ using the expression ICC$(2,1)$ of equation 9.2.3, it is common practice among researchers to want to evaluate the p-value associated with the estimate obtained. Let us assume you have a reference value ρ_0 to which you like to compare the "true" and unknown value of ρ that you are interested in. The question you like to answer is whether ρ exceeds ρ_0. Since you do not have the actual value of ρ, such a comparison will be based on ratings produced by a random sample of subjects, and must be probabilistic. That is, we need to evaluate the likelihood that the observed ratings are consistent with the hypothesis we are interested in. The use of a probabilistic approach comes with a price, which is the error risk that the answer to your research question will carry. The p-value is a probability value that measures the extent to which observed ratings support the claim that ρ exceeds ρ_0.

To compute the p-value, proceed as follows:

(a) Compute all means of squares, MSS, MSR, MSI, and MSE as described in the beginning of section 9.3.1. As mentioned earlier, if there is a single measurement taken per subject (i.e. $m = 1$) then error and interaction effects are blended together, and MSI (renamed as MSE) will represent the mean of squares of the common effect.

(b) Compute the values a, b, and c of equation 9.3.3 using ρ_0 in place of ρ.

(c) Compute the number of degrees of freedom v as shown in equation 9.3.4, using the means of squares of step (a) and the factors a, b, and c of step (b).

(d) Compute F_{obs} using equation 9.3.5 (developed for F), using the terms obtained in previous steps.

(e) The p-value is then defined as the probability that a random variable F that follows the F-distribution with $n - 1$ and v degrees of freedom, exceeds F_{obs}. That is,

$$p\text{-}Value = P\left(F \geq F_{obs}\right). \tag{9.3.6}$$

If the p-value is very small (e.g. below 0.05) then F_{obs}, which is based on ρ_0 can be considered to be much larger than what you would normally expect from the F distribution based on the true value ρ. Therefore, one can conclude that $\rho > \rho_0$ since F of equation 9.3.3 is a decreasing function of ρ.

The p-value can be computed using Excel as follows:

$=$ F.DIST.RT$(F_{obs}, n - 1, v)$ *(for Excel 2010/2011 or a more recent version),*

$=$ FDIST$(F_{obs}, n - 1, v)$ *(for Excel 2007/2008 or an earlier version).*

Example 9.3 ───

In Example 9.1, we calculated the intraclass correlation associated with inter-rater reliability, and obtained $ICC(2,1) = 0.7497$. Based on the observed ratings, this number is our best guess of what the value of ρ is. We next used the same data (Table 9.2) in Example 9.2 to construct the 95% confidence interval $(0.5444, 0.937)$, which we claim contains the true value of ρ with 95% certainty.

Suppose that we now want to test the hypothesis that the true ICC ρ exceeds a reference value 0.65 (i.e. $\rho_0 = 0.65$)[11]. To this end, we will compute the p-value associated with our calculated ICC of 0.7497, and with respect to our hypothesized value $\rho_0 = 0.65$. The first thing to do is compute F_{obs} based on equation 9.3.5, where ρ is replaced with ρ_0. We must re-compute the coefficients a, b and c as follows:

$$a = \frac{4 \times 0.65}{8 \times (1 - 0.65)} = 0.9286, \; b = 1 + \frac{4(8-1) \times 0.65}{8(1-0.65)} = 7.5,$$
$$c = (57/8 - 4) \times 0.65/(1 - 0.65) = 5.8036.$$

Therefore,

$$F_{obs} = \frac{11,701.52}{0.9286 \times 1,523.31 + 7.5 \times 319.1734 + 5.8036 \times 479.3333} = 1.7756.$$

Before we are able to compute the p-value itself, we need to compute v according to equation 9.3.4. v represents the second number of degrees of freedom associated with the F distribution used in the calculation of the p-value.

$$v = \frac{(0.9286 \times 1,523.31 + 7.5 \times 319.1734 + 5.8036 \times 479.3333)^2}{\dfrac{(0.9286 \times 1,523.31)^2}{4-1} + \dfrac{(7.5 \times 319.1734)^2}{(4-1)(8-1)} + \dfrac{(5.8036 \times 479.3333)^2}{57 - 4 \times 8}} = 34.762.$$

The p-value represents the probability that the F distribution with 7 *(i.e. 8-1)* and 34.762 degrees of freedom, exceeds F_{obs}. Using Excel as described above, we obtained p-value $= 0.1246$ (the Excel formula =FDIST(1.7756,8-1,34.762) was used). This p-value is unduly high. Therefore the rating data this analysis is based upon does not support the hypothesis that the "true" value of ρ exceeds 0.65. The widely-accepted rule of thumb is for the p-value to be below 0.05 before considering the data to be consistent with you conjecture.

Table 9.3 shows the p-value as a function of ρ_0, and provides the quantities a, b, c, v, and F_{obs} used in the calculations. If you want to see all the steps involved in the p-value calculation, you may download the Excel spreadsheet,

www.agreestat.com/book4/chapter9examples.xlsx

and look at the "Example 9.3" worksheet.

─────────────────────────────────

[11]Sometimes this problem is formulated as one about testing the research hypothesis $H_1 : \rho > \rho_0$. A more detailed account of statistical hypothesis testing procedures is provided in Gwet (2010*b*)

Table 9.3: Calculation of p-values for different values of ρ_0

ρ_0	a	b	c	F_{obs}	v	p-Value
0.5	0.5	4.5	3.1250	3.1661	35.8178	0.0106
0.55	0.6111	5.2778	3.8194	2.6318	35.4243	0.027
0.6	0.75	6.25	4.6875	2.1733	35.0742	0.061
0.65	0.9286	7.5	5.8036	1.7756	34.7620	0.1246
0.7	1.1667	9.1667	7.2917	1.4273	34.4825	0.2267
0.75	1.5	11.5	9.375	1.1198	34.2313	0.3737
0.8	2.0	15.0	12.5	0.8463	34.0047	0.5575
0.85	2.8333	20.8333	17.7083	0.6015	33.7993	0.7501
0.9	4.5	32.5	28.125	0.3810	33.6125	0.9068
0.95	9.5	67.5	59.375	0.1815	33.4420	0.9874

It follows from Table 9.3 that the p-value is smaller than 0.05 only for a ρ_0 value that is equal to or smaller than 0.55. Consequently, we can claim that ρ exceeds those values.

9.3.2   *Statistical Inference about Intra-Rater Reliability Coefficient γ*

In this section, we want to know how well the expression $\mathrm{ICC}_a(2,1)$ (see equations 9.2.11 and 9.2.12) approximates the theoretical intra-rater reliability γ of equation 9.2.1. This is accomplished using the two precision measures which are the confidence interval, and the p-value.

Constructing a Confidence Interval for γ

As usual, you will need to first specify the level of confidence for your interval, which represents its likelihood to contain the "true" intra-rater reliability value. Let $\alpha = 1 - $ *(Confidence Level)*, a quantity often referred to as the significance level[12]. The confidence interval associated with γ is defined by the range of values between the lower confidence bound LCB, and the upper confidence bound UCB, both of which are defined as follows:

$$\mathrm{LCB} = \frac{A - rnF_2 \cdot \mathrm{MSE}}{A + (M - rn)F_2 \cdot \mathrm{MSE}}, \tag{9.3.7}$$

$$\mathrm{UCB} = \frac{A - rnF_1 \cdot \mathrm{MSE}}{A + (M - rn)F_1 \cdot \mathrm{MSE}}, \tag{9.3.8}$$

where $A = n\mathrm{MSS} + r\mathrm{MSR} + (rn - n - r)\mathrm{MSI}$, and the different means of squares MSS, MSR, MSI, as well as MSE are defined in the beginning of section 9.3.1. F_1 and F_2

---

[12]The significance level represents the likelihood that your confidence interval fails to include the "true" intra-rater reliability coefficient.

are respectively the $100(\alpha/2)^{th}$ and $100(1 - \alpha/2)^{th}$ percentiles of the F distribution with v and $M - rn$ degrees of freedom. The number v of degrees of freedom is given by,

$$v = \frac{(a\text{MSS} + b\text{MSR} + c\text{MSI})^2}{\dfrac{(a\text{MSS})^2}{n-1} + \dfrac{(b\text{MSR})^2}{r-1} + \dfrac{(c\text{MSI})^2}{(r-1)(n-1)}}, \tag{9.3.9}$$

where a, b, and c are defined as,

$$a = \frac{1}{r + \dfrac{M\gamma}{n(1-\gamma)}}, \quad b = \frac{1}{n + \dfrac{M\gamma}{r(1-\gamma)}}, \quad \text{and } c = \frac{rn - n - r}{rn + M\dfrac{\gamma}{1-\gamma}}. \tag{9.3.10}$$

When calculating the confidence bounds, the intraclass correlation γ that appears in the expressions of a, b, and c must be replaced by its calculated value of equation 9.2.11, or 9.2.12. Moreover, F_1 and F_2 may be calculated using MS Excel as described in section 9.3.1.

The confidence interval allows us to know how precise our estimate of the intra-rater reliability coefficient is, which is an important information researchers should always obtain. Sometimes however, you want to know how likely is the intra-rater reliability to exceed a hypothetical value γ_0 ?. This question can be answered using the statistical notion of p-value.

Hypothesis Testing: The p-Value for γ

Let us assume that you want to test the hypothesis that γ is higher than a predetermined value γ_0. Let v be given by equation 9.3.9 (with γ replaced with the hypothetical value γ_0), and F_{obs} given by,

$$F_{obs} = \frac{a\text{MSS} + b\text{MSR} + c\text{MSI}}{\text{MSE}}, \tag{9.3.11}$$

with a, b, and c defined by equation 9.3.10 where γ is replaced by γ_0. The p-value in this case, is defined as the probability that a random variable F that follows the F distribution with v and $M - rn$ degrees of freedom, exceeds F_{obs}. This p-value can be calculated with MS Excel as shown in Example 9.3. As usual, if the p-value is smaller than 0.05 then the hypothesis is considered to be consistent with the ratings.

Example 9.4 ⎯⎯⎯⎯⎯⎯⎯⎯⎯⎯⎯⎯⎯⎯⎯⎯⎯⎯⎯⎯⎯⎯⎯⎯

Using rating data from Table 9.2 (c.f. Example 9.1), I previously calculated the intraclass correlation associated with intra-rater reliability, and obtained $\text{ICC}_a(2,1) = 0.788$ as shown in equation 9.2.13. I now want to use the same rating data to compute the associated confidence interval and p-values.

The lower and upper confidence bounds associated with the intra-rater reliability coefficient are defined in equations 9.3.7 and 9.3.8, and are calculated as follows:

$$\text{LCB} = \frac{A - rnF_2 \cdot \text{MSE}}{A + (M - rn)F_2 \cdot \text{MSE}} = \frac{106,088.82 - 4 \times 8 \times 2.753 \times 479.333}{106,088.82 + (57 - 4 \times 8) \times 2.753 \times 479.333},$$
$$= 0.4592.$$

Note that $A = n\text{MSS} + r\text{MSR} + (rn - n - r)\text{MSI} = 8 \times 11,701.52 + 4 \times 1,523.31 + (4 \times 8 - 8 - 4) \times 319.173 = 106,088.82$. For the 95% confidence interval, F_2 represents the 97.5^{th} percentile of the F distribution with v and $M - rn = 57 - 4 \times 8 = 25$ degrees of freedom, where v of equation 9.3.9 equals 8.888629. To see all the details involved in these calculations, you may want to look at the "Example 9.4" worksheet contained in the following Excel spreadsheet,

www.agreestat.com/book4/chapter9examples.xlsx.

The upper confidence bound on the other hand is calculated as follows:

$$\text{UCB} = \frac{A - rnF_1 \cdot \text{MSE}}{A + (M - rn)F_1 \cdot \text{MSE}} = \frac{106,088.82 - 4 \times 8 \times 0.254 \times 479.333}{106,088.82 + (57 - 4 \times 8) \times 0.254 \times 479.333},$$
$$= 0.936.$$

Therefore, the 95% confidence interval associated with the intra-rater reliability coefficient of 0.788 is $(0.4592; 0.936)$.

As for the p-value, it is generally calculated with respect to a hypothetical value from 0 to 1. Table 9.4 shows the p-value associated with the intra-rater reliability coefficient as a function of γ_0, and provides the quantities a, b, c, v, and F_{obs} used in the calculations. If you want to see all the steps involved in the p-value calculation, you may download the Excel spreadsheet,

www.agreestat.com/book4/chapter9examples.xlsx

and look at the "Example 9.4" worksheet.

Table 9.4: Calculation of p-values for different values of γ_0

γ_0	a	b	c	F_{obs}	v	p-Value
0.25	0.1569	0.0784	0.3922	4.3397	8.8886	0.0022
0.3	0.1418	0.0709	0.3544	3.9222	8.8886	0.0040
0.35	0.1276	0.0638	0.3190	3.5303	8.8886	0.0073
0.4	0.1143	0.0571	0.2857	3.1618	8.8886	0.0129
0.45	0.1017	0.0509	0.2543	2.8145	8.8886	0.0226
0.5	0.0899	0.0449	0.2247	2.4868	8.8886	0.0389
0.55	0.0787	0.0393	0.1967	2.1770	8.8886	0.0656
0.6	0.0681	0.0340	0.1702	1.8836	8.8886	0.1081
0.65	0.0580	0.0290	0.1451	1.6055	8.8886	0.1735
0.7	0.0485	0.0242	0.1212	1.3414	8.8886	0.2695

It follows from Table 9.4 that the p-value is smaller than 0.05 only for a γ_0 value that is equal to or smaller than 0.5. Consequently, we can claim that the observed ratings are consistent with the hypothesis that the "true" intra-rater reliability coefficient as measured by $ICC_a(2,1)$ exceeds any of these values.

9.4   Sample Size Calculations

When designing an intra-rater or an inter-rater reliability study, the researcher often needs to know how many raters and subjects must be recruited to obtain an accurate estimation of the agreement coefficient. An agreement coefficient is accurate if its confidence interval is "reasonably" narrow, or its confidence interval length (denoted by L) is "reasonably" small. More information regarding the use of confidence intervals for this purpose may be found in Giraudeau and Mary (2001), and in Doros and Lew (2010). Now, I expect you to wonder how small is considered reasonably small - a common question asked by researchers. *I suggest to consider a confidence interval length L to be "reasonably" small if it is below* 0.4 *times the magnitude of the intraclass correlation coefficient*[13], *whether it represents the inter-rater or the intra-rater reliability coefficient.*

This section presents methods and techniques for calculating the number of subjects, number of raters, and number of trials required to obtain a prescribed confidence interval length for the intraclass correlation coefficient. Sample size requirements for optimizing the estimation of the inter-rater reliability coefficient will be discussed first in section 9.4.1. A similar discussion devoted to the intra-rater reliability coefficient is deferred to section 9.4.2.

9.4.1   *Sample Size Calculations for Inter-Rater Reliability Studies*

For the purpose of designing an inter-rater reliability study, you must decide about the number of raters, number of subjects, and possibly the number of trials per rater and per subject if replication is an option you want to consider. One reason you may want to consider producing multiple ratings for the same subject is if intra-rater reliability will be analyzed in addition to inter-rater reliability. Another reason for using multiple trials is to increase the number of ratings when the costs associated with the recruitment of subjects are high, and should be minimized.

---

[13]Traditionally in statistics, the mean is considered reasonably accurate if its coefficient of variation (i.e. the variation per unit of measurement, also known as CV) does not exceed 10%, or 0.1 (some practitioners may want it smaller). For a 95% confidence interval, this coefficient of variation can be represented as the ratio of the interval length to 4 times the mean. So, $L/(4\mu) \leq 0.1$ leads to $L \leq 0.4\mu$. Here we replace μ with the intraclass correlation of interest.

However, for a given number of ratings per rater, the strategy that yields the most accurate inter-rater reliability coefficient requires the use of a single trial per subject and per rater. Therefore, I propose to first determine the optimal number of raters and subjects for a given confidence interval length, assuming one rating per rater and per subject. If you want to consider two trials or more per subject while maintaining the same number of ratings, then I will show the different options[14] and their impact on the precision of the inter-rater reliability coefficient.

Assuming that the number of raters is limited to 2, figure 9.4.1 depicts the expected length of the 95% confidence interval as a function of number of subjects, and the "true" inter-rater reliability, measured by the intraclass correlation coefficient (referred to here as ICC). Figures 9.4.2, 9.4.3, and 9.4.4 show similar graphs for 3, 4, and 5 raters respectively. All 4 figures reveal a number of important relationships that should be mentioned:

- For any ICC value, the length the of 95% confidence interval decreases as the number of subjects increases. That is, a larger number of subjects will improve the precision of your inter-rater reliability coefficient.

- For any given number of subjects, larger ICC values lead to a smaller interval length (i.e. more accurate inter-rater reliability coefficients). This suggests that raters with high extent of agreement among raters lead to inexpensive studies. This fact has an important practical implication. Giving your raters some training before the experiment is a good investment that is expected to pay off in terms of a reduced number of subjects required to achieve a certain precision level.

Our investigation has revealed that for a given number of ratings per rater, having more than 5 raters will not improve the precision of the inter-rater reliability in any meaningful way. Once you have recruited 5 raters as part of the experiment, the precision of your inter-rater reliability coefficient will improve faster with a larger number of subjects than with a larger number of raters. Unless the cost of recruiting subjects exceeds that of recruiting raters, I would recommend adding more subjects once the number of raters reaches 5. You may want to review all 4 graphs to find the combination of number of raters and subjects that gives you the desired interval length.

Just looking at figure 9.4.1 for example, you can see that to be able to determine how many raters you need requires you to have two things:

(i) a predicted (or anticipated) value for your inter-rater reliability coefficient,

---

[14]These options involve reducing the number of subjects while increasing the number of trials, and will necessarily result in a loss of precision for the inter-reliability coefficient. Therefore, a compromise is necessary between the number of subjects and the number of trials.

(ii) the desired length for your 95% confidence interval.

Let us us review these two requirements, and see how convenient it is to meet them. A predicted inter-rater reliability coefficient is often obtained from one of two sources. These sources are the pilot and previous studies. The pilot study, often based on an arbitrarily small number of subjects and raters, will yield a crude estimate of the inter-rater reliability, and give you a first look at the extent of agreement among raters. If you cannot obtain any anticipated ICC value, one possibility is to determine your sample size based on a moderate hand-picked initial value, such as 0.5. The only adverse consequence of your choice of value may be an experiment that will not produce and inter-rater reliability as accurate as the design has promised.

As an example, suppose a hospital emergency department is designing an inter-rater reliability study to evaluate the extent of agreement among physicians with respect to the measurement of stroke volume (SV) and heart rate (HR) of patients using the Impedance Cardiography (ICG) technology. We also assume that previous studies revealed an inter-rater reliability measured by the ICC to be 0.86 for SV and 0.8 for HR. We know that the emergency department wants to have only two physicians participate in the experiment, but does not know how many patients should be recruited. You can use Figure 9.4.1 to resolve this problem as follows:

(a) Compute $0.4 \times$ ICC for both variables to obtain the desired 95% confidence interval length. This leads to 0.344 and 0.32 for SV and HR respectively.

(b) Using Figure 9.4.1 (for 2 raters), you can see that the second curve from the bottom is associated with an ICC value of 0.85, which the closest you can get to 0.86 the anticipated ICC for the SV variable. Therefore, this curve will be used to determine the required sample size for the SV variable. The same procedure allows you to determine that the third curve from the bottom (associated with ICC of 0.8) is the one to use for obtaining the required number of subjects for the HR variable.

(c) Using the "ICC=0.85" curve, you can see that approximately 15 subjects will be sufficient to yield a 95% confidence interval with length that close to 0.344. Likewise, using the "ICC=0.80" curve, it appears that approximately 25 subjects will yield a 95% confidence interval with length that is close to 0.32.

Since SV and HR measurements must be taken during the same inter-rater reliability experiment, the right approach would be to recruit a total of 25 patients. While all of them will provide HR measurements, only 15 (ideally randomly chosen) will provide SV measurements.

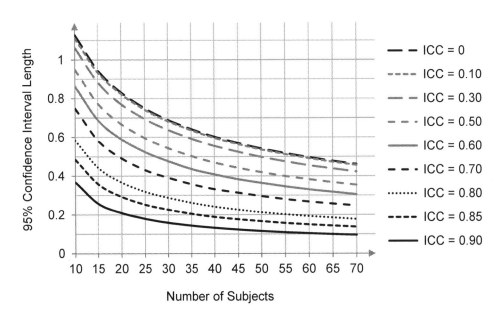

Figure 9.4.1: Expected length of the 95% confidence interval as a function of the number of subjects based on 2 raters.

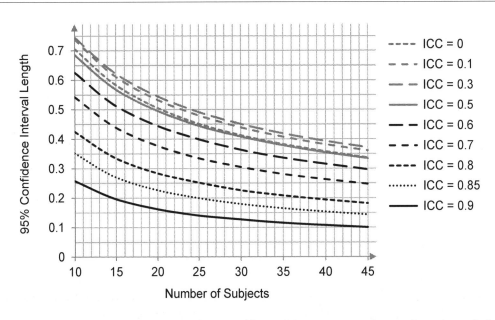

Figure 9.4.2: Expected length of the 95% confidence interval as a function of the number of subjects based on 3 raters.

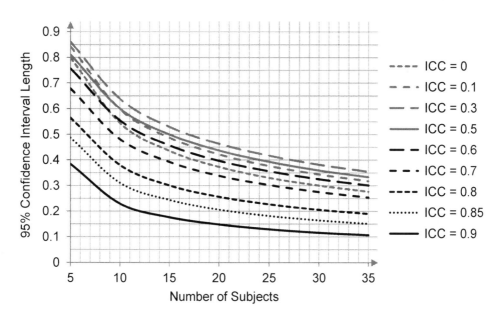

Figure 9.4.3: Expected length of the 95% confidence interval as a function of the number of subjects based on 4 raters.

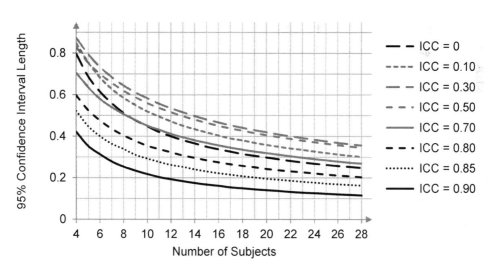

Figure 9.4.4: Expected length of the 95% confidence interval as a function of the number of subjects based on 5 raters.

WHAT IS THE CORRECT NUMBER OF TRIALS?

In this section, I want to briefly consider the problem of replication. Replication consists of conducting multiple trials, or using the same rater to take repeated measurements from the same subject. Replication is essential for computing intra-rater reliability, and may help reduce the required number of subjects in an inter-rater reliability study, albeit some loss of precision. However, some researchers collect repeated measurements before assigning their average value to the subject. The objective here is to assign to each subject a single average score, which is supposedly more accurate than the individual scores. Although this practice is common among researchers, it does not appear to have any solid statistical basis. In fact, there is no evidence that an ICC based on mean ratings has a smaller variance than the ICC based on individual ratings. I recommend the analysis of repeated measurements in their raw form, and not in the form of averages. The use of raw ratings makes the evaluation of the precision associated with the ICC more convenient.

Consider an inter-rater reliability study design that requires 5 raters and 10 subjects to be rated by each of the raters. The question we like to answer is the following: "*instead of using 10 subjects and 1 rating per subject, can we use 5 subjects and 2 ratings per subject?*" The answer to this question is yes we can, if we are willing to accept some loss of precision. Figures 9.4.5, 9.4.6, and 9.4.7 give us the magnitude of the loss of precision due to the use of repeated measurements.

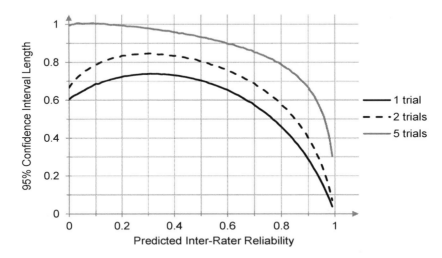

Figure 9.4.5: Expected length of the 95% confidence interval as a function of ICC based on 5 raters and 10 ratings per rater.

Figure 9.4.5 reveals two things:

(*i*) Using 1 trial produces the most precise inter-rater reliability coefficient;

(*ii*) Using 2 trials (hence 5 subjects for the same number of 10 ratings) will increase the length of the 95% confidence interval by approximately 0.1 (note that this increase is smaller when the number of ratings is larger than 10 as seen in figures 9.4.6 and 9.4.7).

All three figures 9.4.5, 9.4.6, and 9.4.7 show that using more than three trials may result in a substantial loss of precision for a given total number of ratings.

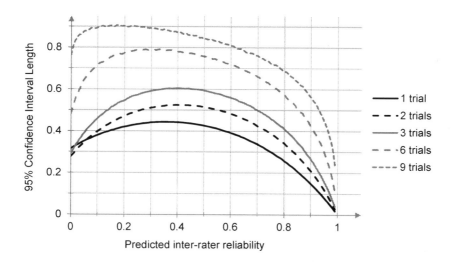

Figure 9.4.6: Expected length of the 95% confidence interval as a function of ICC based on 5 raters and 18 ratings per rater.

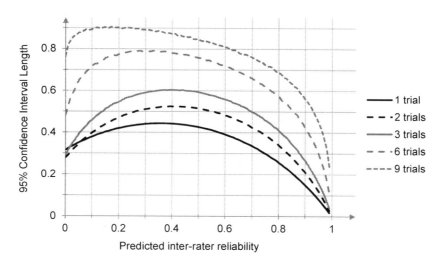

Figure 9.4.7: Expected length of the 95% confidence interval as a function of ICC based on 5 raters and 30 ratings per rater.

9.4.2 *Sample Size Calculations for Intra-Rater Reliability Studies*

We just learned from the previous section that for a given number of ratings, using more than 5 raters will generally not improve the precision of the inter-rater reliability coefficient much. The situation is different when designing an intra-rater reliability study. More raters will generally improve the precision of the intra-rater reliability coefficient in a way that most practitioners will appreciate. The figures 9.4.8 through 9.4.9 can assist you in determining the appropriate number of raters, subjects, and trials when designing an intra-rater reliability study. Let us now see how these graphs could be used.

All 12 figures (9.4.8 through 9.4.19) reveal that in general you will need 4 or 5 trials to obtain the most accurate intra-rater reliability coefficient for a given number of raters and a given number of ratings per rater. That is for 2 raters and 20 ratings per rater for example, the optimal design consists of using 5 subjects and 4 trials or 4 subjects and 5 trials (see Figure 9.4.11). Using only 2 trials can be particularly damaging if the raters involved in the experiment have low reproducibility. However, if you know from a pilot study or from previous studies that the raters used have high reproducibility, but simply want to confirm it with a formal study, you may achieve good results using only 2 trials. If the subjects are human subjects who must endure some discomfort during the trial, then you will want to limit the number of trials per subject and increase the number of subjects instead. Since all study designs generally face specific challenges, the researcher will want to determine the best way to use these graphs.

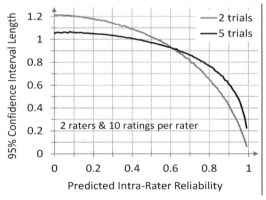

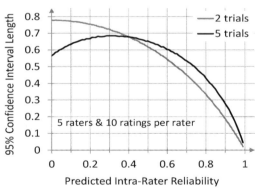

Figure 9.4.8: Interval length by intra-rater reliability (2 raters & 10 ratings per rater).

Figure 9.4.9: Interval length by intra-rater reliability (5 raters & 10 ratings per rater).

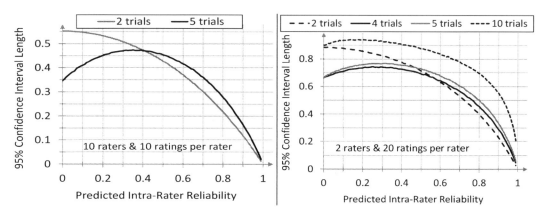

Figure 9.4.10: Interval length by intra-rater reliability (10 raters & 10 ratings per rater).

Figure 9.4.11: Interval length by intra-rater reliability (2 raters & 20 ratings per rater)

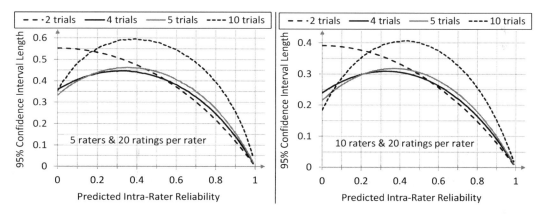

Figure 9.4.12: Interval length by intra-rater reliability (5 raters & 20 ratings per rater).

Figure 9.4.13: Interval length by intra-rater reliability (10 raters & 20 ratings per rater).

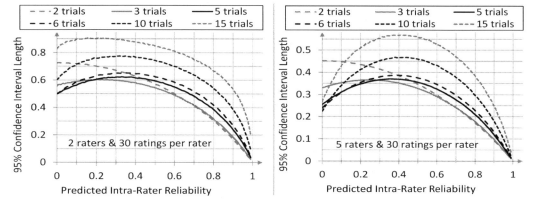

Figure 9.4.14: Interval length by intra-rater reliability (2 raters & 30 ratings per rater).

Figure 9.4.15: Interval length by intra-rater reliability (5 raters & 30 ratings per rater).

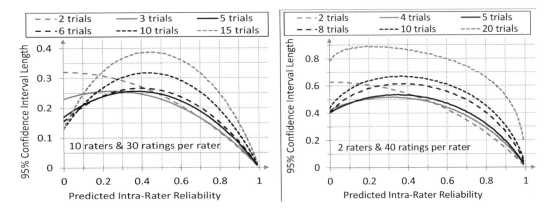

Figure 9.4.16: Interval length by intra-rater reliability (10 raters & 30 ratings per rater).

Figure 9.4.17: Interval length by intra-rater reliability (2 raters & 40 ratings per rater).

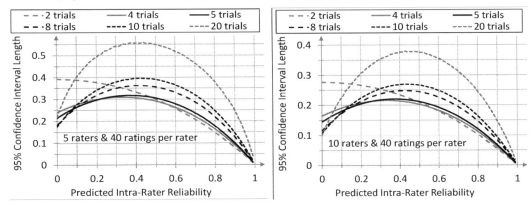

Figure 9.4.18: Interval length by intra-rater reliability (5 raters & 40 ratings per rater).

Figure 9.4.19: Interval length by intra-rater reliability (10 raters & 40 ratings per rater).

9.5 Special Topics

In this section, I want to discuss about two special topics. The first topic is related to the analysis of inter-rater and intra-rater reliability under the random factorial model without interaction. The second topic is about the methods used to create the power curves for determining the different sample sizes, as discussed in the previous section.

9.5.1 *Rater Reliability for a Random Factorial Model Without Interaction*

The inter-rater and intra-rater reliability coefficients were discussed in sections 9.2.1 and 9.2.2 respectively, under the random factorial model with interaction formalized with equation 9.2.1. This model is applicable only if some raters take two measurements or more on some subjects, and if the researcher expects the rater and subject factors to interact. However, some experimental designs are based on a single rating per subject and per rater. Such a design may be recommended if the rating process is very demanding on human subjects. Moreover, in the case of inter-rater reliability there is no clear need to quantify the variation that is due to the subject-rater interaction. The interaction effect can well be blended into the error effect without it affecting the inter-rater reliability coefficient estimation.

Even if repeated measurements are collected for the sake of evaluating intra-rater reliability, the researcher may deem the subject-rater interaction unjustified. However, ignoring the interaction effect when it is present will lead to an understated intra-rater reliability coefficient, which will have a positive side with its smaller variance. However, specifying the interaction effect will produce an approximately unbiased intra-rater reliability coefficient, with the downside of having a higher variance. Therefore, you may not want to increase this variance unnecessarily if interaction is absent.

Let us consider the following reformulation of model 9.2.1:

$$y_{ijk} = \mu + s_i + r_j + e_{ijk}, \tag{9.5.1}$$

where $i = 1, \cdots, n$, $j = 1, \cdots, r$, and $k = 1, \cdots, m_{ij}$ with n being the number of subjects, r the number of raters, and m_{ij} the number of trials associated with subject i and rater j. This model can deal with experiments with repeated measurements and no subject-rater interaction, as well as with experiments with only one rating per subject and per rater (i.e. $m = 1$). Under this model, you can quantify intra-rater reliability only if there are repeated measurements.

The inter-rater reliability coefficient is defined as $\rho = \sigma_s^2/(\sigma_s^2+\sigma_r^2+\sigma_e^2)$. The intra-rater reliability on the other hand is given by $\gamma = (\sigma_s^2+\sigma_r^2)/(\sigma_s^2+\sigma_r^2+\sigma_e^2)$. Although γ can technically be evaluated even without replication (i.e. with a single measurement per subject and per rater), I strongly advise against doing it. Without replication, the random experimental error will be the sole contributing factor to the error variance. Therefore, a high γ value will simply be an indication of a small experimental error, a sign that the experiment was well implemented. There is nothing here suggesting a good intra-rater reliability. With replication however, the random experimental error as well as the intra-rater variation are the two contributing factors to the error variance. In this case, a high γ value can be achieved only if the error variance is relatively small implying that intra-rater variation also is relatively low. That is, intra-rater reliability is high. I will now show how these two coefficients can be calculated from observed ratings.

Using rating data, the estimated value ($\hat{\rho}$) of the inter-rater coefficient is often denoted by ICC(2,1) in the literature. Likewise the estimated value $(\widehat{\gamma})$ of the intra-rater reliability coefficient will be denoted by $\text{ICC}_a(2,1)$. These two quantities as expressed as follows:

$$\text{ICC(2,1)} = \widehat{\sigma}_s^2/(\widehat{\sigma}_s^2 + \widehat{\sigma}_r^2 + \widehat{\sigma}_e^2), \tag{9.5.2}$$

$$\text{ICC}_a(2,1) = (\widehat{\sigma}_s^2 + \widehat{\sigma}_r^2)/(\widehat{\sigma}_s^2 + \widehat{\sigma}_r^2 + \widehat{\sigma}_e^2), \tag{9.5.3}$$

where $\widehat{\sigma}_s^2$, $\widehat{\sigma}_r^2$, and $\widehat{\sigma}_e^2$ are the estimated values of the subject variance, the rater variance, and the error variance respectively. These variance components are calculated as follows:

$$\widehat{\sigma}_e^2 = \frac{\lambda_2(T_{2y} - T_{2s}) + \lambda_1(T_{2y} - T_{2r}) - (T_{2y} - T_{2\mu})}{\lambda_2(M - n) + \lambda_1(M - r) - (M - 1)}, \tag{9.5.4}$$

$$\widehat{\sigma}_s^2 = \left[T_{2y} - T_{2r} - (M - r)\widehat{\sigma}_e^2\right]/(M - k_4), \tag{9.5.5}$$

$$\widehat{\sigma}_r^2 = \left[T_{2y} - T_{2s} - (M - n)\widehat{\sigma}_e^2\right]/(M - k_3), \tag{9.5.6}$$

where M is the total number of ratings generated by the experiment, $\lambda_1 = (M - k_1')/(M - k_4)$, and $\lambda_2 = (M - k_2')/(M - k_3)$. Moreover,

- $k_1' = k_1/M$ where k_1 is the summation of all values $m_{i.}^2$ over all subjects, with $m_{i.}$ being the number of ratings associated with subject i,
- $k_2' = k_2/M$ where k_2 is the summation of all values $m_{.j}^2$ over all raters, with $m_{.j}$ being the number of ratings produced by rater j.
- k_3 is the summation of all values $m_{ij}^2/m_{i.}$ over all subjects and all raters, with m_{ij} being the number of ratings rater j generated for subject i.
- k_4 is the summation of all values $m_{ij}^2/m_{.j}$ over all subjects and all raters.

- T_{2y} is the summation of y_{ijk}^2 values over all subjects, raters, and trials.
- T_{2s} is the summation of $m_{i.}\overline{y}_{i..}^2$ over all n subjects, where $\overline{y}_{i..}$ is the average rating associated with subject i.
- T_{2r} is the summation of $m_{.j}\overline{y}_{.j.}^2$ over all r raters, where $\overline{y}_{.j.}$ is the average rating associated with rater j.
- $T_{2\mu} = M\overline{y}^2$, where $\overline{y}$ is the overall mean rating.

Confidence Interval for the Inter-Rater reliability Coefficient ρ

To obtain the inter-rater reliability confidence interval under the random factorial model (c.f. equation 9.5.1) without interaction, you need to first specify the level of confidence you want to have that your interval will include the "true" inter-rater reliability value. Let $\alpha = 1 - $ *(Confidence Level)*, a quantity often referred to as the significance level. The confidence interval associated with ρ is defined by the range of values between the lower confidence bound LCB, and the upper confidence bound UCB, both of which are defined as follows:

$$\text{LCB} = \frac{n(\text{MSS} - F_2 \cdot \text{MSE})}{n\text{MSS} + F_2\left[r\text{MSR} + (M - n - r)\text{MSE}\right]}, \qquad (9.5.7)$$

$$\text{UCB} = \frac{n(\text{MSS} - F_1 \cdot \text{MSE})}{n\text{MSS} + F_1\left[r\text{MSR} + (M - n - r)\text{MSE}\right]}, \qquad (9.5.8)$$

where the means of squares MSS, MSR, and MSI are defined in the beginning of section 9.3.1. The mean of squares for errors MSE on the other hand, is obtained by first summing the squared differences $(y_{ijk} - \overline{y}_{i..} - \overline{y}_{.j.} + \overline{y})^2$, and by dividing the summation by $(M - r - n + 1)$. Moreover, F_1 and F_2 represent respectively the $100(\alpha/2)^{th}$ and $100(1 - \alpha/2)^{th}$ percentiles of the F distribution with $n - 1$ and v degrees of freedom, where v is given by:

$$v = \frac{(a\text{MSR} + b\text{MSE})^2}{\dfrac{(a\text{MSR})^2}{r - 1} + \dfrac{(b\text{MSE})^2}{M - r - n + 1}}, \qquad (9.5.9)$$

where a and b are defined as,

$$a = \frac{r\rho}{n(1 - \rho)}, \text{ and } b = 1 + \frac{(M - r)\rho}{n(1 - \rho)}. \qquad (9.5.10)$$

Confidence Interval for the Intra-Rater Reliability Coefficient γ

The confidence interval associated with γ is defined by the range of values between the lower confidence bound LCB, and the upper confidence bound UCB defined as follows:

$$\text{LCB} = \frac{n\text{MSS} + r\text{MSR} - (r + n)F_2 \cdot \text{MSE}}{n\text{MSS} + r\text{MSR} + (M - n - r)F_2 \cdot \text{MSE}}, \qquad (9.5.11)$$

$$\text{UCB} = \frac{n\text{MSS} + r\text{MSR} - (r + n)F_1 \cdot \text{MSE}}{n\text{MSS} + r\text{MSR} + (M - n - r)F_1 \cdot \text{MSE}}, \qquad (9.5.12)$$

where the means of squares MSS, MSR, and MSI are defined in the beginning of section 9.3.1. However, the mean of squares for errors MSE in this case is obtained by first summing the squared differences $(y_{ijk} - \overline{y}_{i..} - \overline{y}_{.j.} + \overline{y})^2$, and by dividing the summation by $(M - r - n + 1)$. As for F_1 and F_2, they represent respectively the

$100(\alpha/2)^{th}$ and $100(1-\alpha/2)^{th}$ percentiles of the F distribution with v and $M-r-n+1$ degrees of freedom, where v is defined as follows:

$$v = \frac{(a\text{MSS} + b\text{MSR})^2}{\dfrac{(a\text{MSS})^2}{n-1} + \dfrac{(b\text{MSR})^2}{r-1}}, \tag{9.5.13}$$

with a and b defined as,

$$a = \frac{n}{n + r + M\gamma/(1-\gamma)}, \text{ and } b = \frac{r}{n + r + M\gamma/(1-\gamma)}. \tag{9.5.14}$$

Hypothesis Testing: The p-Value for the Inter-Rater Reliability Coefficient ρ

Let us assume that you want to test the hypothesis that ρ is higher than a predetermined value ρ_0. The p-value needed to perform this test is calculated as follows:

$$p\text{-}value = P\Big(F \geq F_{obs}\Big), \tag{9.5.15}$$

where F is a random variable that follows the F-distribution with $n-1$ and v degrees of freedom, with v given by equation 9.5.9. As for the observed statistic F_{obs}, it is calculated as,

$$F_{obs} = \frac{\text{MSS}}{a\text{MSR} + b\text{MSE}}, \tag{9.5.16}$$

with a, and b defined by equation 9.5.10, where ρ is replaced by ρ_0.

Hypothesis Testing: The p-Value for γ

Assume that we are testing the hypothesis that γ is higher than a predetermined value γ_0. The p-value needed to perform this test is calculated as follows:

$$p\text{-}value = P\Big(F \geq F_{obs}\Big), \tag{9.5.17}$$

where F is a random variable that follows the F-distribution with v and $M-n-r+1$ degrees of freedom, with v given by equation 9.5.13. As for observed statistic F_{obs}, it is calculated as,

$$F_{obs} = \frac{a\text{MSS} + b\text{MSR}}{\text{MSE}}, \tag{9.5.18}$$

with a, and b defined by equation 9.5.14 where γ is replaced by γ_0.

Example 9.5 ──

This example illustrates the analysis of the two tables 9.1 and 9.2 under the assumption of no subject-rater interaction.

Analyzing Table 9.1

Table 9.1 shows ratings from 4 raters that have scored 15 subjects. The experiment that produced this data is based on a single replicate factorial design. With a single rating per subject and per rater, this data would not allow for the analysis of the subject-rater interaction nor the analysis of intra-rater reliability. Therefore, model 9.5.1 must be used, and only for the purpose of analyzing inter-rater reliability.

Figure 9.5.1 shows a graph of the subject mean score difference against the subject mean score, and provides a visual assessment of the extent of agreement among the 4 raters. The subject mean score difference is calculated separately for each subject by averaging all 6 pairwise differences associated with the 6 pairs of raters that can be formed out of the group of 4 raters[15]. This graph can be seen as the multiple-rater version of what is known in the literature as the Bland-Altman plot (see Bland & Altman (1986)). It follows from this graph that the 4 raters agree reasonably well with the exception of an outlier associated with a mean score of 305, and a mean difference of 63.3.

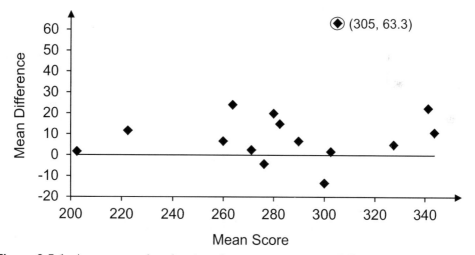

Figure 9.5.1: Agreement plot showing the rater mean score difference against the rater mean score

Figure 9.5.2 on the other hand, depicts the rater standard deviation[16] as a function of their overall mean score. It offers another look at the rater agreement as the score magnitude changes, and is known in the literature as the repeatability plot. (See Bland

───────────────────────────────

[15]How the 2 raters in a given pair are ordered when taking the difference is irrelevant. But the order adopted must remain the same for all subjects.

[16]This standard deviation is that of all scores associated with one subject.

& Altman - 1996 -). This plot is often used for repeated measures, and may also be conveniently used with multiple raters. Both figures 9.5.1 and 9.5.2 tell about the same story showing an overall good agreement with the exception of 1 or 2 outliers.

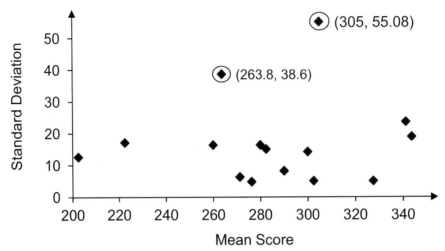

Figure 9.5.2: Repeatability plot showing the rater standard deviation against the rater mean score

The intraclass correlation coefficient ICC(2,1) of equation 9.5.2 is given by,

$$\text{ICC}(2,1) = \frac{1,430.258}{1,430.258 + 57.381 + 410.813},$$
$$= 0.7534.$$

Using equations 9.5.7 and 9.5.8, we can compute the lower and upper bounds of the 95% confidence interval as follows[17]:

$$\text{LCB} = \frac{15(6,131.85 - 1.9616 \times 410.813)}{15 \times 6,131.85 + 1.9616\left[4 \times 1,271.53 + (60 - 15 - 4) \times 410.813\right]},$$
$$= 0.5918.$$
$$\text{UCB} = \frac{15(6,131.85 - 0.4399 \times 410.813)}{15 \times 6,131.85 + 0.4399\left[4 \times 1,271.53 + (60 - 15 - 4) \times 410.813\right]}$$
$$= 0.8784.$$

To compute the p-value, you need to first specify the hypothetical value ρ_0 with respect to which it will be calculated. Although the default hypothetical value of 0 is often used in the context of inter-rater reliability is unjustified.

[17]For more details about these calculations, interested readers may want to download the Excel spreadsheet www.agreestat.com/book4/chapter9examples.xlsx. The "Example 9.5 (Table 9.1 Data)" worksheet shows the step-by-step calculations of ICC(2,1), the confidence interval bounds, and the the p-values, from the input data of Table 9.1 to the final results.

You do not just want to know that there does exist some agreement among raters. Instead, you want to know whether such an agreement is substantial. For a hypothetical value of $\rho_0 = 0.3$, the p-value is obtained from equation 9.5.15 as follows:

$$p - value = P(F \geq 5.0533) = 1.895 \times 10^{-5},$$

where F is random variable that follows the F distribution with $n - 1 = 14$ and $v_0 = 43.0499$ degrees of freedom (see the Excel spreadsheet for more details).

Analyzing Table 9.2

Using ratings from Table 9.2, and assuming the random factorial design without replication described by model 9.5.1, we can analyze both the inter-rater reliability and intra-rater reliability, and obtain the results shown in Tables 9.5 and 9.6[18].

Table 9.5: Inter-Rater Reliability Analysis **Table 9.6**: Intra-Rater Reliability Analysis

ICC(2,1) = 0.77888		ICC$_a$(2,1) = 0.81468	
Confidence Interval	**P-value**	**Confidence Interval**	**P-value**
95% LCB: 0.5334 95% UCB: 0.9358	5.96139×10^{-5}	95% LCB: 0.5935 95% UCB: 0.9481	1.65175×10^{-5}
$a = 1.76122$ $b = 24.33613$ $v = 34.91987$ $F_1 = 0.23056$ $F_2 = 2.68783$	$a_0 = 0.21429$ $b_0 = 3.83929$ $v_0 = 40.24078$ $\rho_0 = 0.3$ $F_{obs} = 6.20$	$a = 0.03047$ $b = 0.01523$ $v = 7.86319$ $F_1 = 0.23323$ $F_2 = 2.57739$	$a_0 = 0.21961$ $b_0 = 0.10980$ $v_0 = 7.86319$ $\rho_0 = 0.3$ $F_{obs} = 6.74$

9.5.2   *How are the Power Curves Obtained?*

In section 9.4, I presented a number of charts that depict the confidence interval length as a function of the intraclass correlation coefficient, and possibly the number of replicates (or trials) used in the experiment. The purpose of this section is to describe how these different curves are obtained. The general approach is based on the Monte Carlo simulation that consists of generating 10,000 confidence intervals (hence 10,000 interval lengths) for each individual ICC value. The average interval length is then associated with the ICC value used, in order to produce one point on the curve. The process is repeated for several ICC values to obtain the whole curve.

---

[18]For more details about these calculations, interested readers will want to download the Excel spreadsheet www.agreestat.com/book4/chapter9examples.xlsx, and review the "Example 9.5 (Table 9.2 Data)" worksheet, which shows the step-by-step calculations of all the numbers shown in both tables.

INTER-RATER RELIABILITY BASED ON ONE TRIAL PER RATER AND PER SUBJECT

When the inter-rater reliability experiment is based on a single trial then the lower and upper confidence bounds are given by equations 9.5.7 and 9.5.8. These equations can be rewritten as follows:

$$\text{LCB} = \frac{n(\text{FSS} - F_2)}{n\text{FSS} + F_2\big[r\text{FSR} + (rn - r - n)\big]},$$

$$\text{UCB} = \frac{n(\text{FSS} - F_1)}{n\text{FSS} + F_1\big[r\text{FSR} + (rn - r - n)\big]},$$

where FSS = MSS/MSE, and FSR = MSR/MSE. Therefore, in order to compute a confidence interval's length for a given value of ρ, we need the two quantities FSS and FSR, and here is how they are obtained:

(a) First determine the set of ρ values for which you want to compute a confidence interval length. For the charts used in this chapter, I used the 100 values $0, 0.1, 0.2, \cdots, 0.99$.

(b) Generate a random variate FSR according to the F distribution with $r - 1$ and $(r - 1)(n - 1)$ degrees of freedom.

(c) Use the FSR value of step (a) to compute v for each of the rho values as follows:

$$v = \frac{(a\text{FSR} + b)^2}{(a\text{FSR})^2/(r - 1) + b^2/\big[(r - 1)(n - 1)\big]},$$

where $a = r\rho/[n(1 - \rho)]$ and $b = 1 + r(n - 1)\rho/[n(1 - \rho)]$ (c.f. equation 9.5.10).

(d) Generate random variates $F^\star$ according to the F distribution with $n - 1$ and v degrees of freedom.

(e) It follows from equation 9.5.16 that one can compute FSS as follows: FSS = $F^\star(a\text{FSR} + b)$.

(f) Using FSS and FSR you can compute one interval length for each of the ρ values defined in step (a). At this stage, you would have obtained an interval length for each of the 100 values, and you may want to save them.

(g) Repeat this process from step (b) a large number of times (e.g. 10,000 times or more).

In the end of this process you will have 10,000 different confidence interval interval lengths for each of the 100 ρ values used in the simulation experiment. For each ρ value, average the 10,000 lengths to obtain a single mean length, which can be used to construct the curve.

INTER-RATER RELIABILITY BASED ON TWO TRIALS
   OR MORE PER RATER AND PER SUBJECT

When an inter-rater reliability experiment involves replication (i.e. two trials or more per subject and per rater), the lower and upper confidence bounds associated with the inter-rater reliability coefficient are given by equations 9.3.1 and 9.3.2. Assuming no missing rating and a constant number of trials m, these two confidence bounds can be re-written as follows:

$$\text{LCB} = \frac{n(\text{FSS} - F_1 \cdot \text{FSI})}{n\text{FSS} + F_1[r\text{FSR} + (rn - n - r)\text{FSI} + rn(m - 1)]},$$

$$\text{UCB} = \frac{n(F_2 \cdot \text{FSS} - \text{FSI})}{nF_2 \cdot \text{FSS} + r\text{FSR} + (rn - n - r)\text{FSI} + rn(m - 1)},$$

where FSS = MSS/MSE, FSR = MSR/MSE, and FSI = MSI/MSE. These three ratios must be obtained before the confidence interval length can be calculated. This can be achieved by implementing the following steps:

(a) First determine the set of ρ values for which you want to compute a confidence interval length. For the charts used in this chapter, I used the following 100 values for ρ: $0, 0.1, 0.2, \cdots, 0.99$.

(b) Generate a random variate FSR according to the F distribution with $r - 1$ and $rn(m - 1)$ degrees of freedom.

(c) Generate a random variate FSI according to the F distribution with $(r - 1)(n - 1)$ and $rn(m - 1)$ degrees of freedom.

(d) For each of the ρ values defined in step (a), use the FSR and FSI values of steps (b) and (c) to compute v as follows:

$$v = \frac{(a\text{FSR} + b\text{FSI} + c)^2}{\dfrac{(a\text{FSR})^2}{r - 1} + \dfrac{(b\text{FSI})^2}{(r - 1)(n - 1)} + \dfrac{c^2}{rn(m - 1)}},$$

where $a = r\rho/[n(1 - \rho)]$, $b = 1 + r(n - 1)\rho/[n(1 - \rho)]$, and $c = r(m - 1)\rho/(1 - \rho)$.

(e) Generate random variates $F^\star$ according to the F distribution with $n - 1$ and v degrees of freedom.

(f) It follows from equation 9.3.5 that one can compute FSS = $F^\star(a\text{FSR} + b\text{FSI} + c)$.

(g) Using FSR, FSI of steps (b) and (c), and FSS of step (f), you can compute one interval length for each of the ρ values defined in step (a). At this stage, you would have obtained an interval length for each of the 100 ρ values, and you should store them in a file.

(*h*) Repeat this process from step (*b*) a large number of times (e.g. 10,000 times or more).

In the end of this process you will have 10,000 different confidence interval interval lengths for each of the 100 ρ values used in the simulation experiment. For each ρ value, average the 10,000 lengths to obtain a single mean length, which can be used to construct the curve.

OPTIMIZING THE INTRA-RATER RELIABILITY ESTIMATION

The lower and upper confidence bounds associated with the intra-rater reliability coefficient are given by equations 9.3.7 and 9.3.8. Assuming no missing rating and a constant number of trials m, these two confidence bounds can be re-written as follows:

$$\text{LCB} = \frac{A^\star F_1 - rn\text{FSE}}{A^\star F_1 + rn(m-1)\text{FSE}},$$

$$\text{UCB} = \frac{A^\star / F_2 - rn\text{FSE}}{A^\star / F_2 + rn(m-1)\text{FSE}},$$

where $A^\star = n\text{FSS} + r\text{FSR} + (rn - n - r)$, $\text{FSS} = \text{MSS/MSI}$, $\text{FSR} = \text{MSR/MSI}$, and $\text{FSE} = \text{MSE/MSI}$. These three ratios must be obtained before the confidence interval length ($\text{UCB} - \text{LCB}$) can be calculated. They can be obtained by implementing the following steps:

(*a*) First determine the set of γ values for which you want to compute a confidence interval length. For the charts presented in this chapter, I used 100 values $0, 0.1, 0.2, \cdots, 0.99$ for γ.

(*b*) Generate a random variate FSS according to the F distribution with $n - 1$ and $(r - 1)(n - 1)$ degrees of freedom.

(*c*) Generate a random variate FSR according to the F distribution with $r - 1$ and $(r - 1)(n - 1)$ degrees of freedom.

(*d*) For each of the γ values, use the FSS and FSR values of steps (*b*) and (*c*) to compute v as follows:

$$v = \frac{(a\text{FSS} + b\text{FSR} + c)^2}{\dfrac{(a\text{FSS})^2}{n-1} + \dfrac{(b\text{FSR})^2}{r-1} + \dfrac{c^2}{(r-1)(n-1)}},$$

where a, b, and c are given by equation 9.3.10.

(*e*) Generate random variates $F^\star$ according to the F distribution with v and $rn(m-1)$ degrees of freedom.

(f) It follows from equation 9.3.11 that FSE $= (a\text{FSS} + b\text{FSR} + c)/F^\star$.

(g) Using FSS, FSR of steps (b) and (c), and FSE of step (f), you can compute one interval length for each of the γ values defined in step (a). At this stage, you would have obtained an interval length for each of the 100 γ values, and you should store them in a file.

(h) Repeat this process from step (b) a large number of times (e.g. 10,000 times or more).

In the end of this process you will have 10,000 different confidence interval interval lengths for each of the 100 ρ values used in the simulation experiment. For each γ value, average the 10,000 lengths to obtain a single mean length, which can be used to construct the curve.

## CHAPTER 10

Intraclass Correlations under the Mixed Factorial Design

OBJECTIVE

This chapter aims at presenting methods for analyzing intraclass correlation coefficients for reliability studies based on a random sample of subjects and a fixed group of raters. Therefore, the rater factor is considered fixed, while the subject factor is considered random. The intraclass correlation coefficient (ICC) used for quantifying intra-rater reliability is a valid measure of reproducibility. However, the ICC used for quantifying inter-rater reliability is a valid measure of consistency, and would be a valid measure of agreement only if there is no systematic bias in the rating process from one rater. This chapter also discusses methods for obtaining confidence intervals and p-values for all types of ICCs under model 3, in addition to presenting a detailed account of the methods used to determine the optimal number of subjects during the experimental design.

CONTENTS

10.1   The Problem

In the previous chapter, I presented methods for computing the intraclass correlation coefficient as a measure of inter-rater or intra-rater reliability, under the random factorial design. The random factorial design treats both the subject and the rater effects as random, which is justified only when the subject and rater samples are randomly selected from larger subject and rater universes. However, the rater effect cannot be treated as random in certain types of reliability experiments. For example, the reliability experiment may use two measuring instruments (an existing one and a new one) to take measurements on subjects. This experiment involves two raters (i.e. the measuring instruments expected to produce comparable measurements), and no other rater is under consideration. The rater effect must be considered fixed in such a situation. A fixed rater effect combined with a random subject effect will lead to an experimental design known as the "Mixed factorial design."

There is a fundamental difference between the random and mixed factorial designs regarding the role the rater effect plays in data analysis. Unlike the random factorial model of the previous chapter, which proceeds with a direct evaluation of the rater variance, the mixed factorial model is essentially based on the analysis of the interaction between raters and subjects. The raters alone do not represent a source of uncertainty to be analyzed since their effect is fixed. The only source of uncertainty involving the raters relies on the subject-rater interaction. A large subject-rater interaction has a negative effect on inter-rater reliability ; but may have a positive effect on intra-rater reliability for a given total variation in the ratings. Note that the subject-rater interaction is high if the score difference between raters varies considerably from subject to subject, and is low otherwise. I will discuss these relationships further in subsequent sections.

If the raters strongly agree then the subject-rater interaction will be small and the mixed factorial design will rightfully yield a high intraclass correlation coefficient. However, a small subject-rater interaction or its complete absence in a well-designed experiment could well yield a high intraclass correlation without the raters being in high agreement. This typically occurs in situations where there is a large and systematic gap (across subjects) between ratings from two raters. Although these situations are unusual in practice, especially with raters having basic training, researchers may want to take a precautionary measure by testing that ratings from all raters come from distributions with a common expected value. If this hypothesis is rejected, then I will not recommend the use of a mixed factorial design for the purpose of analyzing inter-rater reliability. Nevertheless, using a mixed factorial design for the purpose of studying inter-rater reliability is generally an effective approach for quantifying the extent of agreement among raters when the rater effect is fixed. This is due to us not having to worry about the rater variance component that represents raters that did not participate in the reliability experiment.

For the purpose of analyzing intra-rater reliability, the mixed factorial design works well when the rater effect is fixed. For a given total variation in the ratings, having a high subject-rater interaction may be beneficial since it could lead to a higher coefficient of intra-rater reliability. In fact, the error variance under the mixed factorial design includes not only the variance due to random experimental errors, but also the variance due to replication, which actually measures reproducibility. Therefore, a small error variance is an indication of small variance due to replication as well, which in turn is an indication of high reproducibility. Consequently, a high subject-rater interaction for a given total variation is not problematic, and may even be a sign of a relatively small error variance and high reproducibility. The relationship between the subject-rater interaction, inter-rater and intra-rater reliability will be further discussed in subsequent sections.

10.2   Intraclass Correlation Coefficient

The mixed factorial design involves a single group of raters as well as a single group of subjects, all of which are rated by each rater. Note that the word raters in this context could designate a group of 5 individuals (for example) operating the same measuring device, or could also designate 5 trials performed by a single individual operating the same measuring device to score all subjects. The data produced in both situations can be analyzed with the same methods that are discussed in this section. The analysis results may be interpreted differently depending on the context. Therefore, developing an in-depth understanding of the nature of the reliability experiment is essential to properly interpret the data analysis.

The abstract representation of ratings under the mixed factorial design is given by,

$$y_{ijk} = \mu + s_i + r_j + (sr)_{ij} + e_{ijk}, \tag{10.2.1}$$

where y_{ijk} is the kth replicate score[1] that rater j assigned to subject i. The remaining terms in model 10.1 are defined as follows[2]:

▶ μ is the expected value of the y-score.

▶ s_i is the random subject effect, assumed to follow the Normal distribution with 0 mean, and variance σ_s^2.

▶ r_j is the fixed rater effect, assumed to satisfy the condition,

$$\sum_{j=1}^{r} r_j = 0, \tag{10.2.2}$$

---

[1] Many reliability experiments only involves one trial (the first one)
[2] These are standard conditions used in all ANOVA models

where r is the number of raters participating in the experiment.

▶ $(sr)_{ij}$ is the random subject-rater interaction effect, assumed to follow the Normal distribution with mean 0, and variance σ_{sr}^2, and to satisfy the condition,

$$\sum_{j=1}^{r} (sr)_{ij} = 0, \text{ for any subject } i. \qquad (10.2.3)$$

▶ e_{ijk} is the random error effect, assumed to follow the Normal distribution with mean 0, and variance σ_e^2.

The subject, interaction, and error effects are considered mutually independent. That is, the magnitude of one effect does not affect that of another effect. Now, suppose that the reliability experiment involves n subjects, r raters, and m measurements per rater and subject. Later in this section, I will consider the more general situation where the number of measurements m varies by rater and by subject.

Model 10.1 is known in the inter-rater reliability literature as Model 3 (see Shrout & Fleiss, 1979 or McGraw & Wong, 1996), and stipulates that under the mixed factorial design, the different effects are additive (i.e. the subject and rater effects must be added to determine their joint impact on the score). From this model I will derive two intraclass correlation coefficients. One coefficient will be a measure of inter-rater reliability, while the other will be used as a measure of intra-rater reliability.

10.2.1   *Defining Inter-Rater Reliability*

The inter-rater reliability based on model 10.1, is by definition the correlation coefficient between the scores y_{ijk} and $y_{ij'k}$ associated with two raters j and j', the same subject i, and the same trial number k (if any). It follows from equation 10.1 that this inter-rater reliability (denoted by ρ) is defined[3] as,

$$\rho = \frac{\sigma_s^2 - \sigma_{sr}^2/(r-1)}{\sigma_s^2 + \sigma_{sr}^2 + \sigma_e^2} \qquad (10.2.4)$$

Equation 10.2.4 provides the definitional expression of inter-rater reliability based on the idealized model of equation 10.2.1. This coefficient belongs to the family of

---

[3]Note that $\rho = \text{Corr}(y_{ijk}, y_{ij'k}) = \text{Cov}(y_{ijk}, y_{ij'k})/\left[\sqrt{\text{Var}(y_{ijk})}\sqrt{\text{Var}(y_{ij'k})}\right]$. However, the covariance term can be re-written as, $\text{Cov}(y_{ijk}, y_{ij'k}) = \sigma_s^2 + \text{Cov}[(sr)_{ij}, (sr)_{ij'}]$. By taking the variance of both sides of equation 10.2.3, one can prove that $\text{Cov}[(sr)_{ij}, (sr)_{ij'}] = -\sigma_{sr}^2/(r-1)$.

intraclass correlation coefficient (ICC), and the next step in its exploitation is to specify the procedure for calculating it from experimental data. But at this stage, I first need to see whether equation 10.2.4 actually measures the extent of agreement among the r raters that participated in the experiment.

A careful examination of expression 10.2.4 suggests that ρ varies from 0 to 1, and takes a high value closer to 1 only when the subject variance σ_s^2 exceeds the combined variance $\sigma_{sr}^2 + \sigma_e^2$ by a wide margin. That is, ρ will be high when the error and interaction variances are both relatively small. Consequently, you will obtain a high ρ value if the following 3 conditions are satisfied:

(a) The experiment is sufficiently well designed to keep the experimental error low (i.e. σ_e^2 is small),

(b) The subject-rater interaction is limited (i.e. σ_{sr}^2). This variance component particularly, may have a dramatic impact on the intraclass correlation.

(c) The subject variance is substantially larger than the error and interaction variances.

If the raters are in agreement and the experiment well planned, these three conditions will be met. However, there is a problem that stems from the fact that these three conditions could be met without the raters being in agreement. Consider the reliability data of Table 10.1 and the associated graph in Figure 10.2.1. This is a typical example of ratings characterized by total absence of any subject-rater interaction effect (i.e. $\sigma_{st}^2 = 0$). That is the gap between the two graphs associated with raters 1 and 2 remains constant across subjects. This data will nevertheless yield a high ρ value, despite the fact that raters 1 and 2 clearly disagree about the scoring of subjects across the board. This reality has led authors such as Bartko (1976), or McGraw & Wong (1996) to consider ρ of equation 10.4 as a measure of consistency, and not as a measure of agreement.

Table 10.1: Ratings without Subject-Rater Interaction

Subject	Rater (j)	
(i)	Rater1	Rater2
1	9	4
2	6	1
3	8	3
4	7	1
5	10	5
6	6	1

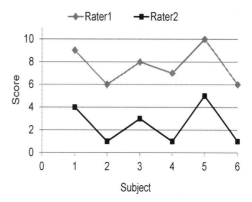

Figure 10.2.1: Table 10.1 Rating Data

Table 10.2: Ratings with Subject-Rater Interaction

Subject	Rater (j)	
(i)	Rater1	Rater2
1	5	4
2	6	5
3	8	9
4	7	8
5	9	7
6	6	7

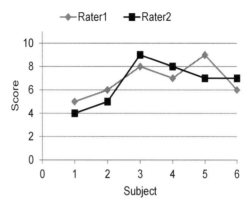

Figure 10.2.2: Table 10.2 Rating Data

Table 10.2 ratings and the associated graph of Figure 10.2.2 show a reasonably good agreement among raters. Because of the (small) subject-rater interaction depicted in this figure (i.e. the gap between the two curves changes from subject to subject) the ρ value of equation 10.2.4 associated with this data will be smaller than that of Table 10.1. Although agreement in Figure 10.2.2 is higher than in Figure 10.2.1, equation 10.2.4 tends to favor Figure 10.2.1. This is due to the observed subject-rater interaction, which penalizes Figure 10.2.2.

The problem I just described regarding Tables 10.1 and 10.2 stems from the systematic rater effect observed in Figure 10.2.1, with rater 1 consistently scoring higher than rater 2. The intraclass correlation coefficient based on a mixed factorial design will be appropriate if the experiment is set up in such a way that some raters do not exhibit any systematic bias towards stringency or leniency. Generally, specific scoring instructions given to raters will minimize the systematic bias in their scoring process. The variation in their scores will depend more on how they interact with subjects.

Equation 10.2.4 will adequately measure the extent of agreement among raters, as long as the raters are not heavily biased when rating subjects. When using the mixed factorial design to analyze inter-rater reliability, researchers may want to first test that the ratings from all raters are distributed around a common expected value. For two raters only, one may use the Mann-Whitney test proposed by Mann and Whitney (1947) or the Wilcoxon rank sum test recommended by Wilcoxon (1949). For three raters or more, one may use the Kruskal-Wallis test proposed by Kruskal (1952), and Kruskal and Wallis (1952) (You may also want to see Gwet, 2010*b*, in section 10.3 for a detailed discussion of this test). If these statistical tests reject the hypothesis that the ratings are distributed around the same expected value, then I would not use the mixed factorial design for analyzing inter-rater reliability.

If the experiment uses a single rater who rates each subject several times, then there will be no rater bias issue, and equation 10.2.4 may be used. Note that if you can use the mixed factorial design, you should always do so. It will generally yield a higher (sometimes much higher) intraclass correlation than the random factorial design of the previous chapter, because of the absence of an explicit rater variance component.

10.2.2   *Defining Intra-Rater Reliability*

The mixed factorial design where the rater effect is fixed can be used for analyzing the inter-rater reliability as discussed in the previous section. But you may use it to analyze intra-rater reliability as well, provided the experiment produces repeated measurements on the same subjects. Usually two trials are sufficient to evaluate intra-rater reliability. As usual, I define the intra-rater reliability coefficient as the correlation coefficient between two ratings y_{ijk} and $y_{ijk'}$ associated with the same rater, the same subject, and two trials k and k'. Using the statistical model described with equation 10.2.1, one can establish that the intra-rater reliability coefficient is defined by,

$$\gamma = \frac{\sigma_s^2 + \sigma_{sr}^2}{\sigma_s^2 + \sigma_{sr}^2 + \sigma_e^2}, \qquad (10.2.5)$$

where σ_s^2, σ_{sr}^2, and σ_e^2 are the variance components due to the subject, subject-rater interaction, and error effects. It follows from this expression that the magnitude of the intra-rater reliability coefficient is essentially determined by the ratio of the error variance to the total of the subject and subject-rater interaction variances. Consequently, if the error variation exceeds the total subject and interaction variation by a wide margin, then the intra-rater reliability coefficient will be small. However, a relatively small error variance will lead to a high intra-rater reliability coefficient. This is what you would normally expect since the error variation is induced by both the replication and of the experimental error. Hence a small error variation implies a small replication variation, which guarantees reproducibility.

Note that a large error variance will automatically lead to a small intra-rater reliability coefficient whether the ratings are actually reproducible or not. This reminds us that intra-rater reliability experiments must be carefully conducted to minimize possible experimental errors, whose presence make any reproducibility of measurements or rater agreement undetectable.

10.2.3   *Calculating Inter-Rater and Intra-Rater Reliability Coefficients*

When your data contains no missing score (i.e. each rater has scored all subjects), then the ICC can be calculated using a simple procedure based on standard means of squares. In practice however, many experimental datasets contain some missing scores, which makes it necessary to have a computational procedure that can handle them properly. The more general procedure that can handle missing scores will work with complete data as well, and involves complex calculations. Shrout & Fleiss (1979) as well as McGraw & Wong (1996) described the simpler procedure for complete data, and without replication (i.e. $m = 1$). I will first present this procedure (slightly adapted to accommodate replicates), before discussing the more general procedure for missing scores.

SPECIAL METHOD FOR BALANCED DATA

If your data is complete, and two measurements or more are taken on each subject (i.e. $m \geq 2$), then the inter-rater reliability coefficient ρ of equation 10.2.4 can be estimated[4] by,

$$\text{ICC}(3, 1) = \frac{(\text{MSS} - \text{MSI}) - (\text{MSI} - \text{MSE})/(r - 1)}{\text{MSS} + r(\text{MSI} - \text{MSE}) + (rm - 1)\text{MSE}}, \qquad (10.2.6)$$

where, MSS, MSI, and MSE represent respectively the mean of squares for subjects, the mean of squares for the subject-rater interaction, and the mean of squares for errors. These means of squares are calculated as follows:

▶ Mean Squares for Subjects (**MSS**)
The MSS is calculated by summing the squared differences $(\overline{y}_{i..} - \overline{y})^2$ over all n subjects, and multiplying the summation by $rm/(n - 1)$. Note that $\overline{y}$ is the overall score average, while $\overline{y}_{i..}$ is the average of all measurements associated with subject i.

▶ Mean Squares for Interaction (**MSI**)
The MSI is calculated by summing the squared differences $(\overline{y}_{ij.} - \overline{y}_{i..} - \overline{y}_{.j.} + \overline{y})^2$ over all n subjects, and r raters, and by multiplying the summation by $m/[(r - 1)(n - 1)]$. The term $\overline{y}_{ij.}$ represents the average of all measurements associated with rater j and subject i. The term $\overline{y}_{.j.}$ on the other hand, is the average of all measurements associated with rater j.

---

[4]The estimated value of ρ based on experimental data is designated by $\text{ICC}(3, 1)$ to keep the notation used in the literature, where number 3 refers to model 3, and number 1 refers to the fact that the unit of analysis is 1 basic measurement as opposed to an average of several measurements.

▶ Mean Squares for Errors (**MSE**)

The MSE is calculated by summing the squared differences $(y_{ijk} - \overline{y}_{ij\cdot})^2$ over all rnm measurements, and by dividing the summation by $rn(m-1)$. Note that this mean of squares can be calculated only if there are 2 measurements or more taken on each subject (i.e. $m \geq 2$). In case the experiment is conducted without replication (i.e. $m = 1$), do not compute this quantity. Instead, compute MSI and rename it as MSE since interaction and error effects will be blended together.

Using observed ratings, the intra-rater reliability coefficient γ of equation 10.2.5 can be estimated data as follows:

$$\text{ICC}_a(3,1) = \frac{\text{MSS} + r\text{MSI} - (r+1)\text{MSE}}{\text{MSS} + r\text{MSI} + (rm - r - 1)\text{MSE}}, \qquad (10.2.7)$$

where the different means of squares are defined as above.

If there is a single measurement taken on each subject (i.e. $m = 1$ or no replication) then you cannot evaluate intra-rater reliability, although inter-rater reliability can be calculated. To compute the inter-rater reliability coefficient with a single measurement per subject, you need to assume a statistical model similar to that of equation 10.2.1 but without the interaction term[5]. Under this restricted model, the inter-rater reliability coefficient is estimated as follows:

$$\text{ICC}(3,1) = \frac{\text{MSS} - \text{MSE}}{\text{MSS} + (r-1)\text{MSE}}, \qquad (10.2.8)$$

where the mean of squares for subjects (MSS), and the mean of squares for errors (MSE) are calculated as follows:

▶ MSS is the summation of all squared differences $(\overline{y}_{i\cdot} - \overline{y})^2$ that is multiplied by $r/(n-1)$. Moreover, $\overline{y}_{i\cdot}$ is the average of all scores associated with subject i, and $\overline{y}$ the overall mean score.

▶ MSE on the other hand, is the summation of all squared differences $(y_{ij} - \overline{y}_{i\cdot} - \overline{y}_{\cdot j} + \overline{y})^2$ that is divided by $(r-1)(n-1)$, where $\overline{y}_{\cdot j}$ is the average of all scores associated with rater j.

The following example illustrates the calculation of the inter-rater and intra-rater reliability of equations 10.2.6 and 10.2.7.

---

[5] Assuming a model without interaction does not mean that you refute the existence of a possible interaction. Instead, it means you will treat the interaction and error effects as a single effect.

Example 10.1

To illustrate the calculation of $ICC(3, 1)$ of equation 10.2.6 when the data is complete, let us consider the data shown in Table 10.3. Four chiropractors evaluated twice the distance along the spine of a particular condition on 16 patients.

Therefore $n = 16$ (number of subjects), $r = 4$ (number of raters or chiropractors), and $m = 2$ (the number of replicates). It follows from equation 10.2.6 that we need to compute the 3 means of squares MSS, MSI, and MSE. These means of squares may be computed following the definitions given above. For more details, you may want to look at the Excel worksheet named "Example 10.1" contained in the downloadable Excel workbook "`www.agreestat.com/book4/chapter10examples.xlx`."

Table 10.3: Chiropractic Assessment of 16 Patients by 4 Chiropractors *(Numbers represent the distance in millimeters along the spine, of a particular condition.)*

	Chiropractor (j)					Chiropractor (j)			
Patient	CC	PK	JA	LM	Patient	CC	PK	JA	LM
1	115	132	22	33	9	140	74	65	66
1	45	34	243	10	9	114	101	185	86
2	191	191	216	193	10	122	56	60	50
2	197	196	223	208	10	98	70	64	53
3	50	29	26	25	11	100	72	122	190
3	27	23	31	26	11	56	114	124	51
4	63	175	29	189	12	120	110	103	32
4	52	93	65	92	12	97	127	38	124
5	195	149	170	155	13	125	86	12	123
5	166	142	164	180	13	131	102	82	91
6	67	160	35	33	14	100	29	36	23
6	170	41	22	159	14	53	35	22	32
7	192	140	138	184	15	42	39	84	50
7	72	120	143	127	15	38	51	59	40
8	153	61	77	172	16	18	120	18	93
8	170	61	72	52	16	54	115	22	24

The three means of squares needed here are given by,

- MSS $= 15,961.333$ • MSI $= 1,852.558$ • MSE $= 1,771.555$.

Consequently, the intraclass correlation of equation 10.2.6 associated with inter-rater reliability is calculated as follows:

$$ICC(3, 1) = \frac{(15,961.333 - 1,852.558) - (1,852.558 - 1,771.555)/(4 - 1)}{15,961.333 + 4 \times (1,852.558 - 1,771.555) + (4 \times 2 - 1) \times 1,771.555},$$
$$= 14,081.77/28,686.23 = 0.4909.$$

As for the intra-rater reliability, the associated intraclass correlation coefficient of equation 10.2.7 is given by,

$$\text{ICC}_a(3,1) = \frac{15,961.33 + 4 \times 1,852.56 - (4+1) \times 1,771.55}{15,961.33 + 4 \times 1,852.56 + (4 \times 2 - 4 - 1) \times 1,771.555},$$

$$= 14,513.82/28,686.24 = 0.5059.$$

GENERAL METHOD FOR UNBALANCED DATA

It is very common in inter-rater and intra-rater reliability studies, for one rater to generate more or less ratings than another rater. This situation may occur because one rater for whatever reason failed to rate one subject that other raters have rated. Even if all raters rate the same number of subjects, one rater may still take more measurements on some subjects than other raters. In both situations, we are dealing with the common problem of missing ratings. Instead of ignoring it as is often the case in the inter-rater reliability literature, I would like to address it adequately by adapting some general statistical techniques previously proposed by Searle (1997, page 474).

For data containing missing ratings, the inter-rater reliability coefficient ICC(3, 1), and the intra-rater reliability coefficient $\text{ICC}_a(3,1)$ are calculated as follows:

$$\text{ICC}(3,1) = \frac{\widehat{\sigma}_s^2 - \widehat{\sigma}_{sr}^2/(r-1)}{\widehat{\sigma}_s^2 + \widehat{\sigma}_{sr}^2 + \widehat{\sigma}_e^2}, \tag{10.2.9}$$

$$\text{ICC}_a(3,1) = \frac{\widehat{\sigma}_s^2 + \widehat{\sigma}_{sr}^2}{\widehat{\sigma}_s^2 + \widehat{\sigma}_{sr}^2 + \widehat{\sigma}_e^2}, \tag{10.2.10}$$

where $\widehat{\sigma}_e^2, \widehat{\sigma}_s^2, \widehat{\sigma}_{sr}^2$ represent the values of the error variance, the subject variance, and the interaction variance estimated from experimental data.

The methods for calculating these variance components are first presented for the situation where two measurements or more were taken on some subjects by the same rater. Next I will address the situation where no more than one measurement is taken on a subject by the same rater. Let m be the maximum number of measurements per subject and per rater.

- If $m \geq 2$ (i.e. 2 or more measurements are taken on some subjects) then these variance components are calculated as follows:

$$\widehat{\sigma}_e^2 = (T_{2y} - T_{2sr})/(M - \lambda_0), \tag{10.2.11}$$

$$\widehat{\sigma}_{sr}^2 = \big[T_{2sr} - \text{RSS} - (\lambda_0 - n - r + 1)\widehat{\sigma}_e^2)\big]/h_6 \tag{10.2.12}$$

$$\widehat{\sigma}_s^2 = \big[T_{2sr} - T_{2r} - (\lambda_0 - r)\widehat{\sigma}_e^2\big]/(M - k_4) - (r-1)\widehat{\sigma}_{sr}^2/r. \tag{10.2.13}$$

where M is the total number of measurements, λ_0 is the number of non-empty subject-rater cells[6] (i, j), while k_4 is calculated by summing the quantities $m_{ij}/m_{\cdot j}$ over all subjects and raters (note that m_{ij} is the number of measurements associated with subject i and rater j, and $m_{\cdot j}$ the number of measurements associated with rater j).

⟹ T_{2y} is the summation of all squared scores y_{ijk}^2.

⟹ T_{2sr} is the summation of the quantities $y_{ij\cdot}^2/m_{ij}$ over all subjects and raters, where $y_{ij\cdot}$ is the sum of all measurements associated with subject i and rater j.

⟹ T_{2r} is the summation of the quantities $y_{\cdot j\cdot}^2/m_{\cdot j}$ over all raters j, with $y_{\cdot j\cdot}$ being the sum of all measurements associated with rater j.

Expressions for RSS and h_6 are complex and are fully specified in section 10.5.

• If $m = 1$ (i.e. no more than one measurement is taken per rater and per subject), then model 10.2.1 can no longer describe the ratings adequately. In this context, the rating associated with subject i and rater j is denoted by y_{ij} and is the result of the additive effect of the expected rating μ (known as the "intercept"), the subject effect s_i, the rater effect r_j, and the error effect e_{ij}. That is,

$$y_{ij} = \mu + s_i + r_j + e_{ij}, \qquad (10.2.14)$$

where the different effects are still subject to the same assumptions listed in the beginning of section 10.2. You may observe that the interaction term that existed in model 10.2.1 has now disappeared. In fact, it is now blended into the error term, since error and interaction become confounding factors when a single measurement is taken.

The intraclass correlation coefficient defining inter-rater reliability is now given by,

$$\rho = \sigma_s^2 / (\sigma_s^2 + \sigma_e^2). \qquad (10.2.15)$$

This ICC is calculated from experimental data as follows:

$$\text{ICC}(3, 1) = \widehat{\sigma}_s^2 / (\widehat{\sigma}_s^2 + \widehat{\sigma}_e^2), \qquad (10.2.16)$$

where $\widehat{\sigma}_e^2$ and $\widehat{\sigma}_s^2$ are given by,

$$\widehat{\sigma}_e^2 = (T_{2y} - \text{RSS})/(M - n - r + 1),$$
$$\widehat{\sigma}_s^2 = \left[\text{RSS} - T_{2r} - (n-1)\widehat{\sigma}_e^2\right]/(M - k_4).$$

---

[6]If the reliability experiment involves 2 raters and 3 subjects for example, then the total number of subject-rater cells would be $3 \times 2 = 6$. Suppose all subjects are rated by both raters, except subject #3 that is rated by rater #1 only. Therefore, the cell associated with subject #3 and rater #2 will be empty and does not count. The number of non-empty cells will then be $\lambda_0 = 5$ (i.e. $6 - 1 = 5$).

See section 10.5 for the calculation of RSS and h_6, and the previous bullet point for the definition of k_4, T_{2y}, and T_{2r}.

Note that intra-rater reliability cannot be evaluated when each rater only takes one measurement on subjects. Therefore $ICC_a(3,1)$ is not calculated in this situation.

10.3 Statistical Inference About the ICC

In the previous section, I defined the intraclass correlation coefficients ρ and γ and later described the procedures for computing them from experimental data using the statistics ICC(3,1) and $\mathrm{ICC}_a(3,1)$ respectively. Note that ICC(3,1) and $\mathrm{ICC}_a(3,1)$ are only two approximations to the two abstract parameters ρ and γ. A key question to be asked now is how close are these approximations to their respective estimands ρ and γ? Can we trust these approximations given the quality of the observed ratings? Two statistical procedures are used to address these important questions: the confidence interval and the test of hypothesis (or the p-value).

For a parameter such as ρ, the confidence interval will be the range of values that lie between a lower confidence bound (LCB) and an upper confidence bound (UCB), expected to contain the true (and unknown) value ρ with a pre-determined probability called the *Confidence Level*. The interest of the confidence interval is based on the fact that if the 2 confidence bounds are close to one another, their magnitude will tell the researcher about how high the true ICC ρ is expected to be. This same reasoning applies to γ the ICC for intra-rater reliability.

Sometimes the researcher wants to use the observed ratings to determine whether one may conclude that the intraclass correlation ρ (or γ) exceeds a hypothetical value[7] ρ_0 (or γ_0). The problem is that of testing the research hypothesis $\rho > \rho_0$. The p-value in this context, estimates how often we can expect an abstract summary statistic that depends on and is inversely proportional[8] to ρ, to exceed its observed value, which is calculated using the observed ratings and the hypothetical value ρ_0. The logic here is that if ρ actually exceeds ρ_0 as surmised, then the summary statistic based on ρ is expected to be below its observed value based on ρ_0, or will exceed it only with a very small probability[9]. Therefore, *a small p-value will be a strong indication that our research hypothesis is likely to be accurate.*

---

[7]Note that ρ_0 is specified by the researcher, and may represent a standard of acceptability in the profession.

[8]Two quantities are inversely proportional to each other when they change in opposite directions. That is when one goes up, the other goes down

[9]The summary statistic used here must be carefully chosen so that its probability distribution can be determined even if the ρ parameter upon which it depends is unknown.

10.3.1   *Confidence Interval for the Inter-Rater Reliability Coefficient*

Let ρ of equation 10.2.4 be the intraclass correlation for which we want to construct a confidence interval at a specified confidence level. Let $\alpha = 1 - $ *(Confidence Level)*. The confidence interval is defined by all values between the lower confidence bound LCB, and the upper confidence bound UCB. Once again I will treat multiple-measurement and single-measurement experiments separately.

MULTIPLE-MEASUREMENT EXPERIMENTS

In a typical multiple-measurement inter-rater reliability experiment, a rater may rate the same subject multiple times. I am assuming here that some subjects were rated multiple times by the same rater. Let M be the total number of ratings produced by all raters. The confidence bounds in this case are defined as follows:

$$\text{LCB} = \frac{\text{MSS} - F_1 \cdot \text{MSI}}{\text{MSS} + F_1 \big[(r-1)\text{MSI} + (M/n - r)\text{MSE} \big]}, \tag{10.3.1}$$

$$\text{UCB} = \frac{\text{MSS} - F_2 \cdot \text{MSI}}{\text{MSS} + F_2 \big[(r-1)\text{MSI} + (M/n - r)\text{MSE} \big]}, \tag{10.3.2}$$

These two confidence bounds involve many terms that we will now define.

▶ MSS is the Mean of Squares for Subjects, and is calculated by summing the squares $m_{i\cdot}(\overline{y}_{i\cdot\cdot} - \overline{y})^2$ over all n subjects, and by dividing the summation by $n - 1$. Note that $m_{i\cdot}$ represents the total number of ratings associated with subject i, and $\overline{y}_{i\cdot\cdot}$ the average rating associated with subject i.

▶ MSI is the Mean of Squares for Interaction, and is calculated by summing the expressions $m_{ij}(\overline{y}_{ij\cdot} - \overline{y}_{i\cdot\cdot} - \overline{y}_{\cdot j\cdot} + \overline{y})^2$ over all raters and subjects that were rated, with the summation being divided by $(r-1)(n-1)$. Moreover, m_{ij}, and $\overline{y}_{ij\cdot}$ are respectively the number of ratings and average rating associated with subject i and rater j.

▶ MSE is the Mean of Squares for Errors, and is calculated by summing the squares $(y_{ijk} - \overline{y}_{ij\cdot})^2$ over all raters and subjects that were rated, and by dividing the summation by $M/n - r$.

In addition to calculating all the means of squares, you will need to calculate the two quantities F_1 and F_2, which depend on the F probability distribution. Let a, and b be defined as follows:

$$a = \frac{1 + (r-1)\rho}{1 - \rho}, \text{ and } b = (M/n - r)\frac{\rho}{1-\rho}, \tag{10.3.3}$$

and v given by,

$$v = \frac{(a\text{MSI} + b\text{MSE})^2}{\dfrac{(a\text{MSI})^2}{(r-1)(n-1)} + \dfrac{(b\text{MSE})^2}{M - rn}} \qquad (10.3.4)$$

The two factors F_1 and F_2, are defined as follows:

▶ F_1 is the $100(1-\alpha/2)^{th}$ percentile of the F distribution with $n-1$ and v degrees of freedom.

▶ F_2 is the $100(\alpha/2)^{th}$ percentile of the F distribution with $n-1$ and v degrees of freedom.

Researchers familiar with anyone of the major statistical packages (e.g. SAS, SPSS, STATA, and others) may use them to calculate F_1 and F_2. For those not familiar with any major statistical software, one of the most convenient ways for obtaining these factors is to use Excel. With Windows/Mac Excel 2010/2011 or a more recent version you can obtain these two factors as follows (assume the confidence level is 95%, which implies that $\alpha = 1 - 0.95 = 0.05$):

$$= \text{F.INV}(1 - 0.05/2, n - 1, v) \quad \textit{(for } F_1\textit{)},$$

$$= \text{F.INV}(0.05/2, n - 1, v) \quad \textit{(for } F_2\textit{)},$$

v being a term that you will need to compute first using equation 10.3.4 along with the estimated value of ρ. The function F.INV, which was introduced with Excel 2010/2011, is not available in earlier versions. If you are using an earlier version of Excel (e.g. Excel 2007/2008 or earlier), then you will need to use the function FINV as follows:

$$= \text{FINV}(0.05/2, n - 1, v) \quad \textit{(for } F_1\textit{)},$$

$$= \text{FINV}(1 - 0.05/2, n - 1, v) \quad \textit{(for } F_2\textit{)}.$$

For readers who may want to understand the statistical theory underlying the confidence interval construction, I suggest to consider the statistic F defined as,

$$F = \frac{\text{MSS}}{a\text{MSI} + b\text{MSE}}. \qquad (10.3.5)$$

This statistic follows the F distribution with $n-1$ and v degrees of freedom. This result follows from the fact that $E(\text{MSS}) = aE(\text{MSI}) + bE(\text{MSE})$ and from Satterthwaite's approximation of the Chi-square distribution (see Satterthwaite (1946)). The F distribution may be derived from this Chi-square distribution, according to some standard results in mathematical statistics that are beyond the scope of this book.

SINGLE-MEASUREMENT EXPERIMENTS

Suppose now that the inter-rater reliability has produced no more than one rating per rater and per subject. Therefore, the two confidence bounds are given by,

$$\text{LCB} = \frac{F_{\text{L}} - 1}{F_{\text{L}} + (r - 1)}, \tag{10.3.6}$$

$$\text{UCB} = \frac{F_{\text{U}} - 1}{F_{\text{U}} + (r - 1)}, \tag{10.3.7}$$

where $F_{\text{L}} = F_{obs}/F_1$, $F_{\text{U}} = F_{obs}/F_2$, and $F_{obs} = \text{MSS}/\text{MSE}$. Moreover, F_1 is the $100(1 - \alpha/2)^{th}$ percentile of the F distribution with $n - 1$ and $(r - 1)(n - 1)$ degrees of freedom, while F_2 is the $100(\alpha/2)^{th}$ percentile of the F distribution with $n - 1$ and $(r - 1)(n - 1)$ degrees of freedom. These quantities can be calculated with Excel using the functions F.INV or FINV as explained above, with v being replaced with $(r - 1)(n - 1)$. The means of squares MSS and MSE are defined as follows:

▶ MSS is the Mean of Squares for Subjects, and is calculated by summing $r_i(\overline{y}_{i\cdot} - \overline{y})^2$ over all n subjects, and dividing the summation by $n - 1$. Moreover, $\overline{y}_{i\cdot}$ represents the average rating associated with subject i.

▶ MSE is the Mean of Squares for Errors, and is calculated by summing $(y_{ij} - \overline{y}_{i\cdot} - \overline{y}_{\cdot j} + \overline{y})^2$ over all raters and subjects that were rated, with the summation being divided by $(r - 1)(n - 1)$.

10.3.2   *Confidence Interval for the Intra-Rater Reliability Coefficient*

The concept of intra-rater reliability was explicitly formulated mathematically with equation 10.2.5. This parameter labeled as γ will generally be estimated from observed ratings with $\text{ICC}_a(3, 1)$ (see equation 10.2.10). Suppose you want to construct a 95% confidence interval around the "true" intra-rater reliability coefficient γ. That is, you want to specify a range of values expected to contain the "true" intra-rater reliability coefficient 95% of times a reliability experiment is performed under the same conditions. As indicated earlier, this range of values is expressed in the form of an interval defined by its lower bound LCB and its upper bound UCB to be defined. 95% is known as the confidence level (CL) associated with the interval.

Let F_1 and F_2 be respectively the $100(\alpha/2)^{th}$ and $100(1 - \alpha/2)^{th}$ percentiles of the F distribution with v and $M - rn$ degrees of freedom, where n is the number of subjects, $\alpha = 1 - $ *(Confidence Interval)*, and v is defined as follows:

$$v = \frac{(a\text{MSS} + b\text{MSI})^2}{\dfrac{(a\text{MSS})^2}{n - 1} + \dfrac{(b\text{MSI})^2}{(r - 1)(n - 1)}}, \tag{10.3.8}$$

with a and b defined as,

$$a = \frac{1}{(r+1) + \dfrac{M\gamma}{n(1-\gamma)}}, \text{ and } b = \frac{r}{(r+1) + \dfrac{M\gamma}{n(1-\gamma)}}. \tag{10.3.9}$$

The two confidence bounds can be defined as follows:

$$\text{LCB} = \frac{\text{MSS} + r\text{MSI} - (r+1)F_2\text{MSE}}{\text{MSS} + r\text{MSI} + [M/n - r - 1]F_2 \cdot \text{MSE}}, \tag{10.3.10}$$

$$\text{UCB} = \frac{\text{MSS} + r\text{MSI} - (r+1)F_1\text{MSE}}{\text{MSS} + r\text{MSI} + [M/n - r - 1]F_1 \cdot \text{MSE}}. \tag{10.3.11}$$

The different means of squares that are part of equations 10.3.10 and 10.3.11 are defined right after equations 10.3.2. The calculation of F_1 and F_2 can be done with Excel or with one of the major statistical packages. When using Excel 2010/2011 or a more recent version, proceed as follows:

$$= \textsf{F.INV}((1 - CL)/2, v, M - rn) \quad \text{(for } F_1\text{)},$$

$$= \textsf{F.INV}(1 - (1 - CL)/2, v, M - rn \quad \text{(for } F_2\text{)}.$$

The following example illustrates the construction of 95% confidence intervals for inter-rater and intra-rater reliability coefficients.

Example 10.2 _____

Let uss consider the observed ratings displayed in Table 10.4. These ratings were produced by 4 judges who rated 5 subjects labeled as {1, 2, 3, 4, 5} multiple times. While some subjects were rated once, others were rated 4 times. Our goal is to use this data to compute both the inter-rater and intra-rater reliability coefficients as well as the associated 95% confidence interval.

Since the rating dataset of Table 10.4 is balanced (i.e. all subjects have the same number ratings), equations 10.2.6 and 10.2.9 will yield the same inter-rater reliability coefficient. Likewise, equations 10.2.7 and 10.10 will yield the same intra-rater reliability coefficient. For simplicity sake, equations 10.2.6 and 10.2.7 will be used for computing the inter-rater and intra-rater reliability coefficients. As for the confidence intervals, the lower and upper confidence bounds will be calculated using equations 10.3.1 and 10.3.2 for inter-rater reliability, and equations 10.3.10 and 10.3.11 for intra-rater reliability.

The three means of squares that we need here are the following:

- MSS = 23.3102,   - MSI = 2.2446,   - MSE = 1.1618.

Readers interessted in getting more details about the calculations shown in this example should look at the Excel worksheet named "Example 10.2" contained in the downloadable Excel workbook "`www.agreestat.com/book4/chapter10examples.xlx`."

Using equation 10.2.6 and the means of squares shown above, one can obtain the estimated inter-rater reliability coefficient of $ICC(3, 1) = 0.5122$. As for the 95% confidence interval, its lower and upper confidence bounds are obtained from equations 10.3.1 and 10.3.2 as LCB = 0.2159, and UCB = 0.9141.

Based on equation 10.2.7 and the means of squares computed above, the estimated intra-rater reliability coefficient can be calculated as $ICC_a(3, 1) = 0.6551$. As for the associated 95% confidence interval, its lower and upper confidence bounds are calculated from equations 10.3.10 and 10.3.11 as LCB = 0.3179, and UCB = 0.9053.

Table 10.4: Ratings of 5 Subjects by 4 Judges

Subject	Judge (j)			
(i)	Judge 1	Judge 2	Judge 3	Judge 4
1	6	1	3	2
1	6.5	3	3	4
1	4	3	5.5	4
5	10	5	6	9
5	9	4.5	5	9
5	9.5	4	6.6	8
4	6	2	4	7
4	7	1	3	6
4	8	2.5	4	5
2	9	2	5	8
2	7	1	2	6
2	8	2	2	7
3	10	5	6	9
3	7	4	6	5
3	8	4	6	8

10.3.3   *p-Value about the Inter-Rater Reliability Coefficient*

In the beginning of section 10.3, I explained the concept of *p*-value, and will now show the steps for computing it. Once again, I will treat multiple-trial and single-trial experiments separately. I assume that the researcher has a reference value ρ_0 to which the "true" intraclass correlation ρ must be compared. More formally, I want to test the research hypothesis that $\rho > \rho_0$ using the p-value.

The p-Value for Multiple-Trial Inter-Rater Reliability Experiments

(a) Compute the three means of squares MSS, MSI, and MSE as described in section 10.3.1 following equation 10.3.2.

(b) Compute the values a and b of equation 10.3.3 where ρ is replaced with ρ_0.

(c) Compute the number of degrees of freedom v as shown in equation 10.3.4, using the numbers computed in the previous two steps.

(d) Compute F_{obs} based on equation 10.3.5 initially developed for F, and using a, b, and the means of squares of the previous steps.

(e) The p-value is calculated as the probability that F exceeds F_{obs}, where F is a random variable that follows the F distribution with $n - 1$ and v degrees of freedom. That is,

$$p\text{-}Value = P\big(F \geq F_{obs}\big).$$

Users who do not have access to a major statistical software to compute this p-value, may still compute it using Excel as follows:

$= \text{F.DIST.RT}(F_{obs}, n - 1, v)$ *(for Excel 2010/2011 or a later version),*

$= \text{FDIST}(F_{obs}, n - 1, v)$ *(for Excel 2007/2008 or an earlier version).*

The p-Value for Single-Trial Inter-Rater Reliability Experiments

The p-value calculation is straightforward in this situation, and can be obtained with fewer steps.

(a) Compute the two means of squares MSS, and MSE as described in section 10.3.1 following equation 10.3.7.

(b) Compute F_{obs} as follows:

$$F_{obs} = \frac{\text{MSS}}{\text{MSE}} \times \frac{1 - \rho_0}{1 + (r - 1)\rho_0}.$$

(e) The p-value is calculated as the probability for F to exceed F_{obs}, with F being a random variable that follows the F distribution with $n - 1$ and $(r - 1)(n - 1)$ degrees of freedom. That is,

$$p\text{-}Value = P\big(F \geq F_{obs}\big).$$

Users without access to a major statistical software may still compute the p-value using Excel as follows:

$= \text{F.DIST.RT}(F_{obs}, n - 1, (r - 1)(n - 1))$ *(Excel 2010/2011 or newer ver.),*

$= \text{FDIST}(F_{obs}, n - 1, (r - 1)(n - 1))$ *(Excel 2007/2008 or earlier version)*

10.3.4   *p-Value about the Intra-Rater Reliability Coefficient*

In this section, I will show how to compute the p-value for testing the hypothesis that the intra-rater reliability coefficient γ exceeds a predetermined value arbitrarily denoted by γ_0. Once you observe your ratings, the question becomes "is the gathered evidence supporting the research hypothesis?" The p-value provides an answer to this question.

The rating-based evidence needed to evaluate the research hypothesis is summarized by a statistic F defined by,

$$F = \frac{a_0 \text{MSS} + b_0 \text{MSI}}{\text{MSE}}, \qquad (10.3.12)$$

where a_0 and b_0 are given by equation 10.3.9 in which γ is replaced with γ_0, and the means of squares defined in the paragraph following equation 10.3.2. This statistic follows the F distribution with v and $M - rn$ degrees of freedom. The strength of this evidence is measured by the probability that this variable exceeds its calculated value based on observed ratings. The procedure for obtaining the p-value is the following:

(a) Compute the three means of squares MSS, MSI, and MSE as described in the beginning of section 10.3.1.

(b) Compute the values a_0 and b_0 as discussed above.

(c) Compute the number of degrees of freedom v of equation 10.3.8 using the a_0 and b_0 values of step (b) in place of a and b.

(d) Compute F_{obs}, the observed value of F of equation 10.3.12.

(e) The p-value is calculated as the probability for F to exceed F_{obs}, with F being a random variable that follows the F distribution with v and $M - rn$ degrees of freedom. That is,

$$p\text{-}Value = P\big(F \geq F_{obs}\big).$$

Users without access to a major statistical software may still compute the p-value using Excel as follows:

$= \text{F.DIST.RT}(F_{obs}, v, M - rn)$ *(for Excel 2010/2011 or a newer version),*

$= \text{FDIST}(F_{obs}, v, M - rn)$ *(for Excel 2007/2008 or an earlier version)*

The purpose of the next example is to illustrate the p-value calculation for both the inter-rater and intra-rater reliability coefficients. The same dataset of Table 10.4 used in example 10.2 will be used again for that purpose.

Example 10.3 _____

Using Table 10.4 data, I want to test the hypothesis that the "true" inter-rater reliability coefficient ρ and the "true" intra-rater reliability coefficient γ both exceed 0.5. That is, both coefficients share the same hypothetical value $\rho_0 = \gamma_0 = 0$.

In Example 10.2, I estimated the inter-rater reliability coefficient ρ using Table 10.4 data as $ICC(3, 1) = 0.5122$, and the intra-rater reliability γ was estimated by $ICC_a(3, 1) = 0.6551$. The fact that the estimated value of ρ exceeds 0.50 by itself does not guarantee that ρ exceeds 0.50. Likewise, the fact that the estimated value of γ based on our specific observed ratings exceeds 0.5 does not guarantee that γ itself exceeds 0.5. It is because the estimated value is subject to random variation due to the selection of subjects. A different subject sample may produce different estimates that could be below 0.5. Therefore, the interpretation of our estimated values must be statistical and should account for the random errors that may cause estimates to exceed the "true" values being estimated.

Table 10.5 shows the p-values associated with inter-rater and intra-rater reliability coefficients for different values of ρ_0 and γ_0. For each value of ρ_0/γ_0, I calculated F_{obs} for both inter-rater and intra-rater reliability coefficients using the means of squares MSS and MSE of Example 10.2. You may want to look at the "Examples 10.3" worksheet in the Excel workbook,

    www.agreestat.com/book4/chapter10examples.xlsx,
for more details regarding how these p-values were obtained.

Note that rating data are deemed consistent with the hypothesis that $\rho > \rho_0$ only if the p-value remains below the widely-accepted threshold of 0.05. Table 10.5 shows that the inter-rater reliability p-value remains below that threshold as long as ρ_0 is 0.2 or smaller. However, the intra-rater reliability p-value is below the threshold of 0.05 if the γ_0 is 0.3 or smaller. Consequently, Table 10.4 rating data do not support the research hypothesis stating that $\rho > 0.50$ or $\gamma > 0.5$.

Table 10.5: p-Values for testing the hypotheses $\rho > \rho_0$ and $\gamma > \gamma_0$

ρ_0/γ_0	Inter-Rater Reliability		Intra-Rater Reliability	
	F_{obs}	p-value	F_{obs}	p-value
0	10.3849	0.000716929	5.5582	0.000160773
0.1	5.4527	0.003899012	4.3881	0.001083587
0.2	3.4215	0.023121064	3.4739	0.005321516
0.3	2.3134	0.081271646	2.7400	0.020180109
0.4	1.6158	0.19516304	2.1378	0.06141524
0.5	1.1361	0.356612668	1.6348	0.153731511
0.6	0.7861	0.542254881	1.2083	0.320731392

10.4   Sample Size Calculations

This section addresses the problem of sample size determination when designing inter-rater and intra-rater reliability studies under the mixed factorial model. It provides guidelines and methods for calculating the number of raters and number of subjects required in order to achieve the prescribed precision level with which inter-rater or intra-rater reliability coefficients must be estimated. Before the proposed methods can be used, the researcher must specify the desired precision level. The precision of the ICC estimate can be specified by the length of the associated 95% confidence interval[10]. More information regarding the use of confidence intervals for this purpose may be found in Giraudeau and Mary (2001), and in Doros and Lew (2010). In the previous chapters, I recommended that the desired confidence interval length (L) be expressed as a fraction of the the ICC value, and suggested $L = 0.4 \times$ ICC as being a reasonable precision level for the intraclass correlation coefficient[11]. You may decide to obtain a more precise ICC estimate by setting a confidence interval length that represents an even smaller fraction of the ICC, such as $0.2 \times ICC$.

Section 10.4.1 is devoted to the inter-rater reliability coefficient, while section 10.4.2 focuses on the intra-rater reliability coefficient. Note that the inter-rater and intra-rater reliability coefficients have conflicting sample size requirements. A good inter-rater reliability study requires fewer raters and more subjects, whereas a good intra-rater reliability study requires more raters and fewer subjects. Consequently, if the same study is designed for both types of coefficients, a compromise will be necessary.

10.4.1   *Sample Size Calculations for Inter-Rater Reliability*

For a given number of ratings per rater, the most efficiency strategy for obtaining an accurate inter-rater reliability coefficient is to maximize the number of subjects by allowing the raters to produce a single rating for each subject. For example, if each rater must produce a total of 14 ratings, rather than producing 2 ratings on each of 7 subjects, the inter-rater reliability coefficient will be more precise if the design is based on 14 subjects and 1 rating per subject. If the recruitment of subjects is costly, then the researcher may want to increase the number of ratings per rater by rating some subjects more than once. This strategy will result in a loss of precision in the estimation of the inter-rater reliability coefficient.

---

[10]The 95% confidence interval associated with an ICC estimate is a range of values expected to contain the "true" value of the ICC 95% of the times.

[11]In the classical context of population mean estimation, this condition would ensure a coefficient of variation that does not exceed 20%.

In this section, I will first assume that there will be a single rating per rater and per subject (i.e. no replication). This will allow you to determine the number of subjects and raters that can yield your desired confidence interval length. If this optimal number of subjects is deemed unduly high, you will be able to explore some options for reducing the number of subjects while maintaining the same number of ratings per rater. This is typically achieved by increasing the number of ratings per subject for each rater. You will see how much you will lose in precision by using this alternative approach, before deciding whether it should be considered or not.

NUMBER OF RATERS AND SUBJECTS - NO REPLICATION

With the mixed factorial design, researchers generally know ahead of time how many raters will be used in the inter-rater reliability study. One retains all the raters willing to be part of the investigation. However, our investigation has revealed that, for a given number of ratings per rater, using more than 5 raters can increase the precision of the inter-rater reliability only marginally. This explains why I have investigated this problem for 2, 3, 4, and 5 raters.

Figure 10.4.1 depicts the length of the 95% confidence interval associated with the inter-rater reliability coefficient as a function of the number of subjects, and the magnitude of the ICC, when the number of raters is limited to 2. An examination of this figure reveals the following facts:

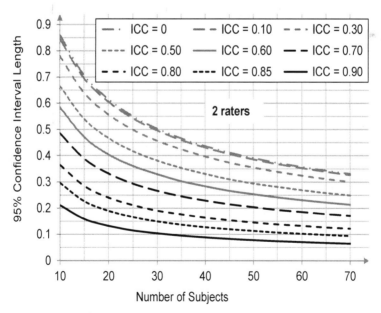

Figure 10.4.1: 95% C.I. Length by Number of Subjects for 2 Raters

- For any given ICC value, the confidence interval length decreases (i.e. precision improves) as the number of subjects increases. That is, having more subjects in the experiment can only improve the quality of the inter-rater reliability coefficient.

- For any given number of subjects, the interval length decreases as the ICC value increases. Consequently, your experiment will yield a more accurate inter-rater reliability coefficient if the extent of agreement among raters is high. This is logical because raters who agree are homogeneous with respect to the way they rate subjects. Therefore, a handful of subjects will generally be sufficient to tell an accurate story regarding the extent to which they agree.

The lesson to be learned here is that giving some training to the raters prior to conducting the experiment is likely to pay off, and the payoff could be big. If ICC=0 indicating total absence of agreement, then achieving a desired precision level may become an impossible task.

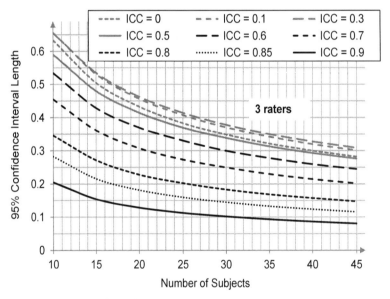

Figure 10.4.2: 95% C.I. Length by Number of Subjects for three Raters

Suppose you know that your study will involve two raters only, and want to know how many subjects to recruit. To be able to use Figure 10.4.1, you will need two things: (*i*) a predicted ICC value (i.e. a predicted inter-rater reliability coefficient), and (*ii*) the desired confidence interval length (e.g. $0.4 \times$ ICC). The predicted ICC often comes from a pilot or a prior study. This initial ICC value is essential and obtaining it is part of the preliminary exploratory analysis necessary for an effective study design. Assume for example that this initial value is $ICC_0 = 0.70$. This leads to our desired 95% confidence interval length of $0.4 \times$ ICC $= 0.4 \times 0.70 = 0.28$.

On figure 10.4.1 you will use the fourth curve from the bottom (the one associated with the ICC value of 0.70) to find that the desired precision can be achieved with approximately 25 subjects.

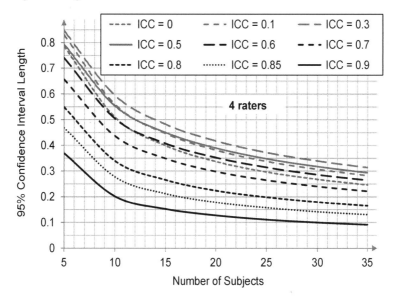

Figure 10.4.3: 95% C.I. Length by Number of Subjects for 4 Raters

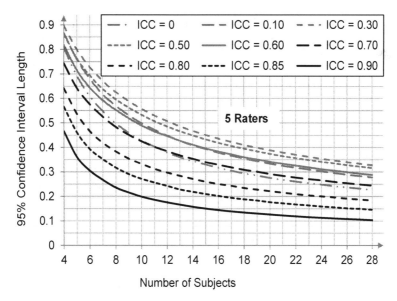

Figure 10.4.4: 95% C.I. Length by Number of Subjects for 5 Raters

Figure 10.4.2 shows that with 3 raters in your experiment, you will need about 21 subjects to achieve the same precision level. Four raters will require about 20 subjects as seen in figures 10.4.3, while five raters requires 19 subjects as seen in figure 10.4.4. That is using more than 4 raters will not further reduce the number of subjects for a given precision level.

NUMBER OF RATERS AND SUBJECTS - WITH REPLICATION

The example previously discussed revealed that an inter-rater reliability experiment based on 2 raters requires 25 subjects to achieve a 95% confidence length of 0.28. The question I want to answer now is the following: can one use fewer subjects and 2 trials per subject and still be able to achieve a reasonable interval length? The figures 10.4.5 through 10.4.12 can help answer this question.

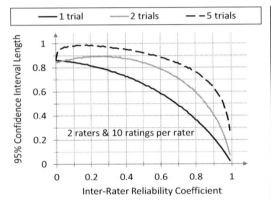 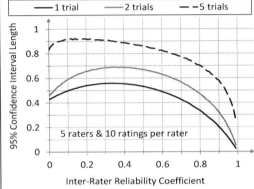

Figure 10.4.5: Interval length by inter-rater reliability & number of trials (2 raters & 10 ratings per rater).

Figure 10.4.6: Interval length by inter-rater reliability & number of trials (5 raters & 10 ratings per rater).

Figure 10.4.5 shows the 95% confidence interval length as a function of the "true" inter-rater reliability coefficient, and the number of trials, for a study that is based on 2 raters and 10 ratings per rater. Since the continuous black curve is associated with 1 trial, it represents an inter-rater reliability experiment with 2 raters, 10 subjects and 1 trial (i.e. $10 \times 1 = 10$ ratings per rater). Likewise the gray curve describes the relationship between the precision of the estimated inter-rater reliability and its actual value for an experiment based on 2 raters, 5 subjects and 2 trials (i.e. $5 \times 2 = 10$ ratings per rater). As for the dotted black line it refers to an experiment with 2 raters, 2 subjects and 5 trials (i.e. $2 \times 5 = 10$ ratings per rater). Figures 10.4.5 through 10.4.12 all indicate that the smaller the number of trials, the more accurate the estimate of the inter-rater reliability coefficient. Using more than 3 trials will likely result in a substantial loss of precision for a given number of ratings per subject.

Figure 10.4.9 shows that an inter-rater reliability experiment that is based on 2 raters, 15 subjects and 2 trials (i.e. $15 \times 2 = 30$ ratings per rater) will yield a 95% confidence interval length of about 0.45. We saw earlier that 25 subjects and 1 trials will yield an interval length of 0.28. Consequently, reducing the number of subjects has a negative impact on the precision of estimates that can be substantial even if the total number of ratings per rater increases.

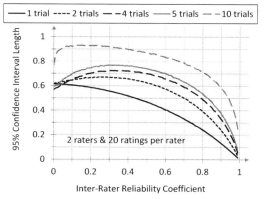

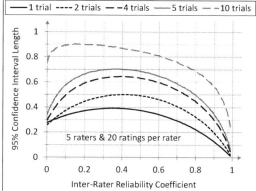

Figure 10.4.7: Interval length by IRR & # of trials (2 raters & 20 ratings per rater).

Figure 10.4.8: Interval length by IRR & # of trials (5 raters & 20 ratings per rater).

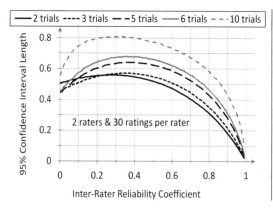

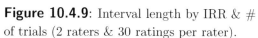

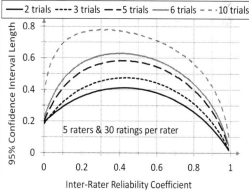

Figure 10.4.9: Interval length by IRR & # of trials (2 raters & 30 ratings per rater).

Figure 10.4.10: Interval length by IRR & # of trials (5 raters & 30 ratings per rater).

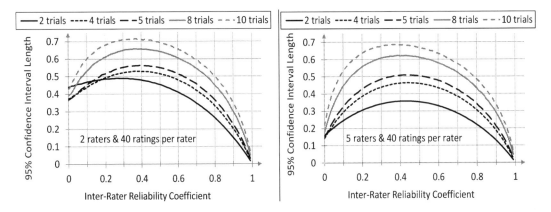

Figure 10.4.11: Interval length by IRR & # of trials (2 raters & 40 ratings per rater).

Figure 10.4.12: Interval length by IRR & # of trials (5 raters & 40 ratings per rater).

10.4.2   *Sample Size Calculations for Intra-Rater Reliability*

The purpose of an intra-rater reliability study is to evaluate the reproducibility of ratings. The researcher quantifies the extent to which the raters can replicate the rating procedures and consistently produce comparable ratings. Under the mixed factorial design, the researcher generally knows how many raters will be tested. However, because of both the subject and subject-rater interaction effects, subjects are expected to have an impact on the reproducibility of ratings. Moreover, the number trials plays a pivotal role in the quantification of reproducibility, since these trials produce a set of ratings associated with the same rater and the same subject. Therefore, the researcher needs to determine the optimal number of subjects and trials to consider for the experiment that will produce the desired confidence interval length.

Here are a few things researchers need to know upfront:

• Using only 2 trials in an intra-rater reliability is a bad thing, unless you know from prior studies or from a pilot study that reproducibility is expected to be high. Reproducibility needs to exceed 0.6 when using 2 raters, and needs to exceed 0.3 when using 3 raters or more, if you want 2 trials to produce an acceptable precision level for the intra-rater reliability coefficient. If reproducibility as measured by the ICC can be below 0.3, then using only 2 trials may lead to poor results, with estimates of intra-rater reliability that are very unreliable.

• For a given number of ratings per rater, the best results are generally obtained with 3, 4, or 5 trials. Using more than 5 trials will generally decrease the precision of the intra-rater reliability coefficient for the same number ratings. Therefore, if you have a fixed number of ratings per rater that you cannot exceed, then I would strongly recommend using 3 or 4 trials, since a good balance must be found between the number subjects and the number of trials.

Figures 10.4.13 through 10.4.36 depict the relationship between the length of the 95% confidence interval and the magnitude of the intra-rater reliability coefficient. The confidence interval is associated with the intra-rater reliability coefficient that will be estimated using observed ratings. Its expected length is what is depicted on the graph. The magnitude of the intra-rater reliability coefficient is generally replaced at the design stage with a surrogate obtained from a pilot study or from old studies.

The figures 10.4.13 through 10.4.36 do not cover all possible scenarios, although they give you a glimpse into what you can expect in terms the precision associated with your intra-rater reliability coefficient. Let us consider figure 10.4.13 for example. It assumes an intra-rater reliability study using 2 raters and 10 ratings per subject. There are 2 possible designs that give you 10 ratings per rater. One possibility is to use 5 subjects and 2 trials, and a second possibility is to use 2 subjects and 5 trials. These 2 possibilities are represented with the continuous black curve (for 5 raters and 2 trials) and the continuous gray curve (for 2 raters and 5 trials). It follows from this chart that if you anticipate high reproducibility represented by an inter-rater reliability coefficient that exceeds 0.8, then using 2 trials is expected to yield the most accurate coefficients. However, if reproducibility is below 0.7 then using only 2 raters will yield a wide confidence interval; therefore an intra-rater reliability coefficient that is very unreliable. An examination of the remaining curves reveals that using more raters or more ratings per rater improve the precision of the intra-rater reliability coefficient.

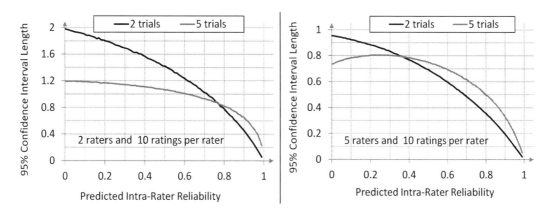

Figure 10.4.13: Interval length by IRR & # of trials (2 raters & 10 ratings per rater). **Figure 10.4.14**: Interval length by IRR & # of trials (5 raters & 10 ratings per rater).

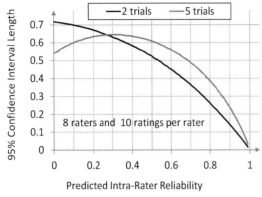

Figure 10.4.15: Interval length by IRR & # of trials (8 raters & 10 ratings per rater)

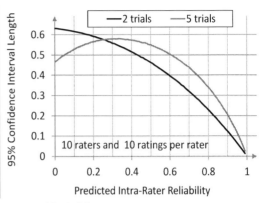

Figure 10.4.16: Interval length by IRR & # of trials (10 raters & 10 ratings per rater)

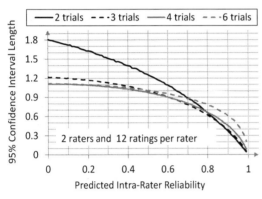

Figure 10.4.17: Interval length by IRR & # of trials (2 raters & 12 ratings per rater)

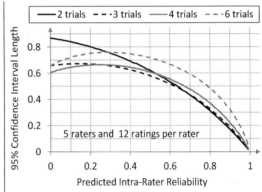

Figure 10.4.18: Interval length by IRR & # of trials (5 raters & 12 ratings per rater)

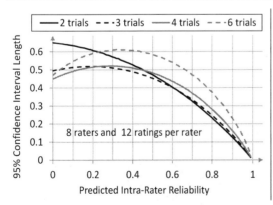

Figure 10.4.19: Interval length by IRR & # of trials (8 raters & 12 ratings per rater)

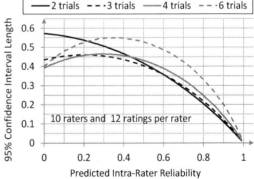

Figure 10.4.20: Interval length by IRR & # of trials (10 raters & 12 ratings per rater)

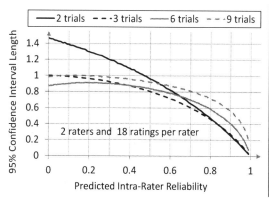

Figure 10.4.21: Interval length by IRR & # of trials (2 raters & 18 ratings per rater)

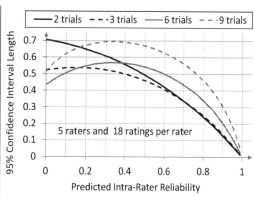

Figure 10.4.22: Interval length by IRR & # of trials (5 raters & 18 ratings per rater)

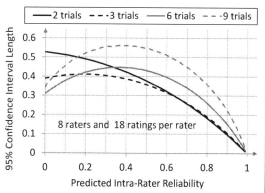

Figure 10.4.23: Interval length by IRR & # of trials (8 raters & 18 ratings per rater)

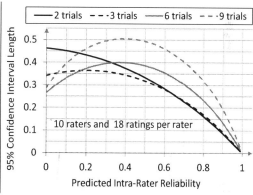

Figure 10.4.24: Interval length by IRR & # of trials (10 raters & 18 ratings per rater)

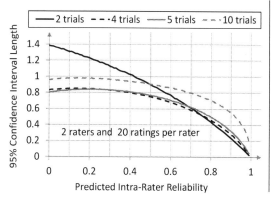

Figure 10.4.25: Interval length by IRR & # of trials (2 raters & 20 ratings per rater)

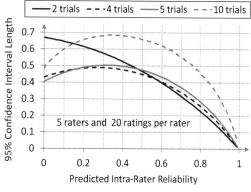

Figure 10.4.26: Interval length by IRR & # of trials (5 raters & 20 ratings per rater)

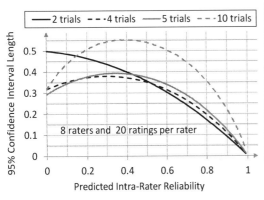

Figure 10.4.27: Interval length by IRR & # of trials (8 raters & 20 ratings per rater)

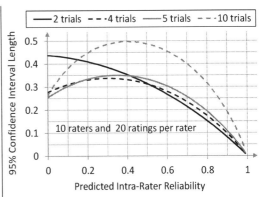

Figure 10.4.28: Interval length by IRR & # of trials (10 raters & 20 ratings per rater)

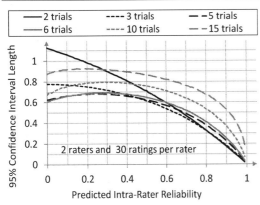

Figure 10.4.29: Interval length by IRR & # of trials (2 raters & 30 ratings per rater)

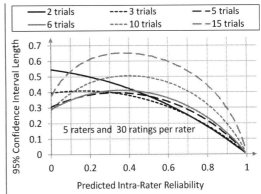

Figure 10.4.30: Interval length by IRR & # of trials (5 raters & 30 ratings per rater)

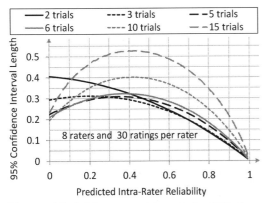

Figure 10.4.31: Interval length by IRR & # of trials (8 raters & 30 ratings per rater)

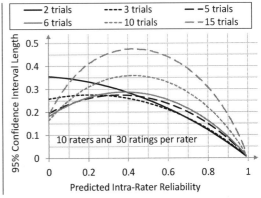

Figure 10.4.32: Interval length by IRR & # of trials (10 raters & 30 ratings per rater)

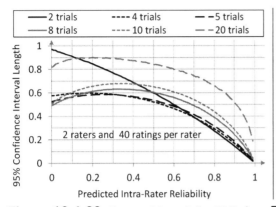

Figure 10.4.33: Interval length by IRR & # of trials (2 raters & 40 ratings per rater)

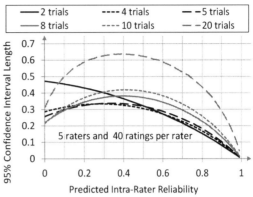

Figure 10.4.34: Interval length by IRR & # of trials (5 raters & 40 ratings per rater)

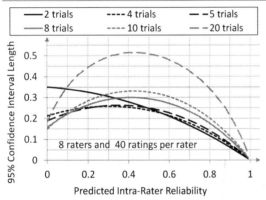

Figure 10.4.35: Interval length by IRR & # of trials (8 raters & 40 ratings per rater)

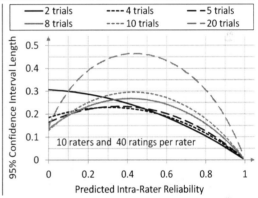

Figure 10.4.36: Interval length by IRR & # of trials (10 raters & 40 ratings per rater)

10.5   Special Topics

10.5.1   *Calculations of RSS and h_6 Related to Equation 10.2.12*

This section is very technical and not needed to understand the material presented in this chapter. Its goal to show the different steps needed to compute the terms RSS and h_6 required for obtaining the ICC of equations 10.2.9 and 10.2.10 when your experimental data contain missing scores. A computer programmer wanting to write a software for calculating $\mathrm{ICC}(3,1)$ or $\mathrm{ICC}_a(3,1)$ when some scores are missing, may find this material useful.

▶ *Creating the $(r-1) \times (r-1)$ matrix $\boldsymbol{F} = \left(f_{jj'}\right)$ for $j, j' = 1, \cdots, r-1$*

Let n be the number of subjects, and r the number of raters that participated in the inter-rater reliability experiment. The $\boldsymbol{F}$ matrix is defined as the sum of n matrices $\boldsymbol{F}_i$ (with $i = 1, \cdots, n$), each of which being of size $(r-1) \times (r-1)$. A typical element $f_{jj'}^{(i)}$ associated with the j-*th* row, and the j'-*th* column of matrix $\boldsymbol{F}_i$, is defined as follows:

$$f_{jj'}^{(i)} = \begin{cases} (m_{ij}^2/m_{i.})(\lambda_i + m_{i.} - 2m_{ij}), & \text{if } j = j', \\ (m_{ij}m_{ij'}/m_{i.})(\lambda_i - m_{ij} - m_{ij'}), & \text{if } j \neq j', \end{cases} \tag{10.5.1}$$

where $j, j' = 1, \cdots, r-1$, and λ_i given by[12]:

$$\lambda_i = \sum_{j=1}^{r} m_{ij}^2/m_{i.}$$

Recall that m_{ij} represents the number of measurements associated with subject i and rater j. If rater j does not rate subject i then we will have $m_{ij} = 0$. On the other hand, $m_{i.}$ is the number of measurements associated with subject i. Calculating the quantities $f_{jj'}^{(i)}$ requires that you use only $r-1$ of the r raters available. It does not matter which subset of $r-1$ raters you use, since all possible sub-groups of $r-1$ raters will yield the same RSS and h_6 values. Each element $f_{jj'}$ of matrix $\boldsymbol{F}$ is defined by,

$$f_{jj'} = \sum_{i=1}^{n} f_{jj'}^{(i)}, \tag{10.5.2}$$

---

[12]Note that for the purpose of calculating λ_i, all r subjects must be used

where $f_{jj'}^{(i)}$ is defined by equation 10.5.1. Although matrix $\boldsymbol{F}$ is the sum of the n matrices $\boldsymbol{F}_i$, there is no need to first create all n matrices $\boldsymbol{F}_i$ before summing them. It is more effective to directly compute each $\boldsymbol{F}$-element $f_{jj'}$ from equation 10.5.2.

▶ *Creating the $(r-1) \times (r-1)$ matrix $\boldsymbol{C} = (c_{jj'})$ for $j, j' = 1, \cdots, r-1$*

The purpose of this step is to create a single matrix $\boldsymbol{C}$, defined as follows:

$$
c_{jj'} = \begin{cases} m_{\cdot j} - \displaystyle\sum_{i=1}^{n} \frac{m_{ij}^2}{m_{i\cdot}}, & \text{if } j = j', \\[2ex] -\displaystyle\sum_{i=1}^{n} \frac{m_{ij}m_{ij'}}{m_{i\cdot}}, & \text{if } j \neq j'. \end{cases}
$$

Note that $m_{\cdot j}$ is the number of measurements associated with rater j. The subset of $r-1$ raters used to create matrix $\boldsymbol{C}$ must be the same as the one used in the previous step to create matrix $\boldsymbol{C}$.

▶ *Creating the r-dimensional vector $\boldsymbol{b} = (b_j)$ for $j = 1, \cdots, r-1$*

For each rater j in the subset of $r-1$ raters defined in the previous steps, b_j is defined by,

$$
b_j = y_{\cdot j\cdot} - \sum_{i=1}^{n} m_{ij} \overline{y}_{i\cdot\cdot},
$$

where $y_{\cdot j\cdot}$ is the summation of all measurements associated with rater j, while $\overline{y}_{i\cdot\cdot}$ is the average of all measurements associated with subject i.

▶ *Calculating RSS*

$$
\text{RSS} = T_{2s} + \boldsymbol{b}^\top \boldsymbol{C}^{-1} \boldsymbol{b},
$$

where T_{2s} is the summation of the terms $y_{i\cdot\cdot}^2/m_{i\cdot}$ over all n subjects, with $y_{i\cdot\cdot}$ being the summation of all measurements associated with subject i. $\boldsymbol{C}^{-1}$ is the inverse of matrix $\boldsymbol{C}$.

▶ *Calculating h_6*

h_6 is calculated as $h_6 = M - k^*$ where k^* is given by,

$$
k^* = \sum_{i=1}^{n} \lambda_i + \text{tr}\left(\boldsymbol{C}^{-1} \sum_{i=1}^{n} \boldsymbol{F}_i \right),
$$

and M the total number of measurements obtained from the experiment. The symbol tr represents the trace (i.e. the sum of all diagonal elements) of the matrix in parentheses.

Because the calculations needed to obtain RSS and h_6 can be complex, I like to recommend simple verification procedures here, which computer programmers can use for testing purposes.

(a) First create a vector b and matrix C using all r raters that participated in the inter-rater reliability experiment. That is, b will be of size r and C of size $r \times r$.

(b) Verify now that all b-values sum to 0, and that each separate column of the C matrix sums to 0. If that is the case, then you know for sure that your calculations are correct.

(c) You may now remove one rater from vector b and the corresponding row and column from matrix C so b is of size r-1 and C of size $(r - 1) \times (r - 1)$. If you chose to remove the last rater, you may simply drop the last element of your vector b vector of step (a), then drop the last row and last column of matrix C of step (a).

Note that if you decide to use all r raters for calculating RSS and h_6 then you will run into serious trouble. It is because matrix C will not have an inverse, because of condition (b) above. Therefore, it is crucial to base all of your calculations for RSS and h_6 only on a subset of $r - 1$ raters of your choice.

10.5.2   *How are the Power Curves Obtained ?*

In section 10.4, I presented a number of charts that depict the confidence interval length as a function of the intraclass correlation coefficient, and possibly the number of replicates (or trials) used in the experiment. I like to describe here how these different curves were obtained. The general approach is based on the Monte Carlo simulation that consists of generating 10,000 confidence intervals (hence 10,000 interval lengths) for each ICC value. The average interval length is then associated with the ICC value used to produce one point on the curve. The process is repeated for several ICC values to obtained a curve.

INTER-RATER RELIABILITY BASED ON ONE TRIAL PER RATER AND PER SUBJECT

When the inter-rater reliability experiment is based on a single trial then the lower and upper confidence bounds are given by equations 10.3.6 and 10.3.7, which can be re-written as follows:

$$\text{LCB} = \frac{\text{FSS}/F_1 - 1}{\text{FSS}/F_1 + (r-1)}, \text{ and UCB} = \frac{\text{FSS} \times F_2 - 1}{\text{FSS} \times F_2 + (r-1)}, \qquad (10.5.3)$$

where FSS = MSS/MSE. Once these two interval bounds are determined, one can compute the interval length as Length = UCB − LCB. But these two bounds are determined only if FSS (which is a function of ρ) is known. To create the power curves, we need a series of points (ρ, Length), which is obtained as follows:

(a) First determine the set of ρ values for which to compute a confidence interval length. For the charts used in this chapter, we used 100 ρ values $0, 0.1, 0.2, \cdots, 0.99$.

(b) Generate a random variate $F^\star$ according to the F distribution with $n-1$ and $(r-1)(n-1)$ degrees of freedom. The discussions in section 10.3.3 revealed that the statistic $\text{FSS}(1-\rho)/[1+(r-1)\rho]$ follows the F distribution with $n-1$ and $(r-1)(n-1)$ degrees of freedom. Therefore, $\text{FSS} = F^\star[1+(r-1)\rho]/(1-\rho)$.

(c) Using the FSS of step (b), compute the two interval bounds and the interval length for each ρ defined in step (a). At this stage, you should have obtained an interval length for each of the 100 ρ values. Store them in a file for use at a later time.

(d) Repeat this process from step (b) a large number of times (e.g. 10,000 times or more).

In the end of this process you will have 10,000 different confidence interval interval lengths for each of the 100 ρ values used in the simulation experiment. For each ρ value, average the 10,000 lengths to obtain a single mean length, which can be used to construct the curve.

INTER-RATER RELIABILITY BASED ON TWO TRIALS OR MORE PER RATER AND PER SUBJECT

When the inter-rater reliability experiment is based on 2 trials or more then the lower and upper confidence bounds are given by equations 10.3.1 and 10.3.2, which can be re-written as follows:

$$\text{LCB} = \frac{\text{FSS} - F_1}{\text{FSS} + F_1[(r-1) + r(m-1)/\text{FSI}]}, \qquad (10.5.4)$$

$$\text{UCB} = \frac{\text{FSS} - F_2}{\text{FSS} + F_2[(r-1) + r(m-1)/\text{FSI}]}, \qquad (10.5.5)$$

where FSS = MSS/MSI, and FSI = MSI/MSE. Once these two interval bounds are determined, you can compute the interval length as Length = UCB − LCB. But these two bounds are determined only if FSS adn FSI, which are functions of ρ are both known. To create the power curves, we need a series of points (ρ, Length), which is obtained as follows:

(a) First determine the set of ρ values for which to compute a confidence interval length. For the charts used in this chapter, we used 100 ρ values $0, 0.1, 0.2, \cdots, 0.99$.

(b) Generate a random variate FSI according to the F distribution with $(r-1)(n-1)$ and $rn(m-1)$ degrees of freedom.

(c) Generate a random variate $F^\star$ according to the F distribution with $n-1$ and v degrees of freedom, v is given by,

$$v = \frac{(a\text{FSI} + b)^2}{\dfrac{(a\text{FSI})^2}{(r-1)(n-1)} + \dfrac{b^2}{rn(m-1)}}, \tag{10.5.6}$$

where $a = [1 + (r-1)\rho]/(1-\rho)$ and $b = r(m-1)\rho/(1-\rho)$.

The discussions in section 10.3.3 revealed that the statistic $\text{FSS}/[a + b/\text{FSI}]$ follows the F distribution with $n-1$ and v degrees of freedom. Therefore, $\text{FSS} = F^\star[a + b/\text{FSI}]$.

(d) Using the FSI of step (b), and FSS of step (c), compute the two interval bounds and the interval length for each ρ defined in step (a). At this stage, you should have obtained an interval length for each of the 100 ρ values. Store them in a file for use at a later time.

(d) Repeat this process from step (b) a large number of times (e.g. 10,000 times or more).

In the end of this process you will have 10,000 different confidence interval interval lengths for each of the 100 ρ values used in the simulation experiment. For each ρ value, average the 10,000 lengths to obtain a single mean length, which can be used to construct the curve.

INTRA-RATER RELIABILITY FOR MIXED FACTORIAL MODELS

Statistical inference about the intra-rater coefficient under the mixed factorial design is based on the assumption that some raters rated subjects more than once. That is, the experiment involves some replication. The lower and upper confidence bounds associated with the intra-rater reliability coefficient γ under the mixed factorial design are given by equations 10.3.10 and 10.3.11, which can be re-written as follows:

$$LCB = \frac{FSS + r - (r + 1)F_2 \cdot FSE}{FSS + r + [r(m - 1) - 1]F_2 \cdot FSE}, \tag{10.5.7}$$

$$UCB = \frac{FSS + r - (r + 1)F_1 \cdot FSE}{FSS + r + [r(m - 1) - 1]F_1 \cdot FSE}, \tag{10.5.8}$$

where FSS = MSS/MSI, and FSE = MSE/MSI. Once these two interval bounds are determined, you can compute the interval length as Length = UCB − LCB. But these two bounds are determined only if FSS and FSE, which are functions of ρ are both known. To create the power curves, we need a series of points (ρ, Length), which is obtained as follows:

(a) First determine the set of γ values for which to compute a confidence interval length. For the charts used in this chapter, we used 100 γ values $0, 0.1, 0.2, \cdots, 0.99$.

(b) Generate a random variate FSS according to the F distribution with $n - 1$ and $(r - 1)(n - 1)$ degrees of freedom.

(c) Generate a random variate $F^\star$ according to the F distribution with v and $rn(m - 1)$ degrees of freedom, v is given by,

$$v = \frac{(a\mathrm{FSS} + b)^2}{\dfrac{(a\mathrm{FSS})^2}{n - 1} + \dfrac{b^2}{(r - 1)(n - 1)}}, \tag{10.5.9}$$

where $a = 1/[r + 1 + rm\gamma/(1 - \gamma)]$ and $b = r/[r + 1 + rm\gamma/(1 - \gamma)])$. The discussions in section 10.3.4 revealed that the statistic $(a\mathrm{FSS} + b)/\mathrm{FSE}$ follows the F distribution with v and $rn(m - 1)$ degrees of freedom. Therefore, $\mathrm{FSE} = (a\mathrm{FSS} + b)/F^\star$.

(d) Using the FSS of step (b), and FSE of step (c), compute the two interval bounds and the interval length for each γ defined in step (a). At this stage, you should have obtained an interval length for each of the 100 γ values. Store them in a file for use at a later time.

(d) Repeat this process from step (b) a large number of times (e.g. 10,000 times or more).

In the end of this process you will have 10,000 different confidence interval interval lengths for each of the 100 γ values used in the simulation experiment. For each γ value, average the 10,000 lengths to obtain a single mean length, which can be used to construct the curve.

PART IV

MISCELLANEOUS TOPICS ON THE ANALYSIS OF
INTER-RATER RELIABILITY EXPERIMENTS

## CHAPTER 11

Inter-Rater Reliability: Conditional Analysis

OBJECTIVE

This chapter introduces a number of measures of validity (as opposed to the measures of reliability discussed in the past few chapters), and describes statistical techniques for analyzing the extent of agreement among raters conditionally upon the subject membership in a specific category. This specific category used in the conditioning, could be the subject's "true" category if it exists, or the category into which one rater classified the subject. Conditional analysis offers the advantage of evaluating the extent of agreement among raters for a subgroup of subjects known to belong to a particular category. This analysis reduces the dependency of the agreement coefficient on trait prevalence and on the distribution of subjects across categories, and can help identify a special group of subjects where agreement is hard to reach. Methods for computing the variances associated with these conditional measures are also discussed.

CONTENTS

11.1 Overview

Scientific inquiries often involve classifying subjects into predefined categories. For example patients in a hospital could be labeled as "NORMAL" or "HIGH" according to their blood pressure level. In an inter-rater reliability experiment, category membership will be characterized either by a clear-cut operational definition establishing a deterministic relationship between subjects and categories, or by the raters' individual preferences. Clear operational definitions allow experts to determine the "true" score, also known in the literature as gold-standard scores, which are associated with each subject. The knowledge of true scores allow researchers to further investigate inter-rater reliability coefficients separately for each category, and to possibly identify problem categories where agreement is hard to reach. In this case, subjects are said to have an "Absolute Category Membership" (or ACM). When the categories are tied to the raters rather than to the subjects, then classification depends more on each rater's preferences. No operational definition exists linking subjects to specific categories. The subjects are then said to have a "Relative Category Membership" (or RCM). Marginal probabilities in this case are often seen as fixed since raters generally have known preferences. Inter-rater reliability coefficients for RCM ratings could be further analyzed by considering only subjects that one rater classified into a specific category.

Let us consider an experiment involving the chart review of women who enter the Emergency Department with an abdominal pain or a vaginal bleeding. Two chart abstractors named "Abstractor 1", and "Abstractor 2" must assign 100 patients to one of the following two categories:

- Ectopic Pregnancy (EP), and
- Intrauterine Pregnancy (IP).

A highly experienced chart reviewer also categorizes the same 100 patients into what is considered to be the "True" categories. The results of this experiment are summarized in Table 11.1, where EP_T and IP_T represent respectively the "True" (or Expert-ascertained) EP and IP categories. Table 11.1 indicates that both abstractors categorized 15 pregnancies as Ectopic, of which 13 are actually "True" Ectopic pregnancies while the other 2 are "True" Intrauterine pregnancies. Moreover, 14 of the 18 pregnancies that abstractor 2 classified as Ectopic are "True" Ectopic pregnancies while the remaining 4 are "True" IPs.

It is natural for a researcher to want to know whether abstractors are more likely to agree while rating a "True" Ectopic pregnancy than while rating a "True" IP. Agreement in this case must be evaluated conditionally upon the true nature of the pregnancy. The statistically notion of conditioning applies in this case by restricting the pool of females subjects to be rated to those who carry a specific pregnancy type of interest. For example, the conditional percent agreement given a true EP is $p_{a|EP} = (13 + 2)/20 = 0.75$. That is, abstractors agreed to classify 13 of the 20 true EPs as EPs, 2 as IPs, and disagreed about the classification of the remaining 5 True EPs. The denominator in this case is 20, because the analysis is limited to the 20 true EPs in the study group as shown in Table 11.1.

Table 11.1: Distribution of 100 Emergency Room Pregnant Women by Abstractor and Type of Pregnancy

Abstractor 1	Abstractor 2						Total		
	EP			IP					
	EP_T	IP_T	Total	EP_T	IP_T	Total	EP_T	IP_T	Total
EP	13	2	**15**	4	3	**7**	17	5	**22**
IP	1	2	**3**	2	73	**75**	3	75	**78**
Total	14	4	**18**	6	76	**82**	20	80	**100**

Although the 2 true EPs classified as IPs by both abstractors would increase reliability, they would not increase validity. They should not be considered as agreement if validity is being measured. Validity will answer a research question such as "*Would abstractors more likely to positively detect true Ectopic pregnancies than they would positively detect true IPs?*" Being able to identifying categories where agreement is more easily reached will identify other categories that should be the focus of further abstractor training. Conditional analysis could also lead to a possible modification of some categories that observers deem unclear. This analysis is carried out by breaking down the inter-rater reliability coefficient $\hat{\kappa}$ into 2 components $\hat{\kappa}_{EP}$, and $\hat{\kappa}_{IP}$ associated with the 2 response categories. These two conditional inter-rater reliability coefficients are discussed in greater details in section 11.2.

Let us turn to reliability experiments where the notion of "True" scores is nonexistent. Consider Tables 11.2 and 11.3 where two raters classified 100 garments into one of two categories "Good" (or **G**) and "Bad" (or **B**). The rating process in this case depends more on the rater's personal taste than on the nature of the object. Even though the garment type still affects the rater's choice, the very relationship between the two remains under the rater's control. Consequently, the rater's marginal probabilities can be considered fixed for a given population of garments, making them sufficiently important to play a pivotal role in the interpretation of the inter-rater reliability magnitude.

Based on the AC_1 coefficient, the extent of agreement between raters A and B is evaluated at 0.597 and that between raters C and D evaluated at 0.31. Although AC_1 indicates that raters A and B are more in agreement than raters C and D by a ratio of almost 2 to 1, a close look at both Tables 11.2 and 11.3 suggests that given the observed marginal probabilities[1], raters A and B have reached the minimum agreement possible while raters C and D have reached the maximum agreement possible. Therefore, one may argue that raters C and D are more in agreement than raters A and B (in a relative sense) given their respective rating propensities.

Table 11.2:
Distributions of 100 Garments by Rater (A/B) & Quality of Garment

Rater A's Scores	Rater B's Scores		
	B	**G**	**Total**
B	70	15	85
G	15	0	15
Total	85	15	100

Table 11.3:
Distributions of 100 Garments by Rater (C/D) & Quality of Garment

Rater C's Scores	Rater D's Scores		
	B	**G**	**Total**
B	50	40	90
G	0	10	10
Total	50	50	100

One objective of this chapter is to present ways to evaluate the extent of agreement among raters conditionally on their marginal probabilities. Conditional analysis of raters' agreement will generally be appropriate if the researcher wants to study the effect of categories on the agreement level, or if comparison between groups of raters is of interest and marginal probabilities can be assumed fixed.

11.2   Conditional Agreement Coefficient for two Raters in ACM Studies

Throughout this section, a k-subject refers to any subject whose "True" response category is k. The rating of subjects is said to be reliable when the raters consistently classify subjects into the same categories; but will be valid only if the subjects are consistently classified into their correct category by the raters. That is,

Validity = Reliability+Exactness.

In this section, I introduce reliability and validity measures. A measure of reliability in the case of two raters for example, represents the frequency with which both raters classify subjects into the same category (whether it is the 'true category or not). A measure of validity on the other hand quantifies the extent to which both raters classify subjects into their true category. Because validity is a more stringent condition than reliability, validity coefficients are expected to be smaller than reliability coefficients. When the pool of subjects used to evaluate reliability or validity is restricted to k-subjects only, one obtains conditional reliability and conditional

---

[1]i.e. the marginal probabilities (0.85 and 0.15 for rater A for instance) are considered fixed.

validity coefficients given category k. The use of all subjects for which ratings have been collected would lead to unconditional coefficients.

Throughout this chapter p_k represents the probability that the true category of a randomly selected subject is k. Referring to the emergency room pregnancy data of Table 11.1, the probability of true Ectopic pregnancy is $p_{EP} = (14 + 6)/100 = 0.20$, while the probability of true Intrauterine Pregnancy is $p_{IP} = (4 + 76)/100 = 0.80$. In the next subsection 11.2.1, I will introduce the basic elements needed for calculating reliability and validity coefficients conditionally upon the true categories.

11.2.1 Basic Conditional Probabilities for ACM Studies

Conditional analysis of ACM data requires the use of various basic conditional probabilities that I will define in this section. To illustrate how they are calculated, I will occasionally use Table 11.1 data. These probabilities are the following:

▶ *Raters' agreement probabilities as a function of the true category*

These agreement probabilities are calculated separately for each true category. For a true category k for example, the main entry $p_{ll}^{(k)}$ of the probability table (see Table C of Figure 11.2.1), represents the probability for a randomly selected subject to have k as its true category, and to be classified into the same category l by both raters. For all practical purposes, this is the relative number of subjects that meet the 2 conditions of being (i) k-subjects, and (ii) being classified into the same category l by both raters.

Table A: Distribution of EP_T Patients

Abstractor 1	Abstractor 2		
	EP	**IP**	**Total**
EP	13	4	17
IP	1	2	3
Total	14	6	20

Table B: Distribution of IP_T Patients

Abstractor 1	Abstractor 2		
	EP	**IP**	**Total**
EP	2	3	5
IP	2	73	75
Total	4	76	80

Table C: Agreement probabilities by true category $p_{ll}^{(k)}$

Selected Pregnancy Type (l)	True Pregnancy Type (k)	
	EP_T	IP_T
EP	0.13	0.02
IP	0.02	0.73

Figure 11.2.1: Calculation of the agreement probabilities by true category

Figure 11.2.1 describes the process for computing agreement probabilities separately for each true category. It starts with the creation of Tables A and B, which are derived directly from Table 11.1. The diagonals of these 2 tables are divided by 100 (the total number of subjects used in the experiment) to get the 2 columns of agreement probabilities in Table C, which are associated with the 2 true categories.

▶ *Raters' marginal probabilities as functions of the true category*

Each rater's marginal probabilities are calculated separately for each true category. For any given true category k, observer 2's marginal probability associated with category l is denoted by $p_{+l}^{(k)}$, and represents the probability that a randomly selected subject is a k-subject and is classified into category l by rater 2. A similar marginal probability for observer 1 is denoted by $p_{l+}^{(k)}$.

Abstractor 1 and abstractor 2 have each, 4 marginal probabilities, which are shown in Table C of Figure 11.2.2. Each of these probabilities is computed by dividing the associated number from Tables A and B by 100, which is the number of subjects that participated in the reliability experiment. It follows from Table C of Figure 11.2.2 that 17% (i.e. 0.17) of all female patients carried a true ectopic pregnancy, and were categorized as such by abstractor 1.

Table A: Distribution of EP_T Patients

Abstractor 1	Abstractor 2		
	EP	**IP**	**Total**
EP	13	4	17
IP	1	2	3
Total	14	6	20

Table B: Distribution of IP_T Patients

Abstractor 1	Abstractor 2		
	EP	**IP**	**Total**
EP	2	3	5
IP	2	73	75
Total	4	76	80

Table C: Raters' marginal probabilities by rater and true category

Selected Pregnancy Type (l)	Abstractor 1 ($p_{l+}^{(k)}$)		Abstractor 2 ($p_{+l}^{(k)}$)	
	EP_T	IP_T	EP_T	IP_T
EP	0.17	0.05	0.14	0.04
IP	0.03	0.75	0.06	0.76

Figure 11.2.2: Calculation of the marginal probabilities by true category

▶ *Raters' marginal probabilities conditionally upon the true category*

Table B of Figure 11.2.3 shows each abstractor's propensity for classification in a particular category given the subject's initial true status. For example abstractor 1 would categorize any true EP pregnancy correctly 85% of the times, and would classify it incorrectly as IP 15% of the times. These conditional marginal probabilities must read column-wise. *In the statistical jargon, one would write $p_{EP+|EP_T} = 0.85$ (should be read as "Given that the pregnancy to be classified is a true Ectopic pregnancy, abstractor 1 will rate it as such with a probability of 0.85"). Because a condition (i.e. the pregnancy as true ectopic) is set prior to the probability being calculated, the value 0.85 is referred to as a conditional probability.*

All conditional marginal probabilities in Table B are calculated based on the (unconditional) marginal probabilities of Table A as depicted in Figure 11.2.3. Note that Table A of Figure 11.2.3 is a replication of Table C of Figure 11.2.2.

Table A: Raters' marginal probabilities by rater and true category

Selected Pregnancy Type (l)	Abstractor 1 ($p_{l+}^{(k)}$)		Abstractor 2 ($p_{+l}^{(k)}$)	
	EP_T	IP_T	EP_T	IP_T
EP	0.17	0.05	0.14	0.04
IP	0.03	0.75	0.06	0.76
True Membership Probability	0.20	0.80	0.20	0.80

| 0.17÷0.20 | 0.03÷0.20 | 0.04÷0.80 | 0.76÷0.80 |

Table B: Conditional marginal probabilities by rater and true category

Selected Pregnancy Type (l)	Abstractor 1 ($p_{l+|k}$)		Abstractor 2 ($p_{+l|k}$)	
	EP_T	IP_T	EP_T	IP_T
EP	0.85	0.0625	0.7	0.05
IP	0.15	0.9375	0.3	0.95

Figure 11.2.3: Calculation of the marginal probabilities conditionally on the true category

▶ *Category Use Frequency Conditionally upon the True Category*

I want to be able to compute the relative number of times a specific category is used by raters when only a restricted group of subjects is selected based on their true category membership. For example, given that only *intrauterine pregnancies* (i.e. condition) are rated, the relative number of pregnancies categorized as Ectopic is denoted by $\pi_{E|I}$. This represents the relative frequency of use of the ectopic pregnancy type when rating only true intrauterine pregnancies. Because of the specific condition imposed on the restricted pool of subjects to be rated, $\pi_{E|I}$ is referred to as the conditional relative frequency of ectopic. If there is no restriction on the pool of subjects to be rated, the relative frequency is said to be unconditional. More generally, let $\pi_{l|k}$ be the relative frequency with which category l is used *when rating k-subjects only*. This quantity is calculated as follows:

$$\pi_{l|k} = \pi_{l(k)}/p_k, \qquad (11.2.1)$$

where $\pi_{l(k)}$ is the relative frequency with which k-subjects are assigned to category l *when rating all subjects*. That is, the conditional relative frequency is calculated as the ratio of the (unconditional) relative frequency of k-subjects in category l to the prevalence of k-subjects in the sample of subjects.

Note that if the raters' marginal probabilities have already been calculated, then they may be used to obtain the relative frequency of k-subjects in category l as follows:

$$\pi_{l(k)} = \left(p_{+l}^{(k)} + p_{l+}^{(k)}\right)/2.$$

Using Table 11.1 data these probabilities can be calculated as shown in Figure 11.2.4 (see the right side of Table B).

Table A: Raters' marginal probabilities by rater and true category

Assigned Pregnancy Type (l)	Abstractor 1 ($p_{l+}^{(k)}$)		Abstractor 2 ($p_{+l}^{(k)}$)	
	EP_T	IP_T	EP_T	IP_T
EP	0.17	0.05	0.14	0.04
IP	0.03	0.75	0.06	0.76
True Membership Probability	0.20	0.80	0.20	0.80

(0.17+0.14)÷2 → EP
(0.03+0.06)÷2
0.045÷0.20
0.155÷0.20

Table B: Calculating conditional relative frequencies

Assigned Pregnancy Type (l)	Relative Frequency of k-Subjects ($\pi_{l(k)}$)		Conditional Relative Frequency ($\pi_{l|k}$)	
	EP_T	IP_T	EP_T	IP_T
EP	0.155	0.045	0.775	0.05625
IP	0.045	0.755	0.225	0.94375

Figure 11.2.4: Calculation of the conditional relative frequencies given the true category

There are 4 conditional rates that are calculated, 2 for each true category. One of the rates is $\pi_{E|E} = 0.775$, which indicates that if a pregnancy is a true ectopic type, it will be categorized (by either abstractor) as such, 77.5% of the times. It follows from the right side of Table B (in Figure 11.2.4), that 0.775 is obtained as the ratio of 0.155 to 0.20, where 0.155 is $\pi_{E(E)}$ (i.e. the prevalence of true ectopic pregnancies, which are also categorized as being of ectopic type), and 0.2 is the overall prevalence of true ectopic pregnancies.

Here is the list of all conditional relative frequencies:

$$\pi_{E|E} = 0.775, \quad \pi_{E|I} = 0.056,$$
$$\pi_{I|E} = 0.225, \quad \pi_{I|I} = 0.944.$$

The conditional frequency $\pi_{I|E}$ for example, is calculated as $\pi_{I|E} = \pi_{I(E)}/p_{EP} = 0.045/0.20 = 0.225$. The other conditional frequencies are calculated the same way.

11.2.2 Conditional Reliability Coefficient between two Raters in ACM Reliability Studies

Unconditional reliability coefficients for ACM studies are identical to the regular inter-rater reliability coefficients covered in part II of this book, and will not be discussed any further in this section. This section will be devoted entirely to the study of conditional reliability coefficients given the subject's "true" membership to a specific category. For example, a conditional reliability coefficient may quantify the extent of agreement among two abstractors under the condition that the woman's "true" pregnancy type is Ectopic. As previously indicated, the primary purpose of conditioning is to have a reliability measure that is not affected by the distribution of women across the different types of pregnancy. Such a conditional reliability coefficient will facilitate comparison between reliability studies based on populations with different prevalence rates of Ectopic pregnancies. It also helps identify the specific categories where agreement is hard to reach.

In this section, I will introduce four conditional agreement coefficients. These are the conditional Gwet's AC_1, Cohen's Kappa, Scott's Pi, and Brennan-Prediger coefficients, given a particular true category k.

▶ Conditional AC_1 Coefficient

Let k be an arbitrary category (e.g. k could designate EP or IP pregnancy). The conditional AC_1 reliability coefficient given a "true" membership category k is denoted by $\kappa_{G|k}$ (where G stands for Gwet (2008) who first proposed this coefficient). It is defined as the ratio of the percent of intrinsic agreement to the likelihood of no chance agreement[2]; both components being evaluated under

---

[2] *Note that the possibility of no chance agreement includes intrinsic agreements, and disagreements of all kinds as well.*

the condition that the true category of the subject being rated is k. More formally,

$$\widehat{\kappa}_{G|k} = \frac{p_{a|k} - p_{e|k}}{1 - p_{e|k}}, \quad \text{where} \quad \begin{cases} p_{a|k} = \sum_{l=1}^{q} p_{ll|k}, \\ p_{e|k} = \frac{1}{q-1} \sum_{l=1}^{q} \pi_{l|k}(1 - \pi_{l|k}), \end{cases} \quad (11.2.2)$$

where $p_{a|k}$ is the likelihood that two raters agree based on the classification of a k-subjects alone, and $p_{e|k}$ the likelihood that two raters agree by pure chance based on the rating of k-subjects alone. Note that $p_{a|k}$ is calculated by summing all conditional probabilities $p_{ll|k}$ associated with any category l, where $p_{ll|k} = p_{ll}^{(k)}/p_k$. The conditional probability $\pi_{l|k}$ was defined in section 11.2.1, and represents for all practical purposes, the conditional frequency of use of category l by observers based on the rating of k-subjects alone.

Let us look more closely and step by step, at the calculation of the conditional AC_1 coefficient using the rating data of Table 11.1. Since this reliability experiment involves two pregnancy types, I will need to compute two conditional AC_1 coefficients, which are $AC_{1|E}$ (for Ectopic), and $AC_{1|I}$ (for Intrauterine).

Figure 11.2.5 depicts the steps necessary for computing the two conditional percent agreement values $p_{a|E} = 0.75$, and $p_{a|I} = 0.9375$ (see the last row of Table B in Figure 11.2.5). The first input values going into these calculations are shown in Table A, and represent the relative number of times the raters agree, calculated separately for each true category and each assigned category. These numbers come from Table C of Figure 11.2.1.

Calculating the conditional percent agreement values

- The value $p_{a|E} = 0.75$ is obtained by summing the two conditional agreement probabilities $p_{EE|E} = 0.65$, and $p_{II|E} = 0.10$. Note that 0.65 represents the conditional relative number times both abstractors would assign a true ectopic pregnancy to the ectopic category, whereas 0.10 is the conditional relative number times both abstractors would assign a true ectopic pregnancy to the intrauterine category.

- The conditional relative frequency $p_{EE|E} = 0.65$ is calculated as the ratio of the (unconditional) relative frequency $p_{EE}^{E} = 0.13$ to the prevalence of true ectopic $p_E = 0.20$. The conditional relative frequency $p_{II|E} = 0.10$ on the other hand, is the ratio of the (unconditional) relative frequency $p_{II}^{E} = 0.02$ to the prevalence of true ectopic $p_E = 0.20$.

The value $p_{a|I} = 0.9375$ can be calculated using the same procedure described above for $p_{a|E} = 0.75$.

Figure 11.2.6 shows the steps for calculating the conditional percent chance agreement for each true category.

- The percent chance agreement conditionally upon the true ectopic type pregnancy is given by, $p_{e|E} = 0.34875$, whereas the percent chance agreement conditionally upon the true intrauterine type pregnancy is given by, $p_{e|I} = 0.106172$. To get these two numbers, one needs to start with the four conditional relative frequencies previously calculated in Table B of Figure 11.2.4, and reported on the left side of Table A in Figure 11.2.6. The right side of Table A is obtained by multiplying each left-side number by its complement.

- The next step is to compute the "Total" row by summing the numbers column-wise. At this stage, the conditional chance agreement probabilities are obtained by dividing the totals by 2-1 (i.e. the number of categories minus 1), which is 1 and will not affect the total values.

Figures 11.2.5 and 11.2.6 provide the two agreement percentages, and the two chance-agreement percentages necessary to compute the conditional AC_1 coefficients named $\widehat{\kappa}_{G|E}$ (for ectopic), and $\widehat{\kappa}_{G|I}$ for intrauterine. Therefore,

$$\widehat{\kappa}_{G|E} = \left(p_{a|E} - p_{e|E}\right)/\left(1 - p_{e|E}\right),$$
$$= (0.75 - 0.34875)/(1 - 0.34875) = 0.616.$$
$$\widehat{\kappa}_{G|I} = \left(p_{a|I} - p_{e|I}\right)/\left(1 - p_{e|E}\right),$$
$$= (0.9375 - 0.106172)/(1 - 0.106172) = 0.93.$$

It follows from these conditional agreement coefficients that based on the AC_1 coefficient, the two abstractors would agree more often if they rate true intrauterine pregnancies ($AC_{1|I} = 0.93$) than if they rate true ectopic pregnancies ($AC_{1|E} = 0.616$). If the abstractors must be given further training, the training session would be more productive if it focuses on improving the rating of true ectopic pregnancies. One should note that the conditional agreement coefficients discussed here measures the extent to which abstractors classify subjects into the same category. These are agreement coefficients. They do not evaluate the extent to which abstractors classify subjects into their correct and true category. Only validity coefficients discussed in the next section will quantify the propensity for raters to agree on the subject's true category.

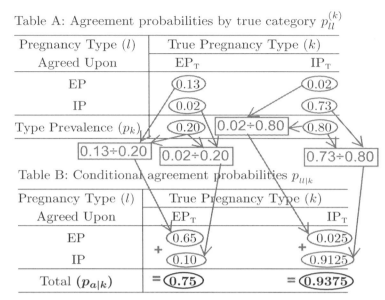

Table A: Agreement probabilities by true category $p_{ll}^{(k)}$

Pregnancy Type (l) Agreed Upon	True Pregnancy Type (k)	
	EP_T	IP_T
EP	0.13	0.02
IP	0.02	0.73
Type Prevalence (p_k)	0.20	0.80

Table B: Conditional agreement probabilities $p_{ll|k}$

Pregnancy Type (l) Agreed Upon	True Pregnancy Type (k)	
	EP_T	IP_T
EP	0.65	0.025
IP	0.10	0.9125
Total $(p_{a|k})$	= 0.75	= 0.9375

Figure 11.2.5: Calculation of the conditional percent agreement based on the true category

Table A: Calculating conditional chance-agreement percentages

Assigned Pregnancy Type (l)	$\pi_{l|k}$: conditional relative frequencies based on k-subjects		$\pi_{l|k} \times (1 - \pi_{l|k})$	
	EP_T	IP_T	EP_T	IP_T
EP	0.775	0.05625	0.174375	0.053086
IP	0.225	0.94375	0.174375	0.053086
Total	1	1	0.34875	0.106172
% chance agreement[a]: $p_{e|k}$	N/A		0.34875	0.106172

[a] *This quantity is calculated as the ratio of Total (c.f. previous row) to the number of categories (in this case 2) minus 1*

Figure 11.2.6: Calculation of the conditional chance-agreement percentages based on the true category

▶ Conditional Kappa Coefficient

The conditional Kappa reliability coefficient given a "true" membership category k is denoted by $\widehat{\kappa}_{\text{C}|k}$ (where C stands for Cohen (1960) who first proposed the general Kappa coefficient), and defined as follows:

$$\widehat{\kappa}_{C|k} = \frac{p_{a|k} - p_{e|k}}{1 - p_{e|k}}, \text{ where } p_{e|k} = \sum_{l=1}^{q} p_{+l|k} p_{l+|k}. \tag{11.2.3}$$

The conditional percent agreement $p_{a|k}$ used for Kappa is the same as that used with AC_1.

▶ **Conditional Scott's Pi Coefficient**

The Conditional Pi reliability coefficient given a "true" membership category k is denoted by $\widehat{\kappa}_{S|k}$, and defined as follows :

$$\widehat{\kappa}_{S|k} = \frac{p_{a|k} - p_{e|k}}{1 - p_{e|k}}, \text{ where } p_{e|k} = \sum_{l=1}^{q} \pi_{l|k}^2, \tag{11.2.4}$$

▶ **Conditional Brennan-Prediger Coefficient**

The Conditional Brennan-Prediger (BP) Coefficient given a "true" membership category k is denoted by $\widehat{\kappa}_{BP|k}$, and defined as follows :

$$\widehat{\kappa}_{BP|k} = \frac{p_{a|k} - p_{e|k}}{1 - p_{e|k}}, \text{ where } p_{e|k} = 1/q, \tag{11.2.5}$$

Table 11.4 shows the numerical values of these conditional agreement coefficients calculated from Table 11.1 data. It follows from Table 11.4 results that conditional AC_1 coefficients exceed the corresponding Pi and Kappa coefficients by a wide margin. This conditional analysis also reveals that abstractors agree more often on Intrauterine pregnancies.

Table 11.4: Conditional and Unconditional Reliability Coefficients for Table 11.1 Pregnancy Data

True		% Chance Agreement ($p_{e|k}$)				Reliability Coefficients			
Category	$p_{a|k}$	AC_1	Pi	Kappa	BP	$AC_1|k$	Pi$|k$	Kappa$|k$	BP$|k$
Ectopic	0.750	0.350	0.650	0.640	0.5	0.616	0.283	0.306	0.500
Intrauterine	0.938	0.106	0.894	0.894	0.5	0.930	0.411	0.412	0.875
All	0.900	0.320	0.680	0.679	0.5	0.853	0.688	0.688	0.800

More details about the calculation of Table 11.4 numbers can be found in the Excel worksheet "Table11.4 Calculations" included in the following Excel workbook: "www.agreestat.com/book4/chapter11examples.xlx."

11.2.3 Unconditional and Conditional Validity Coefficient between two Raters in ACM Reliability Studies

The objective in this section is to quantify the extent to which two raters agree about the subjects' "True" category. The resulting metric will not simply measure how often the raters agree (i.e. reliability), instead it will measure how often the raters agree about the subject's correct membership category. It will be a measure of validity as opposed to a measure of reliability as discussed in the previous section. When all subjects used in the experiment are included into the calculations, the *Unconditional Validity Coefficient* is obtained. This validity measure will also be discussed conditionally upon the true category of the subject. Using only k-subjects in the calculations will lead to the *Conditional Validity Coefficient* given the "true" category k.

Table 11.5 shows equations for several versions of the unconditional validity coefficient, including the AC_1, Pi, Kappa, and BP (i.e. Brennan-Prediger) versions. The (unconditional[3]) probability p'_a that an agreement is reached on the correct category (also called the "percent agreement on the correct category") is common to all validity coefficients. However, the probability p'_e that an agreement is reached by chance on the correct category is specific to each version of the validity coefficient, and its expression shown in column 3 of the table. The last column contains the formulas pertaining to the different unconditional validity coefficients.

Table 11.5:
Equations of Unconditional Validity Coefficients and associated Probabilities

Coefficient	Percent Agreement (p'_a)	Percent Chance Agreement (p'_e)	Validity Coefficient $(\widehat{\kappa}')$
AC'_1	$\displaystyle\sum_{k=1}^{q} p_{kk}^{(k)}$	$\displaystyle\frac{1}{q(q-1)}\sum_{k=1}^{q}\pi_k(1-\pi_k)$	$\widehat{\kappa}'_G = \dfrac{p'_a - p'_e}{1 - p'_e}$
Pi'	$\displaystyle\sum_{k=1}^{q} p_{kk}^{(k)}$	$\displaystyle\sum_{k=1}^{q}\pi_k^2 p_k$	$\widehat{\kappa}'_S = \dfrac{p'_a - p'_e}{1 - p'_e}$
$Kappa'$	$\displaystyle\sum_{k=1}^{q} p_{kk}^{(k)}$	$\displaystyle\sum_{k=1}^{q}p_{k+}p_{+k}p_k$	$\widehat{\kappa}'_C = \dfrac{p'_a - p'_e}{1 - p'_e}$
BP'	$\displaystyle\sum_{k=1}^{q} p_{kk}^{(k)}$	$1/q^2$	$\widehat{\kappa}'_{BP} = \dfrac{p'_a - p'_e}{1 - p'_e}$

---

[3]The word "probability" used with no other specification assumes it to be unconditional, and therefore evaluated with respect to all subjects.

To define the validity coefficients conditionally upon the subject "true" category, let k be a response category (e.g. k :Pregnancy Type = EP, or IP). The conditional validity coefficient $\widehat{\kappa}'_{\bullet|k}$ given a "true" membership category k represents the validity coefficient calculated under the assumption that the subjects rated are all k-subjects. Table 11.6 contains in column 4, the expressions of 4 different versions of the conditional validity coefficient given a "true" category k, the two previous columns 2, and 3 containing respectively the conditional percent agreement on the correct category given a specific true category, and the conditional percent chance agreement on the correct category given the subject's true category k.

Table 11.6: Equations of the Conditional Validity Coefficients and associated Probabilities

Coefficient	$(p'_{a|k})^a$	$(p'_{e|k})^b$	$(\widehat{\kappa}'_{\bullet|k})^c$
$AC'_{1|k}$	$p^{(k)}_{kk}/p_k$	$\dfrac{1}{q(q-1)}\displaystyle\sum_{l=1}^{q}\pi_{l|k}(1-\pi_{l|k})$	$\widehat{\kappa}'_{G|k}=\dfrac{p'_{a|k}-p'_{e|k}}{1-p'_{e|k}}$
$Pi'_{|k}$	$p^{(k)}_{kk}/p_k$	$\pi^2_{k|k}$	$\widehat{\kappa}'_{S|k}=\dfrac{p'_{a|k}-p'_{e|k}}{1-p'_{e|k}}$
$Kappa'_{|k}$	$p^{(k)}_{kk}/p_k$	$p_{+k|k}p_{k+|k}$	$\widehat{\kappa}'_{C|k}=\dfrac{p'_{a|k}-p'_{e|k}}{1-p'_{e|k}}$
$BP'_{|k}$	$p^{(k)}_{kk}/p_k$	$1/q^2$	$\widehat{\kappa}'_{BP|k}=\dfrac{p'_{a|k}-p'_{e|k}}{1-p'_{e|k}}$

[a]Conditional percent agreement on correct category.
[b]Conditional percent chance agreement on correct category.
[c]Conditional validity coefficient.

Using the pregnancy data of Table 11.1, conditional and unconditional validity coefficients have been calculated. These coefficients and associated probabilities are presented in Table 11.7.

It follows from the rightmost portion of Table 11.7 that based on AC_1 the (unconditional) validity coefficient between the two abstractors is 0.833; for patients with Ectopic pregnancy the conditional AC_1 goes down to 0.576 and up to 0.908 when the patients carry an Intrauterine pregnancy. While a different distribution of patients by pregnancy type in another study may lead to different unconditional validity coefficients, conditional validity coefficients will show more stability across studies. All four validity coefficients show higher valid agreement for Intrauterine pregnancies than for ectopic pregnancies, although AC_1 and BP coefficients are consistently higher than Pi and Kappa.

Table 11.7: Conditional and Unconditional[a] Validity Coefficients, and Probabilities based on Table 11.1 Pregnancy Data

True Category	$p'_{a\|k}$	% Chance Agreement (p'_e)				Validity Coefficients			
		AC'_1	Pi$'$	Kappa$'$	BP$'$	$AC'_1\|k$	Pi$'\|k$	Kappa$'\|k$	BP$'\|k$
Ectopic	0.650	0.175	0.600	0.595	0.25	0.576	0.125	0.136	0.533
Intrauterine	0.913	0.053	0.891	0.891	0.25	0.908	0.200	0.200	0.884
All	0.860	0.160	0.592	0.5196	0.25	0.833	0.657	0.709	0.813

[a]Unconditional probabilities and validity coefficients are shown in the last row of this table.

11.3   Validity and Conditional Coefficients for three Raters or More in ACM Studies

This section aims at extending the validity and conditional agreement coefficients of the past few sections to studies involving three raters or more. When the number of raters is three or more, validity coefficients generally quantify the extent of agreement between a roster of raters and the "gold standard" unanimously accepted as the reference to match. These validity coefficients are discussed in section 11.3.1. Section 11.3.2 is devoted to the conditional agreement analysis for multiple raters in ACM studies.

11.3.1   *Validity Coefficients for three Raters or More*

In this section, I will address the problem of comparing multiple raters to a gold standard. The gold standard score is assumed to be true. It may be the score that a body of experts have agreed upon, and that one would normally expect any competent rater to assign to the subject. The purpose of a gold standard is to evaluate both reliability and validity associated with the ratings. Whenever such a standard is available, I would recommend its use.

The general approach for evaluating agreement with the gold standard is based on a pairwise comparison between two raters and the gold standard, using all possible pairs of raters that can be formed from the group of participating raters. I propose two solutions to this problem. The first is an adaptation of Fleiss' generalized kappa to this situation, and the second is based on an adaptation of Gwet's AC_1 coefficient. I want to present these two solutions in a general setting where an arbitrary number

r of raters must rate n subjects, with the possibility that some raters might not rate all subjects. However, the gold-standard score must be available for each subject used in the analysis. Subjects with no gold-standard score must be excluded from analysis. Moreover, I will assume that there is a set of weights associated with the categories to account for partial agreements. As mentioned in previous chapters, for nominal scales where the notion of partial agreement in irrelevant, one may always use identity weights, where all diagonal elements are 1 and all off-diagonal elements are 0.

Let ε_{ik} be a 0-1 dichotomous variable, which takes a value of 1 if k is the gold-standard category associated with subject i, and takes value 0 otherwise. The symbol r_{ik} designates the count of raters that classified subject i into category k, while r_i is the count of raters that scored subject i. Furthermore, n' is the number of subjects scored by two raters or more. For any two categories k and l, w_{kl} represents the weight.

▶ **AC₁ Validity Coefficient**

The AC₁ coefficient of validity is defined as,

$$
\widehat{\kappa}_{\mathrm{G}} = \frac{p_a - p_e}{1 - p_e}, \quad \text{where} \quad
\begin{cases}
p_a = \dfrac{1}{n'} \displaystyle\sum_{i=1}^{n'} \sum_{k=1}^{q} \frac{\varepsilon_{ik} r_{ik} (r_{ik}^{\star} - 1)}{r_i (r_i - 1)}, \\[3mm]
p_e = \dfrac{T_w^{\star}}{q(q-1)} \displaystyle\sum_{k=1}^{q} \pi_k (1 - \pi_k).
\end{cases}
\tag{11.3.1}
$$

In the above equation, $T_w^{\star}$ is defined as follows (assuming $w_{kk} = 1$ for all k):

$$
T_w^{\star} = 2 \sum_{k=1}^{q} w_{k+} p_k - 1,
\tag{11.3.2}
$$

where p_k is the probability that a subject's gold-standard rating is k, w_{k+} is the sum of all weights w_{kl} associated with category k, and π_k the probability that a rater classifies a subject into category k. Moreover, $r_{ik}^{\star}$ is the weighted count of raters that classified subject i into any category affiliated with category k. Note that a category l is considered affiliated with k if the associated weight w_{kl} is nonzero. Two affiliated categories always represent partial agreement. More formally,

$$
r_{ik}^{\star} = \sum_{l=1}^{q} w_{kl} r_{il}, \quad \text{and} \quad \pi_k = \frac{1}{n} \sum_{i=1}^{n} \frac{r_{ik}}{r_i}.
\tag{11.3.3}
$$

THE VARIANCE

The variance associated with the coefficient of validity is calculated as follows:

$$v(\widehat{\kappa}_{\mathrm{G}}) = \frac{1-f}{n} \frac{1}{n-1} \sum_{i=1}^{n} \left(\widehat{\kappa}_{\mathrm{G}|i}^{\star} - \widehat{\kappa}_{\mathrm{G}}\right)^2, \tag{11.3.4}$$

where,

- $\widehat{\kappa}_{\mathrm{G}|i}^{\star} = \widehat{\kappa}_{\mathrm{G}|i} - 2(1 - \widehat{\kappa}_{\mathrm{G}}) \dfrac{p_{e|i} - p_e}{1 - p_e}$,

- $p_{e|i} = \sum_{k=1}^{q} \left[\dfrac{T_w^{\star}(1 - \pi_k)}{q(q-1)} r_{ik}/r_i + (w_{k+} - 1)(\varepsilon_{ik} - p_k)p_e/T_w^{\star} \right]$.

- $\widehat{\kappa}_{\mathrm{G}|i} = \begin{cases} (n/n')(p_{a|i} - p_e)/(1 - p_e), & \textit{if } r_i \geq 2, \\ 0, & \textit{otherwise}, \end{cases}$

- $p_{a|i} = \sum_{k=1}^{q} \dfrac{\varepsilon_{ik} r_{ik}(r_{ik}^{\star} - 1)}{r_i(r_i - 1)}$.

▶ **Fleiss' Validity Coefficient**

Fleiss' Kappa coefficient of validity is defined as,

$$\widehat{\kappa}_{\mathrm{F}} = \frac{p_a - p_e}{1 - p_e}, \text{ where } \begin{cases} p_a = \dfrac{1}{n'} \sum_{i=1}^{n'} \sum_{k=1}^{q} \dfrac{\varepsilon_{ik} r_{ik}(r_{ik}^{\star} - 1)}{r_i(r_i - 1)}, \\ p_e = \sum_{k=1}^{q} \pi_k p_k (2\pi_k^{\star} - \pi_k), \end{cases} \tag{11.3.5}$$

where $r_{ik}^{\star}$ and π_k are defined as in equation 11.3.3, and

$$\pi_k^{\star} = \sum_{l=1}^{q} w_{kl} \pi_l. \tag{11.3.6}$$

THE VARIANCE

The variance associated with Fleiss' coefficient of validity is calculated as follows:

$$v(\widehat{\kappa}_{\mathrm{F}}) = \frac{1-f}{n} \frac{1}{n-1} \sum_{i=1}^{n} \left(\widehat{\kappa}_{\mathrm{F}|i}^{\star} - \widehat{\kappa}_{\mathrm{F}}\right)^2, \tag{11.3.7}$$

where,

- $\widehat{\kappa}_{\mathrm{F}|i}^{\star} = \widehat{\kappa}_{\mathrm{F}|i} - (1 - \widehat{\kappa}_{\mathrm{F}}) \dfrac{(p_{e|i}^{\star} - p_e) + 2(p_{e|i}^{\star\star} - p_e)}{1 - p_e}$,

$$\bullet\ \widehat{\kappa}_{\mathrm{F}|i} = \begin{cases} (n/n')(p_{a|i} - p_e)/(1 - p_e), & if\ r_i \geq 2, \\ 0, & otherwise, \end{cases}$$

$$\bullet\ p_{e|i}^{\star} = \sum_{k=1}^{q} \varepsilon_{ik} \pi_k (2\pi_k^{\star} - \pi_k), \quad \bullet\ p_{e|i}^{\star\star} = \sum_{k=1}^{q} \Big[\pi_k r_{ik}^{\star} + (\pi_k^{\star} - \pi_k) r_{ik}\Big] p_k / r_i.$$

▶ **Brennan-Prediger Validity Coefficient**

The Brennan-Prediger validity coefficient can be defined as $\widehat{\kappa}_{\mathrm{BP}} = (p_a - p_e)/(1 - p_e)$, where the percent agreement p_a is defined by equation 11.3.1, and the percent chance agreement given by $p_e = T_w^{\star}/q^2$ with $T_w^{\star}$ defined by equation 11.3.2. Its variance can be calculated as follows:

$$v(\widehat{\kappa}_{\mathrm{BP}}) = \frac{1 - f}{n} \frac{1}{n - 1} \sum_{i=1}^{n} \big(\widehat{\kappa}_{\mathrm{BP}|i}^{\star} - \widehat{\kappa}_{\mathrm{BP}}\big)^2, \tag{11.3.8}$$

where,

- $\widehat{\kappa}_{\mathrm{BP}|i}^{\star} = \widehat{\kappa}_{\mathrm{BP}|i} - 2(1 - \widehat{\kappa}_{\mathrm{BP}}) \dfrac{u_i}{1 - p_e}$,

- $\widehat{\kappa}_{\mathrm{BP}|i} = \begin{cases} (n/n')(p_{a|i} - p_e)/(1 - p_e), & if\ r_i \geq 2, \\ 0, & otherwise, \end{cases}$

- $u_i = \sum_{k=1}^{q} (w_{k+} - 1)(\varepsilon_{ik} - p_k)/q^2.$

Equations 11.3.1 and 11.3.5 suggest that the coefficient of validity will generally be smaller than the regular coefficient of reliability. It is because an agreement reached by raters on the wrong category will not be accounted for when computing validity coefficients. Therefore these "spurious" agreements are expected to lower the magnitude of the validity coefficient.

11.3.2 *Conditional Agreement Coefficients for three Raters or More*

In this section, I will discuss the AC_1, Fleiss Kappa, and Brennan-Prediger reliability and validity coefficients conditionally upon the true category k_0. That is, reliability and validity are examined with respect to a restricted group of subjects whose true category is k_0.

CONDITIONAL AC_1 COEFFICIENTS

- *Conditional AC_1 Reliability Coefficient*

Suppose you want to compute the AC_1 or AC_2 reliability coefficient conditionally on a given category labeled as k_0. This essentially means that you want to evaluate the extent of agreement among r raters if the true category of the subject being rated is k_0. Note that in practice, the pool of subjects whose true category is k_0 is rarely known. However, one can often compute the probability that a subject belongs to that category. The conditional AC_1 coefficient given category k_0 is given by,

$$\widehat{\kappa}_{G|k_0} = \frac{p_{a|k_0} - p_{e|k_0}}{1 - p_{e|k_0}} \quad \text{where} \quad \begin{cases} p_{a|k_0} = \frac{1}{p_{k_0}}\left[\frac{1}{n'}\sum_{i=1}^{n'}\frac{r_{ik_0}(r_{ik_0}^{\star} - 1)}{r_i(r_i - 1)}\right], \\[3mm] p_{e|k_0} = \frac{T_w}{q(q-1)}\sum_{k=1}^{q}\pi_{k|k_0}(1 - \pi_{k|k_0}), \end{cases} \quad (11.3.9)$$

and $\pi_{k|k_0}$ is the conditional probability that a subject is classified into category k given that its true category is k_0, and is formally defined as,

$$\pi_{k|k_0} = \frac{1}{np_{k_0}}\sum_{i=1}^{n}\varepsilon_{ik_0}r_{ik}/r_i. \quad (11.3.10)$$

Variance of Conditional AC_1 Reliability Coefficient

The variance associated with the AC_1 coefficient of reliability is calculated as follows:

$$v(\widehat{\kappa}_{G|k_0}) = \frac{1 - f}{n}\frac{1}{n - 1}\sum_{i=1}^{n}\left(\widehat{\kappa}_{G|k_0}^{\star(i)} - \widehat{\kappa}_{G|k_0}\right)^2, \quad (11.3.11)$$

where,

$\diamond$ $\widehat{\kappa}_{G|k_0}^{\star(i)} = \widehat{\kappa}_{G|k_0}^{(i)} - 2(1 - \widehat{\kappa}_{G|k_0})\dfrac{p_{e|k_0}^{(i)} - p_{e|k_0}}{1 - p_{e|k_0}}$,

$\diamond$ $p_{e|k_0}^{(i)} = \dfrac{T_w^{\star}}{q(q-1)}\displaystyle\sum_{k=1}^{q}a_{ik|k_0}(1 - \pi_k)$,

$\diamond$ $a_{ik|k_0} = \left(\varepsilon_{ik_0}r_{ik}/r_i - \pi_{k|k_0}(\varepsilon_{ik_0} - p_{k_0})\right)/p_{k_0}$,

$\diamond$ $\widehat{\kappa}_{G|k_0}^{(i)} = \begin{cases} (n/n')\left(p_{a|k_0}^{(i)} - p_{e|k_0}\right)/(1 - p_{e|k_0}), & \text{if } r_i \geq 2, \\[2mm] \qquad\qquad\qquad\qquad\qquad 0, & \text{otherwise,} \end{cases}$

$\diamond$ $p_{a|k_0}^{(i)} = \dfrac{1}{p_{k_0}}\left(\dfrac{r_{ik_0}(r_{ik_0}^{\star} - 1)}{r_i(r_i - 1)} - (\varepsilon_{ik_0} - p_{k_0})p_{a|k_0}\right)$.

Next, I like to discuss the AC_1 coefficient of validity.

- *Conditional AC_1 Validity Coefficient*

As for the conditional AC_1 validity coefficient, it can be calculated as follows:

$$\widehat{\kappa}_{G|k_0} = \frac{p_{a|k_0} - p_{e|k_0}}{1 - p_{e|k_0}} \text{ where } \begin{cases} p_{a|k_0} &= \frac{1}{p_{k_0}}\left[\frac{1}{n'}\sum_{i=1}^{n'}\frac{r_{ik_0}(r_{ik_0}^\star - 1)}{r_i(r_i - 1)}\right], \\ p_{e|k_0} &= \frac{T_{w|k_0}}{p_{k_0}q(q-1)}\sum_{k=1}^{q}\pi_{k|k_0}(1 - \pi_{k|k_0}), \end{cases}$$

(11.3.12)

where $T_{w|k_0}$ is defined as follows:

$$T_{w|k_0} = 2w_{+k_0} - 1,$$

(11.3.13)

with w_{+k_0} representing the summation of the weights w_{kk_0} for all categories $k = 1, \cdots, q$.

Variance of Conditional AC_1 Validity Coefficient

The variance associated with the AC_1 coefficient of validity is calculated as follows:

$$v(\widehat{\kappa}_{G|k_0}) = \frac{1-f}{n}\frac{1}{n-1}\sum_{i=1}^{n}\left(\widehat{\kappa}_{G|k_0}^{\star(i)} - \widehat{\kappa}_{G|k_0}\right)^2,$$

(11.3.14)

where,

$\diamond\ \widehat{\kappa}_{G|k_0}^{\star(i)} = \widehat{\kappa}_{G|k_0}^{(i)} - (1 - \widehat{\kappa}_{G|k_0})\dfrac{2\varepsilon_{ik_0}\left(p_{e|k_0}^{(i)} - p_{e|k_0}\right) - (\varepsilon_{ik_0} - p_{k_0})p_{e|k_0}}{(1 - p_{e|k_0})p_{k_0}},$

$\diamond\ p_{e|k_0}^{(i)} = \dfrac{T_w}{q(q-1)p_{k_0}}\sum_{k=1}^{q}\dfrac{r_{ik}}{r_i}(1 - \pi_{k|k_0}),$

$\diamond\ \widehat{\kappa}_{G|k_0}^{(i)} = \begin{cases} (n/n')\left(p_{a|k_0}^{(i)} - p_{e|k_0}\right)/(1 - p_{e|k_0}), & \text{if } r_i \geq 2, \\ 0, & \text{otherwise,} \end{cases}$

$\diamond\ p_{a|k_0}^{(i)} = \dfrac{1}{p_{k_0}}\left(\dfrac{r_{ik_0}(r_{ik_0}^\star - 1)}{r_i(r_i - 1)} - (\varepsilon_{ik_0} - p_{k_0})p_{a|k_0}\right).$

The conditional Fleiss' reliability and validity coefficients and their associated variances will be discussed next.

CONDITIONAL FLEISS' COEFFICIENT

- *Conditional Fleiss Reliability Coefficient*

Fleiss' reliability coefficient conditionally upon the "true" category k_0 is defined by,

$$\widehat{\kappa}_{F|k_0} = \frac{p_{a|k_0} - p_{e|k_0}}{1 - p_{e|k_0}} \quad \text{where} \quad \begin{cases} p_{a|k_0} = \dfrac{1}{p_{k_0}}\left[\dfrac{1}{n'}\sum_{i=1}^{n'} \dfrac{r_{ik_0}(r_{ik_0}^{\star} - 1)}{r_i(r_i - 1)}\right], \\[3mm] p_{e|k_0} = \displaystyle\sum_{k=1}^{q} \pi_{k|k_0}\pi_{k|k_0}^{\star}, \end{cases} \quad (11.3.15)$$

with p_{k_0} being the probability that a subject's true category is k_0, $\pi_{k|k_0}$ the conditional probability defined by equation 11.3.10, and $\pi_{k|k_0}^{\star}$ the weighted conditional probability defined by,

$$\pi_{k|k_0}^{\star} = \sum_{l=1}^{q} w_{kl}\pi_{l|k_0}. \quad (11.3.16)$$

Variance of Conditional Fleiss Reliability Coefficient

The variance associated with Fleiss' coefficient of reliability is calculated as follows:

$$v(\widehat{\kappa}_{F|k_0}) = \frac{1-f}{n}\frac{1}{n-1}\sum_{i=1}^{n}\left(\widehat{\kappa}_{F|k_0}^{\star(i)} - \widehat{\kappa}_{F|k_0}\right)^2, \quad (11.3.17)$$

where,

$$\diamond \quad \widehat{\kappa}_{F|k_0}^{\star(i)} = \widehat{\kappa}_{F|k_0}^{(i)} - 2(1 - \widehat{\kappa}_{F|k_0})\frac{\varepsilon_{ik_0}\left(p_{e|k_0}^{(i)} - p_{e|k_0}\right)/p_{k_0}}{1 - p_{e|k_0}},$$

$$\diamond \quad p_{e|k_0}^{(i)} = \sum_{k=1}^{q} \pi_{k|k_0}^{\star} r_{ik}/r_i,$$

$$\diamond \quad \widehat{\kappa}_{F|k_0}^{(i)} = \begin{cases} (n/n')\left(p_{a|k_0}^{(i)} - p_{e|k_0}\right)/(1 - p_{e|k_0}), & \text{if } r_i \geq 2, \\[3mm] 0, & \text{otherwise}, \end{cases}$$

$$\diamond \quad p_{a|k_0}^{(i)} = \frac{1}{p_{k_0}}\left(\frac{r_{ik_0}(r_{ik_0}^{\star} - 1)}{r_i(r_i - 1)} - (\varepsilon_{ik_0} - p_{k_0})p_{a|k_0}\right).$$

The conditional Fleiss' validity coefficient and its associated variance will be discussed next.

- *Conditional Fleiss Validity Coefficient*

Fleiss' validity coefficient conditionally upon the "true" category k_0 is defined by,

$$\widehat{\kappa}_{\text{F}|k_0} = \frac{p_{a|k_0} - p_{e|k_0}}{1 - p_{e|k_0}} \text{ where } \begin{cases} p_{a|k_0} = \frac{1}{p_{k_0}}\left[\frac{1}{n'}\sum_{i=1}^{n'}\frac{r_{ik_0}(r^{\star}_{ik_0} - 1)}{r_i(r_i - 1)}\right], \\ p_{e|k_0} = \pi_{k_0|k_0}(2\pi^{\star}_{k_0|k_0} - \pi_{k_0|k_0}). \end{cases} \quad (11.3.18)$$

Variance of Conditional Fleiss Validity Coefficient

The variance associated with Fleiss' coefficient of validity is calculated as follows:

$$v(\widehat{\kappa}_{\text{F}|k_0}) = \frac{1 - f}{n}\frac{1}{n - 1}\sum_{i=1}^{n}\left(\widehat{\kappa}^{\star(i)}_{\text{F}|k_0} - \widehat{\kappa}_{\text{F}|k_0}\right)^2, \quad (11.3.19)$$

where,

⋄ $\widehat{\kappa}^{\star(i)}_{\text{F}|k_0} = \widehat{\kappa}^{(i)}_{\text{F}|k_0} - 2(1 - \widehat{\kappa}_{\text{F}|k_0})\dfrac{\varepsilon_{ik_0}u_{i|k_0}/p_{k_0}}{1 - p_{e|k_0}},$

⋄ $u_{i|k_0} = \pi_{k_0|k_0}(r^{\star}_{ik_0}/r_i - \pi^{\star}_{k_0|k_0}) + (\pi^{\star}_{k_0|k_0} - \pi_{k_0|k_0})(r_{ik_0}/r_i - \pi_{k_0|k_0}),$

⋄ $\widehat{\kappa}^{(i)}_{\text{F}|k_0} = \begin{cases} (n/n')\left(p^{(i)}_{a|k_0} - p_{e|k_0}\right)/(1 - p_{e|k_0}), & \text{if } r_i \geq 2, \\ 0, & \text{otherwise,} \end{cases}$

⋄ $p^{(i)}_{a|k_0} = \dfrac{1}{p_{k_0}}\left(\dfrac{r_{ik_0}(r^{\star}_{ik_0} - 1)}{r_i(r_i - 1)} - (\varepsilon_{ik_0} - p_{k_0})p_{a|k_0}\right).$

CONDITIONAL BRENNAN-PREDIGER COEFFICIENT

The conditional Brennan-Prediger (BP) agreement and validity coefficients are similar to Fleiss' coefficients discussed above, with the exception of the conditional percent chance agreement. For the conditional Brennan-Prediger validity coefficient, the associated conditional percent chance agreement is given by,

$$p_{e|k_0} = T_{w|k_0}/q^2, \quad (11.3.20)$$

where $T_{w|k_0}$ is given by equation 11.3.13. For the conditional Brennan-Prediger reliability coefficient, the associated conditional percent chance agreement is given by,

$$p_{e|k_0} = T_w/q^2, \quad (11.3.21)$$

where T_w is the summation of all q^2 weights. It follows from these two equations above that the percent chance agreement is a constant and is therefore not subject to any sampling variation. Therefore, the BP conditional reliability and validity coefficients share the same variance formula given by,

$$v(\widehat{\kappa}_{\mathrm{BP}|k_0}) = \frac{1-f}{n}\frac{1}{n-1}\sum_{i=1}^{n}\left(\widehat{\kappa}_{\mathrm{BP}|k_0}^{(i)} - \widehat{\kappa}_{\mathrm{BP}|k_0}\right)^2, \qquad (11.3.22)$$

where,

$$\diamond\ \widehat{\kappa}_{\mathrm{BP}|k_0}^{(i)} = \begin{cases} (n/n')\left(p_{a|k_0}^{(i)} - p_{e|k_0}\right)/(1 - p_{e|k_0}), & \text{if } r_i \geq 2, \\ 0, & \text{otherwise,} \end{cases}$$

$$\diamond\ p_{a|k_0}^{(i)} = \frac{1}{p_{k_0}}\left(\frac{r_{ik_0}(r_{ik_0}^{\star}-1)}{r_i(r_i-1)} - (\varepsilon_{ik_0} - p_{k_0})p_{a|k_0}\right).$$

The only difference between the two variances associated with the validity and reliability coefficients comes from the conditional percent chance agreement $p_{e|k_0}$ that is part of the definition of $\widehat{\kappa}_{\mathrm{BP}|k_0}^{(i)}$. For the validity coefficient $p_{e|k_0}$ is given by equation 11.3.20, and is given by equation 11.3.21 for the reliability coefficient.

11.4   Conditional Agreement Coefficient for two Raters in RCM Studies

As previously indicated the notion of "true" category is nonexistent in RCM reliability studies. Conditional analysis is still made possible by conditioning not on the subject's true category, but rather on the category the subject has been assigned to. In this context, Light(1971) defines inter-rater reliability conditionally upon a response category k as the extent of agreement between two raters "for only those items which one observer placed into the kth specific category." Therefore two-rater reliability studies involving two raters A and B may lead to three different conditional inter-rater reliability coefficients on a category k:

▶ The condition could be that "rater A classified the subject into category k." In this case, only those subjects that rater A classified in category k will be taken into consideration, regardless of where rater B classified them.

▶ The condition could be that "rater B classified the subject into category k." In this case, only those subjects that rater B classified in category k will be analyzed, regardless of where rater A classified them.

▶ The condition could be that rater A or rater B classified the subject into category k. In this case, only those subjects that at least one of the two raters A and B classified into category k will be retained for analysis.

Reliability data is typically reported in one of the two forms shown in Tables 11.8 or 11.9. Table 11.8 contains raw data with no loss of information, where g_{ij} equals one of the categories $1, \cdots, q$, and represents the category where rater j classified subject i. Table 11.9 on the other hand, summarizes the content of Table 11.8 and shows the distribution of subjects by rater and category. In this table, p_{kl} is the proportion of subjects that raters 1 and 2 classified into categories k and l respectively. Moreover, p_{k+} represents rater 1's marginal probability of classification in category k, while p_{+l} represents rater 2's marginal probability of classification in category l. Although Table 11.9 does not indicate the specific category into which a given subject was classified, it contains sufficient information for the calculation of all agreement coefficients discussed in this chapter. However, the raw data of Table 11.8 are needed to compute the variances.

The coefficients $\widehat{\kappa}_{C|k+}$, $\widehat{\kappa}_{C|+k}$, and $\widehat{\kappa}_{C|k}$ respectively denote the conditional Kappa given the subjects that rater 1, rater 2, and rater 1 or 2 classified into category k. Similar conditional coefficients related to the AC_1 are denoted as $\widehat{\kappa}_{G|k+}$, $\widehat{\kappa}_{G|+k}$, and $\widehat{\kappa}_{G|k}$. All versions of the conditional inter-rater reliability discussed here are based upon the same conditional percent agreement probability $p_{a|k} = p_{kk}$.

Table 11.8:
Raw Ratings

Subject	Rater 1	Rater 2
1	g_{11}	g_{12}
2	g_{21}	g_{22}
$\vdots$	$\vdots$	$\vdots$
i	g_{i1}	g_{i2}
$\vdots$	$\vdots$	$\vdots$
n	g_{n1}	g_{n2}

Table 11.9:
Distribution of n Subjects by Rater & Category

Rater 1	Rater 2					Total
	1	$\cdots$	l	$\cdots$	q	
1	p_{11}	$\cdots$	p_{1l}	$\cdots$	p_{1q}	p_{1+}
2	p_{21}	$\cdots$	p_{2l}	$\cdots$	p_{2q}	p_{2+}
$\vdots$	$\vdots$		$\vdots$		$\vdots$	$\vdots$
k	p_{k1}	$\cdots$	p_{kl}	$\cdots$	p_{kq}	p_{k+}
$\vdots$	$\vdots$		$\vdots$		$\vdots$	$\vdots$
q	p_{q1}	$\cdots$	p_{ql}	$\cdots$	p_{qq}	p_{q+}
Total	p_{+1}	$\cdots$	p_{+l}	$\cdots$	p_{+q}	1

In the past few chapters the symbol π_k designated the probability that a randomly selected rater classifies a randomly selected subject into category k. In this chapter conditional versions of this probability are needed to define the Pi and AC_1 coefficients conditionally on a response category. Let $\pi_{l|k+}$ be the probability that a subject is classified into category l if selected from the pool of subjects that rater 1 has classified in category k. The probability $\pi_{l|+k}$ could be defined in a similar manner with the subject being randomly selected from the pool of subjects that rater 2 previously classified into category k. If the subject is randomly selected from the pool of subjects that one of the two raters (1 or 2) previously classified into category k, the resulting probability will be denoted by $\pi_{l|k}$.

Here is how the random experiment these conditional probabilities are based upon works. Assume for example that the conditioning is done with respect to rater 1 and a given category k. Both raters first classify all subjects into various categories. Then a subject is randomly selected from the pool of subjects that rater 1 has classified into category k, and one of the two raters (1 or 2) is randomly chosen with the same probability $1/2$. Then l represents the category into which the chosen rater had classified the selected subject. All the conditional probabilities are defined as follows:

$$\pi_{l|k+} = \begin{cases} (1+p_{+k})/2 & \textit{if } l=k, \\ p_{+l}/2 & \textit{if } l \neq k. \end{cases} \textit{, and } \pi_{l|+k} = \begin{cases} (1+p_{k+})/2 & \textit{if } l=k, \\ p_{l+}/2 & \textit{if } l \neq k. \end{cases} \quad (11.4.1)$$

$$\pi_{l|k} = \begin{cases} \pi_k/p_{2k} & \textit{if } l=k, \\ \dfrac{p_{kl}+p_{lk}}{2p_{2k}} & \textit{if } l \neq k. \end{cases} \textit{ where } p_{2k} = p_{k+} + p_{+k} - p_{kk} \quad (11.4.2)$$

To illustrate the calculation of the conditional probabilities of Equations 11.4.1 and 11.4.2, I will use hypothetical data shown in Table 11.10 and summarized in Table 11.11. This data represents the preferences (GOOD or BAD) of two judges A and B with respect to 12 visiting places. Table 11.12 contains the conditional probabilities $\pi_{l|+k}$ that a place randomly selected among those judge B classified into category k, is classified into category l by one of the 2 judges selected randomly.

It follows that if judge B rates a place as "GOOD", it is likely to be rated as "BAD" with probability 0.125, and as "GOOD" with probability 0.875. Likewise a place rated as "BAD" by judge A is likely to be rated as "GOOD" with probability 0.333 as shown in Table 11.13. Table 11.14 indicates that if it is known that a place was classified as "BAD" by either rater, then it is likely to be classified as "BAD", or "GOOD" with probabilities 0.875, and 0.125 respectively by a randomly selected rater.

11.4.1   *Conditional Kappa Statistic of Light (1971)*

Light (1971) introduced two conditional Kappa coefficients. The first Kappa coefficient denoted by $\widehat{\kappa}_{L|k+}$ is defined conditionally upon subjects that rater 1 classified into category k. The second coefficient $\widehat{\kappa}_{L|+k}$ on the other hand, is defined conditionally upon subjects that rater two classified in category k. These two Kappa coefficients are defined as follows :

$$\widehat{\kappa}_{L|k+} = \frac{p_{kk} - p_{+k}p_{k+}}{p_{k+}(1 - p_{+k})} = \frac{p_{a|k+} - p_{+k}}{1 - p_{+k}}, \tag{11.4.3}$$

$$\widehat{\kappa}_{L|+k} = \frac{p_{kk} - p_{+k}p_{k+}}{p_{+k}(1 - p_{k+})} = \frac{p_{a|+k} - p_{k+}}{1 - p_{k+}}, \tag{11.4.4}$$

where $p_{a|k+} = p_{kk}/p_{k+}$ and $p_{a|+k} = p_{kk}/p_{+k}$. I propose another conditional Kappa $\widehat{\kappa}_{L|k}$, defined conditionally upon subjects that either rater classified into category k. It is defined as follows :

$$\widehat{\kappa}_{L|k} = \frac{p_{kk} - p_{+k}p_{k+}}{p_{2k} - p_{+k}p_{k+}} = \frac{p_{a|k} - p_{e|k}}{1 - p_{e|k}}, \tag{11.4.5}$$

where p_{2k} is the percent of subjects classified into category k, and given by:

$$p_{2k} = p_{k+} + p_{+k} - p_{kk}, \quad p_{a|k} = p_{kk}/p_{2k}, \text{ and } \quad p_{e|k} = p_{k+}p_{+k}/p_{2k}. \tag{11.4.6}$$

For comparison, we would recall that Cohen's unconditional Kappa coefficient discussed in earlier chapters is given by:

$$\widehat{\kappa}_{\kappa} = \frac{p_a - p_{e\kappa}}{1 - p_{e\kappa}}, \text{ where } p_a = \sum_{k=1}^{q} p_{kk}, \text{ and } p_{e\kappa} = \sum_{k=1}^{q} p_{+k}p_{k+}. \tag{11.4.7}$$

Table 11.10: Rating by Judges A & B, of 12 US Places

Place	Judge A	Judge B
1	Good	Good
2	Good	Good
3	Good	Good
4	Good	Bad
5	Good	Good
6	Bad	Bad
7	Good	Good
8	Good	Good
9	Good	Good
10	Bad	Bad
11	Good	Good
12	Bad	Bad

Table 11.11: Distribution of US Places by Judge And Attractiveness (Good vs. Bad)

Judge A	Judge B		
	Bad	Good	Total
Bad	3	0	3
Good	1	8	9
Total	4	8	12

Table 11.12: Conditional Probabilities $\pi_{l|+k}$ given Judge B's Score

Category	Judge B $(+k)$	
(l)	Bad	Good
Bad	0.625	0.125
Good	0.375	0.875
Total	1	1

Table 11.13: Conditional Probabilities $\pi_{l|k+}$ given Judge A's Score

Category	Judge A $(k+)$	
(l)	Bad	Good
Bad	0.667	0.167
Good	0.333	0.833
Total	1.000	1.000

Table 11.14: Conditional Probabilities $\pi_{l|k}$ given Judges A/B's Score

Category	Judge A or B (k)	
(l)	Bad	Good
Bad	0.875	0.056
Good	0.125	0.944
Total	1.000	1.000

Example 11.1

To illustrate the calculation conditional Kappa coefficients, let us consider the reliability data of Table 11.10. Table 11.15 shows Kappa conditionally upon judge A's rating ($\widehat{\kappa}_{\text{L}|k+}$), Kappa conditionally upon judge B's rating ($\widehat{\kappa}_{\text{L}|+k}$), and Kappa conditionally upon judges A and B's ratings ($\widehat{\kappa}_{\text{L}|k}$). The regular (i.e. unconditional) Kappa coefficient is given by: $\widehat{\kappa}_{\text{C}} = (0.917 - 0.583)/(1 - 0.583) = 0.800$.

Table 11.15: Kappa Agreement Coefficients Conditionally upon the Category used by Judges A, B, and A or B Respectively

Category	Judge A's Rating			Judge B's Rating			Judges A or B		
(k)	$p_{a|k+}$	$p_{e|k+}$	$\widehat{\kappa}_{\text{L}|k+}$	$p_{a|+k}$	$p_{e|+k}$	$\widehat{\kappa}_{\text{L}|+k}$	$p_{a|k}$	$p_{e|k}$	$\widehat{\kappa}_{\text{L}|k}$
Bad	1.000	0.333	1.000	0.750	0.250	0.667	0.750	0.250	0.667
Good	0.889	0.667	0.667	1.000	0.750	1.000	0.889	0.667	0.667

▶ Table 11.15 indicates that if judge A characterizes a place as Bad then the extent of agreement with judge B as evaluated by Kappa is 1. That is $\widehat{\kappa}_{\text{L}|\text{BAD}+} = 1$. If it is judge B who characterizes a place as Bad, then the extent of agreement with judge A becomes 0.667.

▶ If either one of the two judges characterizes a place as BAD, the Kappa extent of agreement among judges will be $\widehat{\kappa}_{\text{L}|\text{BAD}} = 0.667$. This Kappa values remains the same under the condition that one of the two judges considers a place as GOOD.

11.4.2   *k-Conditional Coefficient of Fleiss (1971)*

In addition to proposing a multiple-rater version of the Pi coefficient, Fleiss (1971) also suggested a conditional π-statistic on category k using an overall agreement probability of p_{kk}/π_k and a chance-agreement probability π_k. I believe that the basis for using π_k as chance-agreement probability is questionable. Instead, I suggest three conditional coefficients labeled as $\widehat{\kappa}_{\text{F}|k+}$, $\widehat{\kappa}_{\text{F}|+k}$, and $\widehat{\kappa}_{\text{F}|k}$ that are defined conditionally upon the subjects classified into category k by rater 1, rater 2, or either one of them respectively. These coefficients are formally defined as follows:

$$\widehat{\kappa}_{\text{F}|k+} = \frac{p_{kk}/p_{k+} - p_{e|k+}}{1 - p_{e|k+}}, \text{ where } p_{e|k+} = \pi_k^2, \tag{11.4.8}$$

$$\widehat{\kappa}_{\text{F}|+k} = \frac{p_{kk}/p_{+k} - p_{e|+k}}{1 - p_{e|+k}}, \text{ where } p_{e|+k} = \pi_k^2, \tag{11.4.9}$$

$$\widehat{\kappa}_{\text{F}|k} = \frac{p_{kk}/p_{2k} - p_{e|k}}{1 - p_{e|k}}, \text{ where } p_{e|k} = \pi_k^2, \tag{11.4.10}$$

where $p_{2k} = p_{k+} + p_{+k} - p_{kk}$ is the probability that a randomly selected subject is classified into category k by either rater. These conditional agreement coefficients are more in line with the unconditional coefficient of Fleiss (1971).

Example 11.2

The conditional coefficients of equations 11.4.8, 11.4.9, and 11.4.10 are illustrated in Table 11.16 using the reliability data of Table 11.10. These results are close to those of the conditional Kappa coefficients of Table 11.15. Fleiss' unconditional coefficient is given by $\widehat{\kappa}_{\text{F}} = (0.917 - 0.587)/(1 - 0.587) = 0.798$ for comparison.

Table 11.16: Pi-Agreement Coefficients Conditionally upon the Category used by Judges A, B, and A or B Respectively

Category	Judge A			Judge B			Judges A or B		
(k)	$p_{a|k+}$	$p_{e|k+}$	$\widehat{\kappa}_{\text{F}|k+}$	$p_{a|+k}$	$p_{e|+k}$	$\widehat{\kappa}_{\text{F}|+k}$	$p_{a|k}$	$p_{e|k}$	$\widehat{\kappa}_{\text{F}|k}$
Bad	1.000	0.085	1.000	0.750	0.085	0.727	0.750	0.085	0.727
Good	0.889	0.502	0.777	1.000	0.502	1.000	0.889	0.502	0.777

11.4.3 k-Conditional AC_1-Statistic

In this section, I propose three conditional AC_1 agreement coefficients denoted by $\widehat{\kappa}_{\text{G}|k+}$, $\widehat{\kappa}_{\text{G}|+k}$, and $\widehat{\kappa}_{\text{G}|k}$. The first coefficient $\widehat{\kappa}_{\text{G}|k+}$ represents the conditional AC_1 coefficient given the subjects that rater 1 classified into category k. The second coefficient $\widehat{\kappa}_{\text{G}|+k}$ represents the conditional AC_1 coefficient given the subjects that rater two classified into category k, and the third coefficient $\widehat{\kappa}_{\text{G}|k}$ is the conditional AC_1 coefficient given the subjects that either one of the 2 raters classified into category k. More formally, these coefficients are defined as follows:

$$\widehat{\kappa}_{\text{G}|k+} = \frac{p_{kk}/p_{k+} - p_{e|k+}}{1 - p_{e|k+}}, \text{ where } p_{e|k+} = \frac{1}{q-1} \sum_{l=1}^{q} \pi_{l|k+}(1 - \pi_{l|k+}), \tag{11.4.11}$$

$$\widehat{\kappa}_{\mathrm{G}|+k} = \frac{p_{kk}/p_{+k} - p_{e|+k}}{1 - p_{e|+k}}, \quad \text{where } p_{e|+k} = \frac{1}{q-1} \sum_{l=1}^{q} \pi_{l|+k}(1 - \pi_{l|+k}), \qquad (11.4.12)$$

$$\widehat{\kappa}_{\mathrm{G}|k} = \frac{p_{kk}/p_k - p_{e|k}}{1 - p_{e|k}}, \quad \text{where } p_{e|k} = \frac{1}{q-1} \sum_{l=1}^{q} \pi_{l|k}(1 - \pi_{l|k}), \qquad (11.4.13)$$

where the conditional probabilities $\pi_{l|k+}$, $\pi_{l|+k}$, and $\pi_{l|k}$ are given by equations 11.4.1 and 11.4.2.

Example 11.3

The conditional AC_1 coefficients are illustrated in Table 11.17 using the same reliability data of Table 11.10. These coefficients are consistently high except when judge B considers a place to be Bad. In this case, the conditional AC_1 denoted by $AC_1|_{+\mathrm{BAD}}$ decreases to 0.529. The "unconditional" AC_1-coefficient is given by $\widehat{\kappa}_{\mathrm{G}} = (0.917 - 0.413)/(1 - 0.413) = 0.858$.

Table 11.17: AC_1 Statistics Conditionally upon the Category k, used by Judges A, B, and A or B

Category	Judge A			Judge B			Judges A or B		
(k)	$p_{a|k+}$	$p_{e|k+}$	$\widehat{\kappa}_{\mathrm{G}|k+}$	$p_{a|+k}$	$p_{e|+k}$	$\widehat{\kappa}_{\mathrm{G}|+k}$	$p_{a|k}$	$p_{e|k}$	$\widehat{\kappa}_{\mathrm{G}|k}$
Bad	1.000	0.444	1.000	0.750	0.469	0.529	0.750	0.219	0.680
Good	0.889	0.278	0.846	1.000	0.219	1.000	0.889	0.105	0.876

11.4.4 k-Conditional Brennan-Prediger Statistic

In this section, I propose three conditional Brennan-Prediger agreement coefficients denoted by $\widehat{\kappa}_{\mathrm{BP}|k+}$, $\widehat{\kappa}_{\mathrm{BP}|+k}$, and $\widehat{\kappa}_{\mathrm{BP}|k}$. The first coefficient $\widehat{\kappa}_{\mathrm{BP}|k+}$ represents the conditional BP coefficient given the subjects that rater 1 classified into category k. The second coefficient $\widehat{\kappa}_{\mathrm{BP}|+k}$ represents the conditional BP coefficient given the subjects that rater 2 classified into category k, and the third coefficient $\widehat{\kappa}_{\mathrm{BP}|k}$ is the conditional BP coefficient given the subjects classified into category k (by either rater). More formally, these coefficients are defined as follows :

$$\widehat{\kappa}_{\mathrm{BP}|k+} = \frac{p_{kk}/p_{k+} - p_{e|k+}}{1 - p_{e|k+}}, \quad \text{where } p_{e|k+} = 1/q^2, \qquad (11.4.14)$$

$$\widehat{\kappa}_{\mathrm{BP}|+k} = \frac{p_{kk}/p_{+k} - p_{e|+k}}{1 - p_{e|+k}}, \quad \text{where } p_{e|+k} = 1/q^2, \qquad (11.4.15)$$

$$\widehat{\kappa}_{\text{\tiny BP}|k} = \frac{p_{kk}/p_{2k} - p_{e|k}}{1 - p_{e|k}}, \text{ where } p_{e|k} = 1/q^2, \tag{11.4.16}$$

where q is the number of response categories.

Example 11.4 _____

The conditional BP coefficients are illustrated in Table 11.18 using reliability data of Table 11.10. These coefficients consistently exceed 0.6. The "unconditional" BP-coefficient is given by $\widehat{\kappa}_{\text{\tiny BP}} = (0.917 - 0.5)/(1 - 0.5) = 0.834$.

Table 11.18: BP Agreement Coefficients Conditionally upon Category k by Judges A, B, and A or B Respectively

Category	Judge A			Judge B			Judges A or B		
(k)	$p_{a\|k+}$	$p_{e\|k+}$	$\widehat{\kappa}_{\text{\tiny BP}\|k+}$	$p_{a\|+k}$	$p_{e\|+k}$	$\widehat{\kappa}_{\text{\tiny BP}\|+k}$	$p_{a\|k}$	$p_{e\|k}$	$\widehat{\kappa}_{\text{\tiny BP}\|k}$
Bad	1.000	0.25	1.000	0.750	0.25	0.667	0.750	0.25	0.667
Good	0.889	0.25	0.852	1.000	0.25	1.000	0.889	0.25	0.852

11.5   Concluding Remarks

Although chance-corrected inter-rater reliability coefficients represented by a single index have been widely-accepted by researchers, they have also been criticized for being difficult to interpret. The difficulty in interpreting agreement coefficients stems from the dependency of inter-rater reliability coefficients on trait prevalence, or in general on the actual distribution of subjects by response category. It is the need to resolve this problem that led to the development of conditional agreement coefficients.

The notion of actual distribution of subjects by response category assumes for each subject the existence of a unique and specific category to which he can be classified objectively. I considered such subjects to have an Absolute Category Membership (ACM), and refer to them as ACM subjects. Reliability experiments involving ACM subjects were referred to as ACM studies, and agreement coefficients have been conditioned on the subjects' true category. I was able to quantify the extent of agreement among raters under the condition that the subjects belong to a certain category. These conditional agreement coefficients are expected to show more stability over time in addition to allowing comparison between different reliability studies. While rating an ACM subject, two raters may agree either about the correct category or about a wrong one. Although in both cases there will be agreement, I suggested that the extent of agreement about the true category be analyzed with validity coefficients and the extent of agreement about any category be analyzed with reliability coefficients. Both types of coefficients were also studied conditionally upon the subject's true membership category. Conditioning allows researchers to identify specific groups of subjects that prevent raters from reaching higher agreement levels.

As previously indicated, some reliability experiments are based on subjects that do not possess an Absolute Category Membership. For example experiments involving human subjects who express their preferences in the form of response categories. These subjects possess what I referred to as the Relative Category Membership (RCM). While agreement coefficients in ACM studies can be conditioned on the subject's true category, conditioning in RCM studies is typically done on the category into which one or more raters classified the subject. The AC_1 coefficient for example may quantify the extent of agreement conditionally upon subjects that rater 1 classified in category k. Such a coefficient in the context of two raters is denoted by $\widehat{\kappa}_{G|k+}$. I have limited the conditional analysis in RCM studies to two raters only. This is due to the fact that the interest of practitioners for this type of analysis on RCM subjects is yet to be confirmed. Moreover, in a two-rater experiment the other rater is always special since it is necessarily the reference for comparison. In a multiple-rater experiment choosing one rater as reference for comparison might not always be justified. Although reliability coefficients are adjusted for chance agreement, conditioning works well if each rater can be assumed to have a reasonably stable rating pattern for a given subject population.

Practitioners would note that one limitation inherent to all conditional analyzes stems from the difficulty to have a precise evaluation of the various conditional probabilities. For ACM studies, a precise evaluation of the conditional probabilities would require the knowledge of each subject's true membership category in the subject universe. Although experts may at times provide that information, in most practical applications that information will not be available. In RCM studies, a precise evaluation of the conditional probabilities requires the knowledge of raters' marginal probabilities. That is the category into which each rater would classify each population subject. Because of the limited information available following a reliability experiment, the conditional probabilities are generally estimated using sample information with the risk of increasing the sampling error associated with the agreement coefficients.

CHAPTER 12

Measures of Association and Item Analysis

OBJECTIVE

The main objective of this chapter is to review some special agreement coefficients that are used in item analysis, or used to quantify the extent of agreement among raters with respect to the rankings of subjects. I discuss Cronbach's alpha, known to measure internal consistency of items in scale development. I also discuss widely-used measures of association such as the Kendall's coefficient of concordance, the Spearman's correlation coefficient, among others. I present the assumptions underlying these techniques as well as the practical situations in which their use is recommended.

CONTENTS

12.1 Overview

In this chapter, I will review the Cronbach's alpha coefficient frequently used in item analysis. Also discussed are other measures of association aimed at evaluating the extent of agreement among raters with respect to the ranking of subjects. These special agreement coefficients do not fall into the category of chance-corrected measures such as Kappa, nor into the category of intraclass correlation coefficients. Nevertheless, they are often used by practitioners to address specific inter-rater reliability problems that cannot be resolved with the methods discussed in previous chapters.

The Cronbach's alpha, which is discussed in section 12.2, is deemed useful by researchers involved in scale development. It allows you to select an adequate set of questions for developing a scale needed to measure a particular construct of interest. In sections 12.3, 12.4, and 12.5 I present additional methods, which are recommended for evaluating the extent of agreement among raters when the subject's rank relative to other subjects is more relevant than its actual score. In many inter-rater reliability problems, the exact score assigned to subjects is not needed. What matters, is how each subject ranks with respect to other subjects. I previously gave an example of government examiners scoring proposals submitted by contractors in response to a pre-solicitation notice. Although each individual proposal is scored, it is the ranking that determines the winner. Any inter-rater reliability experiment designed to improve the extent of agreement among government examiners for example, will produce data that should be analyzed with rank-based methods.

12.2 Cronbach's Alpha

Cronbach's Alpha[1] (α) is a measure of internal consistency that is popular in the field of psychometrics. This measure was originally developed in a context where a set of questions (also called items) are asked to a group of individuals with the objective of measuring a specific construct such as risk aversion, extraversion or introversion. The extent to which all questions contribute positively towards measuring the same concept is known as internal consistency. This is a key element for evaluating the quality of the overall score. Cronbach's alpha is one of the most widely-used measure of internal consistency.

Items that are internally consistent can be seen as raters that agree about the

---

[1]The term alpha (α) is used very often in the study of reliability as we saw in the past few chapters. We previously investigated Krippendorff's alpha as well as Aickin's alpha. Cronbach's alpha however, proposed by Cronbach (1951) does not have much in common with the previous alpha coefficients.

"true" value of the construct associated with the subjects that participated in the experiment. In that sense, Cronbach's alpha could be seen as an agreement coefficient, although some authors refer to it as a measure of association, or simply a measure of reliability. The terms agreement and association are generally used in this context in a lousy sense.

12.2.1   Defining Cronbach's Alpha

Table 12.1 contains the responses that 15 employees provided to 6 questions aimed at measuring the quality of leadership in the company they work for. Each of these questions must be answered on a five-level Likert scale[2] defined as 1= "Strongly Disagree", 2="Disagree", 3="Undecided", 4="Agree", 5="Strongly Agree." The 5 questions are the following:

1A I know my organization's mission (what it is trying to accomplish).

1B I know my organization's vision (where it is trying to go in the future).

1C My senior (top) leaders use our organization's values to guide us.

1D My senior leaders create a work environment that helps me do my job.

1E My organization's leaders share information about the organization.

1F My organization asks what I think.

Let k be the number of items (or questions), s_i^2 the variance associated with item i, and s_T^2 the variance associated with the total (or sum) of all k item scores. Cronbach's alpha is mathematically defined as follows:

$$\alpha = \frac{k}{k-1}\left(1 - \frac{1}{s_T^2}\sum_{i=1}^{k} s_i^2\right) \qquad (12.2.1)$$

Referring to Table 12.1, one can see that $k = 6$ (the number of questions), which leads to 6 item variances from s_1^2 to s_6^2. Each of the 6 item variances may be calculated as the sample variance using the data in each item's column. Then the total variance s_T^2 may be calculated using data in the Total column.

---

[2]Likert's scales are attributed to Rensis Likert (1931), and are further discussed by McIver and Carmines (1981)

12.2.2 How Does Cronbach's Alpha Evaluate Internal Consistency?

A fundamental question to ask is whether the α coefficient as defined by equation 12.2.1 accomplishes its mission, which is to evaluate internal consistency. In my opinion, the answer is that this mission is well accomplished to a large extent. To see this, I need to re-write equation 12.2.1 as follows:

$$\alpha = \frac{\overline{c}/\overline{v}}{1/k + (1 - 1/k)\overline{c}/\overline{v}}, \tag{12.2.2}$$

where $\overline{c}$ is the average of all $k(k-1)$ pairwise covariances associated with the k items under investigation, and $\overline{v}$ the average of all k item variances s_i^2 (i varying from 1 to k). The ratio $\overline{c}/\overline{v}$ (let's call it $\overline{r}^\star$) can be seen as a proxy measure of correlation between two arbitrary items taken from the set of k items. If the k items are internally consistent (meaning they are highly correlated), then you would expect $\overline{r}^\star$ to be close to 1. In the extreme situation of perfect correlation among the k items, the correlation coefficient $\overline{r}^\star$ will be 1, which in turn leads to an alpha coefficient of 1. If the k items are inconsistent (i.e. are weakly correlated) then $\overline{r}^\star$ is expected to be close to 0. If the k items are totally independent, then their correlation coefficient $\overline{r}^\star$ will be 0, leading to a 0 alpha coefficient. Because of all these properties, the alpha coefficient is seen as a measure of internal consistency that varies between 0 and 1 (i.e. between low consistency and high consistency).

Table 12.1: Leadership Data from 15 Respondents

Respondent	Questions/Items						Total
	1A	1B	1C	1D	1E	1F	
1	5	5	3	3	2	2	20
2	4	4	3	5	4	4	24
3	4	5	4	4	4	4	25
4	5	3	4	4	2	2	20
5	4	3	5	4	3	3	22
6	5	2	1	1	1	1	11
7	5	5	4	4	4	4	26
8	4	4	3	2	1	1	15
9	5	5	1	1	1	1	14
10	5	4	1	2	2	1	15
11	4	4	3	4	3	2	20
12	3	2	3	4	3	4	19
13	5	5	5	1	4	1	21
14	5	5	3	2	4	4	23
15	5	4	3	2	4	2	20

Equation 12.2.2 also indicates that the larger the number of items, the higher the alpha coefficient. That is, questionnaires based on more items are perceived to be more reliable all other factors being the same.

Example 12.1 _____

To illustrate the calculation of Cronbach's alpha, let us consider the data in Table 12.1. As previously mentioned, the number of items being studied is $k = 6$. The 6 item-level variances are given by $s_1^2 = 0.4095$, $s_2^2 = 1.1429$, $s_3^2 = 1.6381$, $s_4^2 = 1.8381$, $s_5^2 = 1.4571$, and $s_6^2 = 1.6857$. The variance associated with the total score is $s_T^2 = 18.3810$. I calculated these variances using Excel and the appropriate variance function. Since the sum of the item-level variances is 8.1714, the alpha coefficient is calculated as follows:

$$\alpha = (6/(6-1)) \times (1 - 8.1714/18.3810) = 0.6665.$$

Is there a threshold that α must exceed before we can conclude that the items are internally consistent ? The answer is that there is no official and widely-accepted threshold. A rule of thumb that has been advocated in the literature (c.f. Nunnaly, 1978) is to require α to equal 0.70 or exceed it before the items are considered internally consistent.

_____

There are a few important comments about Cronbach's alpha that are worth making:

- The α coefficient as defined by equation 12.2.1 is expected to always fall between 0 and 1. In reality, that will not always be the case, especially when the number subjects participating in the experiment is small. The alpha coefficient could indeed take a negative value. The cause of this odd situation is some negative between-item covariances with a large absolute value. The only thing known with certainty is that α does not exceed 1.

- Cronbach's alpha is the generalization of the Kuder-Richardson Formula 20 (often referred to in the literature as KR-20), which was proposed for dichotomous items by Kuder and Richardson (1937). Although the KR-20 is still being mentioned in the literature, it no longer plays an important role in the study of reliability other than being a special case of Cronbach's alpha.

- **Standardized Cronbach's alpha**

  When the k items under investigation use different measurement units, then summing the variances s_i^2 becomes problematic since they would also be expressed in different units. The same issue appears with the calculation of the total variance s_T^2.

  This problem has been resolved by using the *Standardized Cronbach's Alpha* coefficient, which is defined as follows:

$$\alpha_S = \frac{k\bar{r}}{1 + (k-1)\bar{r}},$$

(12.2.3)

where $\bar{r}$ is the average of all distinct $k(k-1)/2$ pairwise correlation coefficients between the k items. Note that the correlation coefficient between two items can always be calculated whether they are both expressed with the same units or with different units.

To illustrate the calculation of the standardized Cronbach's alpha, let us consider the leadership data of Table 12.1 once again. For this dataset, Cronbach's alpha was estimated to be 0.6665.

Example 12.2 _____

Since the leadership test is based on 6 items (or questions), there are $6 \times (6-1)/2 = 15$ different pairwise correlation coefficients that can be calculated. All 15 correlation coefficients are shown in Table 12.2. The average correlation coefficient is given by $\bar{r} = 0.1838$, which leads to a standardized alpha of,

$$\alpha_S = \frac{6 \times 0.1838}{1 + (6-1) \times 0.1838} = 0.5747.$$

Table 12.2: Item Pairwise Correlation Coefficients from Table 12.1 Data

	1A	1B	1C	1D	1E
1B	0.4176				
1C	-0.2209	0.1566			
1D	-0.5708	-0.1478	0.4583		
1E	-0.1295	0.3321	0.6103	0.4190	
1F	-0.4470	0.0515	0.4126	0.7223	0.6927

It appears that the standardized Cronbach's alpha is smaller that the raw coefficient. This is not an indication of the superiority of the raw alpha coefficient. These two coefficients are based on two different computation techniques, and each needs specific benchmarks for interpreting the extent of internal consistency.

• Length of the Test

The test length measured by the number of items, affects the magnitude of Cronbach's alpha as previously indicated. That is, alpha increases as the number k of items goes up. Consequently, a good test must have an adequate number of items in order to achieve a reasonable internal consistency as evaluated with Cronbach's alpha.

Moreover, many test developers want the magnitude of alpha to be an attribute of the test. This will be the case only if alpha is calculated based on a sample of test takers that is representative of the universe they were selected from. Even in this case, alpha would be an attribute of the test and the target population of potential test takers. However, if the sample of test takers is not representative of any target population, then alpha becomes an attribute of both the test and the specific sample used, with limited value beyond.

12.2.3 *Use of Cronbach's Alpha*

In the previous sections, I introduced alpha as a measure of internal consistency. But is the test of internal consistency what matters? Many researchers are primarily concerned with the unidimensionality[3] of the test. However, it is the Factor Analysis that identifies the test dimensions, and not Cronbach's alpha. If the test is unidimensional then its items will be highly correlated and Cronbach's alpha will have a high value. However, a high alpha value is not an indication of unidimensionality. It merely represents internal consistency, which is an appealing property in its own right.

If factor analysis reveals the existence of two dimensions or more, then alpha must be calculated separately for each dimension rather than for all dimensions. Therefore, calculating alpha after factor analysis had identified the factors appears to be the appropriate analysis procedure. Combining all factors will artificially increase the magnitude of alpha due to a larger number of items used in the calculation.

What to do with a low alpha?

A low value for alpha may result from the following three sources:

- **Small Number of Items**

  It is unclear what the optimal number of items should be for a given test. Such an optimal number will depend on various factors that cannot be controlled, including the sample of test takers, and the very nature of the test. However, if alpha is to be used for measuring internal consistency, the number of items will surely need to exceed 2 if you want alpha to have a reasonable magnitude.

- **Multidimensionality**

  If the tests includes several factors, then computing alpha for each factor may increase its value with a higher item pairwise correlation coefficients. As mentioned earlier factor analysis can help identify a multidimensional test.

---

[3]A test is said to be unidimensional if all of its items are important contributors to the value of a single latent trait or construct.

- **Poor Item Correlation**

A low alpha is always the result of low correlation between items, which in turn may be due to a multidimensional test or a non-representative sample of test takers. In either case, problem items could be revised or discarded. These problem items are identified by computing the item-total correlation[4]. One may also compute the alpha coefficient without the designated item in order to determine its impact.

Example 12.3

The purpose of this example is to analyze the effect that each of the 6 items of the leadership test of Table 12.1 has on various statistics related to the instrument reliability. As it appears, item 1A has considerable influence based on the magnitude of all the statistics being investigated. For example, the correlation between 1A and the total score without 1A is negative (-0.303). This may be an indication that 1A and the remaining items do not measure the same construct. The situation is about the same for item 1B with a low item-total correlation of 0.186. When each of these items is removed from the test, the resulting alpha value increases substantially (0.757 when 1A is removed, and 0.689 when 1B is removed).

The impact of 1A and 1B can also be observed on the magnitude of the scale mean (i.e. the mean of the total score) and the scale variance. It also appears from the definition of these items that 1A and 1B both relate to the knowledge by employees of their organization's mission and vision. These two questions do not specifically refer to the organization's leadership, and may not be measuring the same construct as the other items.

Table 12.3: Some Statistics when the Designated Item is Deleted

Item #	Scale Mean	Scale Variance	Item-Total Correlation	Alpha
1A	15.133	19.695	-0.303	0.757
1B	15.667	15.667	0.186	0.689
1C	16.600	11.829	0.558	0.560
1D	16.800	12.457	0.427	0.614
1E	16.867	10.838	0.766	0.476
1F	17.267	11.210	0.631	0.527
N/A[a]	19.667	18.381	1.000	0.667

[a]This refers to the case where no item is deleted (i.e. all items included)

---

[4]The item-total correlation represents the correlation coefficient between the designated item and the total score of the other items

12.3   Pearson & Spearman Correlation Coefficients

In this section, I will present two related bivariate measures of association named the Pearson Product-Moment Correlation Coefficient (better known as Pearson Correlation), and the Spearman's Rank-Order Correlation Coefficient (better known as Spearman Correlation). Each of these two measures can only evaluate the extent to which ratings from two raters are related. The Pearson correlation requires stringent conditions to be met to ensure its validity. When these conditions are not met, Spearman's correlation is often the alternative of choice.

Table 12.4 is an extract of Table 9.1 of chapter 9, and represents lung function measurements of 15 children from Rater 1 and Rater 2. The relationship between the two series of ratings is depicted in Figure 12.3.1, where one may see a linear trend. This data will be used to illustrate the calculation of the two correlation coefficients discussed in this section. Let r designate the Pearson correlation coefficient, and r_s the Spearman's correlation. Let X_1 and X_2 represent the abstract ratings associated with raters 1 and 2 respectively.

Table 12.4: 15 children lung function measurements representing the peak expiratory flow rates (PEFR), and taken by raters 1 and 2

Subject (i)	1	2	3	4	5	6	7	8	9	10	11	12	13	14	15
Rater 1	190	220	260	210	270	280	260	275	280	320	300	270	320	335	350
Rater 2	220	200	260	300	265	280	280	275	290	290	300	250	330	320	320

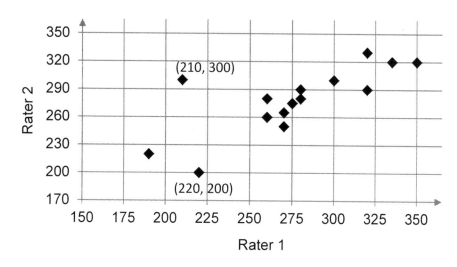

Figure 12.3.1: Lung function measurements of 15 children by Rater 1 and Rater 2

12.3.1 *Pearson's Correlation Coefficient*

The Pearson's correlation is one of the best known coefficients in statistical science, and has been widely used across many fields of research since it was introduced by Pearson (1896, 1900). It is calculated as follows:

$$r = \frac{cov(X_1, X_2)}{\sqrt{v(X_1)}\sqrt{v(X_2)}},$$

(12.3.1)

where $cov(X_1, X_2)$ is the covariance between the ratings X_1 and X_2 associated with raters 1 and 2 respectively, while $v(X_1)$ and $v(X_2)$ are the variances. The variance $v(X_1)$ is a statistical measure that tells you how far you can expect any given rating from rater 1 to stray from the overall average. The covariance $cov(X_1, X_2)$ on the other hand is based on the differences from the ratings to their overall means for both raters 1 and 2, which are multiplied at the individual level. The covariance tells you how large you may expect the product of these individual differences to be. A positive number is an indication that both series of ratings change in the same direction. A negative number on the other hand is an indication that the ratings change in opposite directions.

The correlation coefficient of equation 12.3.1 can be calculated with MS Excel using the function CORREL(). All standard statistical packages have functions for calculating the same coefficient. Using MS Excel, I calculated the correlation coefficient associated with Table 12.4 as follows:

$$r = \frac{1,242.5}{\sqrt{2,065.0}\sqrt{1,301.7}} = 0.758.$$

Note that r determines the extent to which a *linear relationship* exists between the ratings. This coefficient cannot measure agreement as such, since its value may still be high even though one series of ratings is systematically twice higher than the other (a situation that we must admit, is very uncommon for rating data). It is essential to know that Pearson's correlation coefficient assumes that a linear function best describes the relationship between the two series of ratings. If however, that assumption was false then the value of r may not indicate the actual nature of the relationship between the variables. In other words, r would indicate perfect agreement only if both raters agree and that they relationship is linear. Given the importance of the linearity condition, it is essential to first draw a scatterplot as shown in Figure 12.1 in order to perform an initial graphical analysis of the relationship between the 2 series. Only if the graph shows a linear structure should we consider computing the Pearson's correlation coefficient.

Practitioners are not always aware that the validity of the Pearson's correlation coefficient requires a specific list of conditions to be satisfied. Here are these conditions:

(a) The sample of n subjects is randomly selected from the population it represents.

(b) The measurement level associated with each series of ratings is interval or ratio data.

(c) Each of the series of ratings follows the Normal distribution.

Other conditions irrelevant for rating data, are often required to ensure the validity of the Pearson's correlation coefficient.

Computing the p-Value for Pearson's Correlation Coefficient

Let t be a statistic defined as follows:

$$t = \frac{r\sqrt{n-2}}{\sqrt{1-r^2}},$$

(12.3.2)

where n is the number of subjects that participated in the reliability experiment, and r the Pearson's coefficient. The statistic t of equation 12.3.2 follows the Student's distribution[5] with $n-2$ degrees of freedom. The p-value, which measures the statistical significance of the Pearson's correlation coefficient can be calculated using MS Excel as follows:

"=T.DIST.2T(ABS(t),$n-1$)", *for Excel 2010/2011 or a more recent version,*

"=TDIST(ABS(t),$n-1$,2)", *for Excel 2007/2008 or an earlier version.*

Note that the notation Excel 2010/2011 refers to the 2010 Windows version and 2011 Mac version of Excel. Because the last two validity conditions (b) and (c) associated with the Pearson's correlation coefficient are often violated, practitioners frequently use the Spearman's correlation coefficient (also known in the literature as the Spearman's "Rank-Order" Correlation Coefficient).

12.3.2 *Spearman's Correlation Coefficient*

 The Spearman's correlation coefficient is a bivariate measure of correlation, which requires rank-order input data, and which quantifies the extent to which a monotonic relationship exists between 2 sets of ratings. Because it is based on the ranks associated with the ratings, and not on the ratings themselves, Spearman's correlation coefficient is more appropriate for evaluating inter-rater reliability than

---

[5]Readers who need to know more about the Student's law of probability may want to read an introductory statistics book (e.g. Gwet (2010b)).

the Pearson's coefficient. This is due to the fact that if the two series of ratings are in agreement with respect to the ranking of subjects, then their relationship needs not be linear for Spearman's correlation to be high. Agreement on the raw ratings will automatically create a linear relationship between the two series of rankings associated with the raw ratings.

Calculating Spearman's Correlation

The calculation procedure for the Spearman's correlation is best shown with an example. Table 12.5 shows the children lung function data that we analyzed earlier in this section. The "Rank 1" row represents the rankings associated with Rater 1's ratings, while row "Rank 2" contains similar rankings for Rater 2. The rank differences (i.e. Rank 1 - Rank 2) and their squared values calculated in rows d and d^2 are used in the calculation of Spearman's correlation (denoted by r_S) as shown in the following equation:

$$r_S = 1 - \frac{6 \sum_{i=1}^{n} d_i^2}{n(n^2 - 1)}, \tag{12.3.3}$$

where n is the number of subjects (in Table 12.5, $n = 15$), and d_i the rank difference associated with subject i. Based on the information shown in Table 12.5, the Spearman's correlation coefficient is obtained as,

$$r_S = 1 - \frac{6 \times 145}{15 \times (15^2 - 1)} = 0.741.$$

Validity Conditions

Spearman's correlation was developed by Spearman (1904), and can be used if one of the following conditions is satisfied:

(a) The data for both series of ratings are in a rank-order format.

(b) The original data are in a rank-order format for one set of ratings and in an interval/ratio for the second (this latter variable will then have to be converted to ranks before Spearman's correlation is calculated.

(c) The data for both series of ratings have been transformed into a rank-order format from an interval/ratio because the validity conditions associated with the Pearson's coefficient may not be satisfied.

The p-value associated with Spearman's correlation coefficient can be calculated the exact same way it is calculated for Pearson's correlation coefficient.

Table 12.5: Spearman's correlation calculation based on Table 12.4 children lung function measurements

Subject	1	2	3	4	5	6	7	8	9	10	11	12	13	14	15	Total
Rater 1	190	220	260	210	270	280	260	275	280	320	300	270	320	335	350	
Rater 2	220	200	260	300	265	280	280	275	290	290	300	250	330	320	320	
Rank 1	1	3	4.5	2	6.5	9.5	4.5	8	9.5	12.5	11	6.5	12.5	14	15	
Rank 2	2	1	4	11.5	5	7.5	7.5	6	9.5	9.5	11.5	3	15	13.5	13.5	
d	-1	2	0.5	-9.5	1.5	2	-3	2	0	3	-0.5	3.5	-2.5	0.5	1.5	
d^2	1	4	0.25	90.25	2.25	4	9	4	0	9	0.25	12.25	6.25	0.25	2.25	145

Treatment of Ties

If one of the two series of ratings being analyzed contains ties (i.e. repeated ratings or repeated ranks) then it is recommended to compute a tie-adjusted Spearman correlation (denoted by $r_S^\star$), which is given by,

$$
r_S^\star = \frac{A_1 + A_2 - \sum_{i=1}^{n} d_i^2}{2\sqrt{A_1 A_2}},
\tag{12.3.4}
$$

where A_1 and A_2 are now defined. A tie series is defined as a set of ranks that has identical values. It appears from Table 12.5 that each of the two raters has produced 4 tie series containing two scores each. For example, the first tie series from Rater 1 contains the ranks $\{4.5, 4.5\}$ associated with the scores $\{260, 260\}$. Let i be a particular tie series and t_i the associated number of scores. Consider the following quantities:

- T_1 = summation of the differences $t_i^3 - t_i$ for all tie series produced by Rater 1, and $A_1 = (n^3 - n - T_1)/12$. Using Table 12.5 data, T_1 can be calculated as $T_1 = 4 \times (2^3 - 2) = 24$ (note that there are 4 tie series from Rater 1 that contains 2 scores each). Therefore, $A_1 = (15^3 - 15 - 24)/12 = 278$.

- T_2 = summation of the differences $t_i^3 - t_i$ for all tie series produced by Rater 2, and $A_2 = (n^3 - n - T_2)/12$. It follows from Table 12.5 that $T_2 = 4 \times (2^3 - 2) = 24$ (note that there are 4 tie series from Rater 2 that contains 2 scores each). Therefore, $A_2 = (15^3 - 15 - 24)/12 = 278$.

Consequently, the tie-adjusted Spearman correlation is obtained as follows:

$$
r_S^\star = \frac{278 + 278 - 145}{2 \times \sqrt{278 \times 278}} = 0.7392.
$$

12.4   Kendall's Tau

Tau is a Greek character such as alpha, and its symbol τ is used to designate the bivariate measure of association proposed by Kendall (1938). This coefficient is discussed here because a number of researchers have used it to quantify the degree of agreement between rankings from two judges. Kendall's tau is a bivariate coefficient, which is based on rank-order data such as Spearman's correlation. The question then becomes, why Kendall tau when Spearman's correlation was proposed earlier? Although tau requires a more tedious computation procedure, it appears to possess some interesting statistical properties such as unbiasedness that the Spearman's correlation is lacking. Moreover, Lindeman *et a.* (1980) indicated that the Normal distribution provides a good approximation to the sampling distribution of tau for small sample sizes. These appear to be the main reasons some researchers prefer tau to Spearman's correlation.

Kendall's tau can be seen as a measure of the extent of agreement between two sets ranks with respect to the relative ordering of all possible pairs of subjects. That is, for any pair of subjects (i, j) one can determine their rankings (A_i, A_j), and (B_i, B_j) with respect to the two raters A and B. If the sign of the difference $A_i - A_j$ is the same as the sign of the difference $B_i - B_j$, then the pair (i, j) is said to be concordant, otherwise it is said to be discordant. Kendall's tau is essentially the difference between the proportion of concordant pairs and the proportion of discordant pairs.

12.4.1   *Computing Kendall's Tau in the Absence of Ties*

We can claim that there is no tie in the two sets of ratings (and therefore in the associated rankings) when no pair of subjects has two identical values. In this case, any pair of subjects will be either concordant or discordant. The method for dealing with ties will be discussed in the next section.

Let n_C be the number of concordant pairs of subjects, and n_D the number of discordant pairs. If n is the total number of subjects that participated in the experiment, then Kendall's tau is calculated as follows:

$$\tau = \frac{n_C - n_D}{n(n-1)/2}.$$

(12.4.1)

Note that $n(n-1)/2$ is the total number of distinctive pairs of subjects. The following example illustrates the calculation of Kendall's tau using a small sample of 6 subjects.

Example 12.4 _____

Table 12.6 shows 6 subjects and their raw ratings from two judges named Judge1 and Judge2. Rank1 and Rank2 represent the rankings in ascending order of Judge1's and Judge2's ratings. The calculation of Kendall's tau will be based entirely on these rankings as shown in Table 12.7.

Table 12.6: Ratings and Rankings of Six Subjects Scored by Judge 1 and Judge 2

Subject	Judge1	Judge2	Rank1	Rank2
1	9	2.7	5	4
2	6.6	1.4	2	2
3	8	4	4	5
4	7.1	1	3	1
5	10	5.8	6	6
6	6	2	1	3

The first row of Table 12.7 labeled as "Subject #" contains the subject names or labels, the "Rank1" and "Rank2" rows represent the rankings associated with the judges 1 and 2 respectively. The numbers on the table diagonal are Judge 2's rankings. The letters C and D indicate concordant and discordant pairs of subjects formed by the column and row labeled as "Subject #." The first letter C of row $\boxed{1}$ for example, is associated with the pair of subjects $(1, 2)$. This pair is concordant because the associated pairs of ranks (i.e. $(5, 2)$ from Judge1, and $(4, 2)$ from Judge2) change in the same direction (i.e. $5 - 2 = 3 > 0$ and $4 - 2 = 2 > 0$). The first D letter in that same row is associated with the pair of subjects $(1, 3)$. The 2 associated pairs of rankings vary in opposite direction. Therefore, $(1, 3)$ is a discordant pair of subjects. The remaining rows of the table are obtained in the same manner. For example the first C letter of row (ii) is associated with the pair of subjects $(2, 3)$.

Table 12.7: Ratings and Rankings of Six Subjects Scored by Judge 1 and Judge 2

Subject #	$\boxed{1}$	$\boxed{2}$	$\boxed{3}$	$\boxed{4}$	$\boxed{5}$	$\boxed{6}$		
Rank1	5	2	4	3	6	1		
Rank2	4	2	5	1	6	3	n_C	n_D
Subject #								
$\boxed{1}$	4	C	D	C	C	C	4	1
$\boxed{2}$		2	C	D	C	D	2	2
$\boxed{3}$			5	C	C	C	3	0
$\boxed{4}$				1	C	D	1	1
$\boxed{5}$					6	C	1	0
$\boxed{6}$						3	0	0
Concordant & Discordant Pairs							11	4

The symbols n_C and n_D represent the number of concordant and discordant pairs of subjects. It follows from the last row of Table 12.7 that the total number of concordant pairs is 11, while the number of discordant pairs is 4. Using equation 12.4.1, we can compute Kendall's tau as,

$$\tau = \frac{11 - 4}{6 \times (6 - 1)/2} = \frac{7}{15} = 0.4667.$$

12.4.2 Computing Kendall's Tau in the Presence of Ties

When the judges produce ties, then the Kendall's tau coefficient must be properly adjusted. The definition of concordant and discordant pairs of subjects is incompatible with the existence of ties. To see this, consider a pair of subjects (i, j) and the associated ranks $(3.5, 3.5)$ and $(1, 2)$ from 2 judges 1 and 2. This pair of subjects is neither concordant nor discordant since only the second set of ranks changes, the first one remaining unchanged. The tie-adjusted Kendall's tau allows you to exclude pairs with ties from the number of concordant and discordant pairs, and to adjust the denominator accordingly. This tie-adjusted tau coefficient $\tau^\star$ is calculated as follows:

$$\tau^\star = \frac{2(n_C - n_D)}{\sqrt{n(n-1) - T_1} \times \sqrt{n(n-1) - T_2}}. \qquad (12.4.2)$$

To define T_1 and T_2, let i be a specific set of ties, and t_i the number of subjects associated with that set. Then T_1 is the summation of all values $(t_i^3 - t_i)$ for all sets of ties produced by Judge 1. Likewise, T_2 is the summation of all values $(t_i^3 - t_i)$ for all sets of ties produced by Judge 2. The following example illustrates the calculation of the tie-adjusted Kendall's tau coefficient.

Example 12.5

Table 12.8 shows the ratings of 6 subjects by Judge1 and Juge2, as well as the associated rankings labeled as Rank1 and Rank2. Judge1 assigned score 8 to both subjects 2 and 3. This led to the common rank 3.5 being assigned to both subjects. This common rank of 3.5 is obtained as the average of 3 and 4, the two ranks that should normally have been assigned to the two subjects. Likewise the score of 1 that Judge 2 assigned to subjects 1, 2, and 4 led to the rank of 2 being assigned to all 3 subjects (i.e. $2 = (1 + 2 + 3)/3$).

Table 12.9 shows the steps for calculating the tie-corrected Kendall's tau. The procedure is very similar to that of Example 12.4 with the exception that any pair of subjects that possesses ties from either judge will be assigned concordance status of

0. This means that the designated pair of subjects will be excluded from the count of concordant and discordant pairs of subjects.

Table 12.8: Ratings and Rankings of Six Subjects Scored by Judge 1 and Judge 2

Subject	Judge1	Judge2	Rank1	Rank2
1	9	1	5	2
2	8	1	3.5	2
3	8	4	3.5	5
4	7	1	1.5	2
5	10	5.8	6	6
6	7	2	1.5	4

Table 12.9: Computing Tie-Corrected Kendall's Tau Coefficient

Subject#→	1	2	3	4	5	6		
Rank1	5	3.5	3.5	1.5	6	1.5		
Rank2	2	2	5	2	6	4	n_C	n_D
Subject#↓ 1	2	0	D	0	C	D	1	2
2		2	0	0	C	D	1	1
3			5	C	C	C	3	0
4				2	C	0	1	0
5					6	C	1	0
6						4	0	0
Concordant & Discordant Pairs							7	3

It follows from Table 12.9 that the total counts of concordant and discordant pairs of subjects are respectively given by, $n_C = 7$ and $n_D = 3$. Moreover, the series of ratings from judge 1 has 2 sets of ties {3.5,3.5} and {1.5,1.5} with 2 numbers in each. Consequently, $T_1 = (2^3 - 2) + (2^3 - 2) = 12$. On the other hand, the series of ratings from judge 2 shows a single set of ties {2,2,2} with 3 numbers in it. Therefore, $T_2 = (3^3 - 3) = 24$. Using equation 12.4.2, we can compute the tie-corrected Kendall's tau as follows:

$$\tau^\star = \frac{2 \times (7 - 3)}{\sqrt{6 \times (6 - 1) - 12} \times \sqrt{6 \times (6 - 1) - 24}} = 0.7698.$$

The adjusted tau is substantially higher than the unadjusted one. This is due to the relatively high percent of ties in the ratings.

12.4.3   *p-Value for Kendall's Tau*

Let z be a statistic defined as follows:

$$z = \frac{3\tau\sqrt{n(n-1)}}{\sqrt{2(2n+5)}}, \tag{12.4.3}$$

where τ is the sample-based Kendall's tau, and n the number of subjects that participated in the experiment. Under the assumption that the "true" value of τ is actually 0, the statistic z of equation 12.4.3 follows the standard Normal distribution, and can be used for computing the p-value.

The p-value, which represents the probability that the absolute value of the random variable z exceeds its observed value, can be calculated with Excel as follows:

=2*(1-NORM.S.DIST(z_{obs},TRUE)), *for Excel 2010/2011 or a more recent version,*

=2*(1-NORMSDIST(z_{obs})), *for Excel 2007/2008 or an earlier version.*

Equation 12.4.3 will generally be valid for sample sizes as small as 10, and may be used with Kendall's tau whether it is tie-adjusted or not.

Although the number of subjects in Example 12.4 is only 6, using equation 12.4.3 for illustration purposes will yield an observed z-value of,

$$z_{obs} = \frac{3 \times 0.4667\sqrt{6 \times (6-1)}}{2 \times (2 \times 6 + 5)} = 1.3152.$$

This observed z-value leads to a p-value of = 2*(1-NORM.S.DIST(1.3152,TRUE)) = 0.1885, which is too high for Kendall's tau to be considered statistically significant[6]. Kendall's tau, Spearman's and Pearson's correlations are all bivariate measures of association that I discussed in the past few sections. In the next section, I will expand the study of measures of association to include the analysis of three raters or more. The two (very similar) measures to be described are the Kendall's Coefficient of Concordance (KCC), and the Friedman's Chi-Square Statistic (KCS).

12.5   Kendall's Coefficient of Concordance (KCC)

Kendall's coefficient of concordance (KCC) quantifies the extent of agreement among three raters or more with respect to their ranking of the same group of

---

[6]Note that tau would be considered statistically significant in this context, if the p-value is below 0.05. This would mean that the "true" value of tau with no sampling errors can be considered to exceed 0 in absolute 0.

subjects. It is often denoted by W and varies from 0 to 1, 0 representing total absence of agreement and 1 representing complete agreement. The fact that W never takes a negative value is not a problem, as long as the KCC is used to measure agreement among three raters or more. The notion of negative association or negative correlation (i.e. ratings changing in opposite directions) does not apply to a group of three raters or more, even though it is often relevant in the case of 2 raters.

Throughout this section I will assume that the ratings to be analyzed are organized columnwise as shown in Table 12.10. This table shows numeric scores that 4 judges assigned to 6 subjects.

Table 12.10: Ratings of Six Subjects by Judge1, Judge2, Judge3, and Judge4

Subject	Judge1	Judge2	Judge3	Judge4
A	9	2	5	8
B	6	1	3	2
C	8	4	6	8
D	7	1	2	6
E	10	5	6	9
F	6	2	4	7

To formally define Kendall's coefficient of concordance, I assume that n subjects were rated by k judges (for Table 12.10, $n = 6$, and $k = 4$). Since KCC is a measure that is based on ranks, each column of Table 12.10 (except the first column of subject labels) must first be ranked in ascending order from 1 to the number of subjects. Each rating in a particular tie series will receive the same average rank. For example the "Judge1" column of Table 12.10 contains the tie series $\{6, 6\}$, and these numbers are the 2 lowest of all ratings by Judge1. Their respective ranks would normally be 1, and 2, leading to an average rating of $(1 + 2)/2 = 1.5$. For the purpose of calculating the KCC, both numbers will receive the same ranking of 1.5. Let R_{ij} be the abstract rank associated with subject i and rater j.

The KCC represents the ratio of the variance associated with the subject marginal sums of ranks R_i to the maximum possible variance given the number of subjects and the number of judges. More formally, the KCC denoted by W is calculated using one of the following two equations[7]:

$$W = \frac{12S}{k^2 n(n^2 - 1) - kT},$$

(12.5.1)

---

[7]Both ways of calculating Kendall's coefficient of concordance are found in textbooks, and lead to the same result. However, some statistical tables often used to evaluate the statistical significance of KCC are based on the value of S, which cannot be obtained from equation 12.5.2

$$W = \frac{12S^\star - 3k^2 n(n+1)^2}{k^2 n(n^2-1) - kT}, \qquad (12.5.2)$$

where S is the sum over all subjects, of the squared differences from the marginal sums of ranks R_i $(i = 1, \cdots, n)$ to their overall mean $\overline{R}$ (i.e. $(R_i - \overline{R})^2$), and $S^\star$ the sum over all subjects, of the squared R_i (i.e. R_i^2). T is the tie-correction factor that is defined as follows:

$$T = \sum_{l=1}^{m} (t_l^3 - t_l), \qquad (12.5.3)$$

where m is the number of tie series in the data table (e.g. there are 5 tie series having 2 subjects each, in Table 12.10), and t_l is the number of subjects associated with a specific tie series l (e.g. for each tie series l of Table 12.10, $t_l = 2$). The following example illustrates the calculation of Kendall's coefficient of concordance using Table 12.10 data.

Example 12.6

Table 12.11 shows 6 subjects and their rankings by 4 judges based on Table 12.10 ratings. The ratings are ranked independently for each judge. The "R_i" column contains the subject marginal sums of ranks (or row sums), while the "R_i^2" column contains the associated squared values. The "S" row contains the column sum of squared differences $(R_i - \overline{R})^2$, while T shows the result of equation 12.5.3 for each column and for all columns combined.

Table 12.11: Ratings of Six Subjects by Judge1, Judge2, Judge3, and Judge4

Subject	Judge1	Judge2	Judge3	Judge4	R_i	R_i^2
1	5	3.5	4	4.5	17	289
2	1.5	1.5	2	1	6	36
3	4	5	5.5	4.5	19	361
4	3	1.5	1	2	7.5	56.25
5	6	6	5.5	6	23.5	552.25
6	1.5	3.5	3	3	11	121
Total	21	21	21	21	84	1415.5
S	17	16.5	17	17	239.5	
T	6	12	6	6	30	

Using equation 12.5.1, you can compute Kendall's coefficient of concordance as follows:

$$W = \frac{12 \times 239.5}{4^2 \times 6 \times (6^2 - 1) - 4 \times 30} = 0.887.$$

The same result would be obtained using equation 12.12 as follows,

$$W = \frac{12 \times 1,415.5 - 3 \times 4^2 \times 6 \times (6+1)^2}{4^2 \times 6 \times (6^2 - 1) - 4 \times 30} = 0.887.$$

In this example, Kendall's coefficient of concordance is high and close to 1, which suggests high inter-judge reliability among the 4 judges.

Kendall's coefficient of concordance was developed independently by Kendall and Babington-Smith (1939) and Wallis (1939), and has a close relationship with the Spearman's correlation, which is formulated by the following equation:

$$W = \bar{r} - (\bar{r} - 1)/k, \tag{12.5.4}$$

where $\bar{r}$ is the average of all distinct pairwise Spearman's correlation coefficients. Equation 12.5.4 shows that as the number of raters grows, Kendall's coefficient of concordance tends to get closer to the average of the pairwise Spearman correlations.

p-Value of Kendall's Coefficient of Concordance

To compute the p-value associated with Kendall's coefficient of concordance, one must first compute the following statistic:

$$\chi^2 = k(n-1)W, \tag{12.5.5}$$

where W is the KCC computed with equation 12.5.1 or equation 12.5.2. The statistic χ^2 follows the chi-square distribution with $n - 1$ degrees of freedom. The p-value represents the probability that the random variable χ^2 exceeds its observed value (usually denoted by χ^2_{obs}). It can be computed with MS Excel as follows:

=CHISQ.DIST.RT($\chi^2_{obs}, n - 1$), *for EXCEL 2010/2011 or a more recent version,*

=CHIDIST($\chi^2_{obs}, n - 1$), *for EXCEL 2007/2008 or an earlier version.*

Using the numbers from Example 12.6, the observed statistic χ^2_{obs} is calculated as follows:

$$\chi^2_{obs} = k(n-1)W_{obs} = 4 \times (6 - 1) \times 0.887 = 17.74,$$

which leads to a p-value of =CHISQ.DIST.RT(17.74,6-1) = 0.00329. Since this value is below 0.05, one may conclude that the KCC is statistically significant. That is, the "true" error-free coefficient it approximates is considered positive based on the observed ratings. The magnitude of the calculated inter-judge agreement cannot be due to sampling errors alone.

If the number of raters or the number of subjects appears to be too small for the chi-square distribution to provide an adequate approximation to the the sampling distribution of the statistic χ^2, then one may consider some of the methods suggested by Marascuilo and McSweeney (1977) or Siegel and Castellan (1988) who evaluate the significance of W with an adjusted chi-square value.

Relationship with Friedman's Chi-Square Statistic

The Friedman's Chi-Square statistic (denoted by χ_r^2) proposed by Friedman (1937) is sometimes mentioned in studies of inter-judge reliability. But this is essentially due to its close mathematical relationship with Kendall's coefficient (W). Friedman's statistic was developed primarily to test the hypothesis that the ratings assigned to subjects under investigation come from the same statistical population. This is an indirect way of evaluating the extent of agreement among raters.

Kendall's coefficient of concordance may be derived from Friedman chi-square statistic using the following equation:

$$W = \frac{\chi_r^2}{n(k-1)}. \tag{12.5.6}$$

Note that the above equation is valid only if χ_r^2 is calculated first, then used to compute W. If W is calculated first, then it could be used to obtain Friedman's chi-square statistic as,

$$\chi_r^2 = k(n-1)W. \tag{12.5.7}$$

This is due to the fact that in Friedman and Kendall models, k and n play reverse roles.

12.6   Concluding Remarks

In this chapter, I discussed several alternative agreement coefficients that may be more appropriate in special situations where traditional chance-corrected agreement measures or intraclass correlation coefficients are not recommended. These agreement coefficients were discussed along with methods for calculating associated p-values.

The first agreement coefficient presented was Cronbach's alpha, used primarily in the field of psychometrics. Its main objective is to quantify the extent to which a group of items (e.g. items could be questions in a test questionnaire) contribute positively towards the measurement of the same construct such as the proficiency of a nursing student in a particular aspect of patient care. There is no need to worry about agreement by pure chance in this context. Therefore, chance-corrected agreement coefficients will not resolve this problem. Even if the scores are continuous the intraclass correlation coefficient will not be useful since none of the statistical models discussed in the Part III chapters of this book apply. Consequently, the researcher is dealing with a special situation here that requires a special method.

I also presented the well-known Pearson's correlation coefficient. It was not designed to measure agreement among raters at all. Instead, it measures the extent to which the relationship between two series of scores is linear. Although agreement implies a linear relationship, a linear relationship does not imply agreement. The main benefit for using the Pearson's correlation coefficient in the context of agreement analysis lies in its simplicity, and the easiness with which it can be obtained. If this correlation coefficient is low, you know immediately that there is no agreement among raters. On the other hand, if it is high, then you may need to proceed with the use of more appropriate agreement coefficients.

In order to address the issue of agreement among raters with respect to the ranking of subjects, and not with respect to the exact scores, I discussed two coefficients: (i) Spearman's correlation coefficient, and (ii) Kendall's Tau. Both coefficients are designed to quantify the extent to which two raters agree with respect to the ranking of subjects. Although Spearman's correlation is older than Kendall's Tau, the latter coefficient is preferred by some researchers due to some interesting statistical properties it possesses. To quantify the extent of agreement among three raters or more with respect to the ranking of subjects, I also discussed Kendall's coefficient of concordance, and the related Friedman's Chi-square statistic. For the purpose of evaluating agreement with respect to rankings, the use of these coefficients is justified. It is because a disagreement over the scoring of two subjects, which results in the same rankings is considered an agreement. Spearman's correlation, Kendall's Tau, and Kendall's coefficient of concordance will work best with continuous scores, with which chance agreement is less problematic. If raters have a limited number of scores to choose from, the likelihood of chance agreement will increase, leading to an unduly high number of ties. A large number of ties in the rankings must be avoided, as it is expected to reduce the reliability of these ranking-based coefficients.

PART V

APPENDICES

Appendix A

Data Tables

This appendix contains several tables of ratings. Some of these tables were used in examples throughout the book. The reader is encouraged to use them for practice.

Table A.1:
86 Questions and Associated Difficulty Level Scores Assigned by 3 Raters R1, R2, and R3 (Raw Scores 1-5)

Question	R1	R2	R3	Question	R1	R2	R3	Question	R1	R2	R3
1	1	1	1	30	2	3	4	59	3	4	3
2	1	1	1	31	2	3	4	60	3	4	3
3	1	1	3	32	3	3	2	61	3	4	3
4	1	1	3	33	3	3	2	62	3	4	3
5	1	1	3	34	5	3	2	63	3	4	3
6	1	1	3	35	1	4	2	64	3	4	3
7	3	1	1	36	3	4	2	65	3	4	3
8	3	1	1	37	3	4	2	66	3	4	3
9	3	1	2	38	3	4	2	67	3	4	3
10	3	1	2	39	3	4	4	68	3	4	3
11	3	1	2	40	3	4	4	69	3	4	3
12	3	1	2	41	3	4	4	70	3	4	5
13	3	1	2	42	3	4	4	71	3	4	5
14	3	1	2	43	3	4	3	72	3	4	5
15	3	1	2	44	3	4	3	73	3	4	5
16	4	2	2	45	3	4	3	74	3	4	5
17	4	2	2	46	3	4	3	75	3	4	5
18	4	2	3	47	3	4	3	76	3	4	5
19	1	3	2	48	3	4	3	77	3	4	5
20	1	3	2	49	3	4	3	78	4	4	5
21	1	3	2	50	3	4	3	79	4	4	5
22	2	3	2	51	3	4	3	80	4	4	4
23	2	3	2	52	3	4	3	81	3	5	4
24	2	3	2	53	3	4	3	82	4	5	4
25	2	3	2	54	3	4	3	83	5	5	5
26	2	3	2	55	3	4	3	84	5	5	5
27	2	3	4	56	3	4	3	85	5	5	5
28	2	3	4	57	3	4	3	86	5	5	5
29	2	3	4	58	3	4	3				

Table A.2:

86 Questions and Associated Difficulty Level Scores Assigned by 3 Raters R1, R2, and R3 (Distribution of Raters by Question and by Score)

Question	1 2 3 4 5	Question	1 2 3 4 5	Question	1 2 3 4 5
1	3 0 0 0 0	30	0 1 1 1 0	59	0 0 2 1 0
2	3 0 0 0 0	31	0 1 1 1 0	60	0 0 2 1 0
3	2 0 1 0 0	32	0 1 2 0 0	61	0 0 2 1 0
4	2 0 1 0 0	33	0 1 2 0 0	62	0 0 2 1 0
5	2 0 1 0 0	34	0 1 1 0 1	63	0 0 2 1 0
6	2 0 1 0 0	35	1 1 0 1 0	64	0 0 2 1 0
7	2 0 1 0 0	36	0 1 1 1 0	65	0 0 2 1 0
8	2 0 1 0 0	37	0 1 1 1 0	66	0 0 2 1 0
9	1 1 1 0 0	38	0 1 1 1 0	67	0 0 2 1 0
10	1 1 1 0 0	39	0 0 1 2 0	68	0 0 2 1 0
11	1 1 1 0 0	40	0 0 1 2 0	69	0 0 2 1 0
12	1 1 1 0 0	41	0 0 1 2 0	70	0 0 1 1 1
13	1 1 1 0 0	42	0 0 1 2 0	71	0 0 1 1 1
14	1 1 1 0 0	43	0 0 2 1 0	72	0 0 1 1 1
15	1 1 1 0 0	44	0 0 2 1 0	73	0 0 1 1 1
16	0 2 0 1 0	45	0 0 2 1 0	74	0 0 1 1 1
17	0 2 0 1 0	46	0 0 2 1 0	75	0 0 1 1 1
18	0 1 1 1 0	47	0 0 2 1 0	76	0 0 1 1 1
19	1 1 1 0 0	48	0 0 2 1 0	77	0 0 1 1 1
20	1 1 1 0 0	49	0 0 2 1 0	78	0 0 0 2 1
21	1 1 1 0 0	50	0 0 2 1 0	79	0 0 0 2 1
22	0 2 1 0 0	51	0 0 2 1 0	80	0 0 0 3 0
23	0 2 1 0 0	52	0 0 2 1 0	81	0 0 1 1 1
24	0 2 1 0 0	53	0 0 2 1 0	82	0 0 0 2 1
25	0 2 1 0 0	54	0 0 2 1 0	83	0 0 0 0 3
26	0 2 1 0 0	55	0 0 2 1 0	84	0 0 0 0 3
27	0 1 1 1 0	56	0 0 2 1 0	85	0 0 0 0 3
28	0 1 1 1 0	57	0 0 2 1 0	86	0 0 0 0 3
29	0 1 1 1 0	58	0 0 2 1 0		

Table A.3:

Classification of 29 Stickleback Fishes' Color
Displays into 5 Intensity Levels, by 4 Experienced Raters

Fish	Rater 1	Rater 2	Rater 3	Rater 4
1	5	5	5	5
2	3	1	3	1
3	5	5	5	5
4	3	1	3	1
5	5	5	4	5
6	1	2	3	3
7	3	1	1	1
8	1	1	1	3
9	3	3	4	4
10	1	3	1	1
11	5	5	5	5
12	1	1	1	1
13	1	1	1	1
14	1	1	1	1
15	3	3	4	3
16	1	3	3	4
17	4	4	5	5
18	5	5	5	5
19	5	3	3	3
20	3	2	3	3
21	5	3	5	5
22	3	3	3	4
23	1	1	1	1
24	1	1	1	1
25	1	1	3	3
26	3	3	3	1
27	3	3	1	1
28	3	3	1	1
29	3	3	2	5

Table A.4:

Distribution of Raters by Fish and their Degree
of Nuptial Coloration

Fish	1	2	3	4	5	Total
1	0	0	0	0	4	4
2	2	0	2	0	0	4
3	0	0	0	0	4	4
4	2	0	2	0	0	4
5	0	0	0	1	3	4
6	1	1	2	0	0	4
7	3	0	1	0	0	4
8	3	0	1	0	0	4
9	0	0	2	2	0	4
10	3	0	1	0	0	4
11	0	0	0	0	4	4
12	4	0	0	0	0	4
13	4	0	0	0	0	4
14	4	0	0	0	0	4
15	0	0	3	1	0	4
16	1	0	2	1	0	4
17	0	0	0	2	2	4
18	0	0	0	0	4	4
19	0	0	3	0	1	4
20	0	1	3	0	0	4
21	0	0	1	0	3	4
22	0	0	3	1	0	4
23	4	0	0	0	0	4
24	4	0	0	0	0	4
25	2	0	2	0	0	4
26	1	0	3	0	0	4
27	2	0	2	0	0	4
28	2	0	2	0	0	4
29	0	1	2	0	1	4

Table A.5: Classification of 100 Pregnant Women by two Abstractors (1 and 2), into Two Pregnancy Type Categories - Ectopic (ECP) and Intrauterine (IUP).

Patient	Abstractor 1	Abstractor 2	TC(*)	Patient	Abstractor 1	Abstractor 2	TC	Patient	Abstractor 1	Abstractor 2	TC
1	IUP	IUP	IUP	35	ECP	ECP	ECP	68	IUP	IUP	IUP
2	ECP	ECP	ECP	36	IUP	IUP	IUP	69	IUP	IUP	IUP
3	IUP	IUP	IUP	37	IUP	IUP	IUP	70	IUP	IUP	IUP
4	IUP	IUP	IUP	38	ECP	ECP	ECP	71	IUP	IUP	IUP
5	ECP	ECP	ECP	39	ECP	ECP	IUP	72	IUP	IUP	IUP
6	IUP	IUP	IUP	40	IUP	IUP	IUP	73	IUP	ECP	IUP
7	ECP	ECP	ECP	41	IUP	IUP	IUP	74	IUP	IUP	IUP
8	IUP	IUP	IUP	42	IUP	IUP	IUP	75	IUP	IUP	IUP
9	IUP	IUP	IUP	43	ECP	ECP	ECP	76	IUP	ECP	ECP
10	ECP	ECP	ECP	44	IUP	IUP	IUP	77	IUP	IUP	IUP
11	IUP	IUP	IUP	45	IUP	IUP	IUP	78	IUP	IUP	ECP
12	ECP	IUP	ECP	46	IUP	IUP	IUP	79	IUP	IUP	IUP
13	IUP	IUP	IUP	47	IUP	IUP	IUP	80	ECP	ECP	IUP
14	IUP	IUP	IUP	48	IUP	IUP	IUP	81	IUP	IUP	IUP
15	IUP	IUP	IUP	49	ECP	IUP	ECP	82	IUP	IUP	IUP
16	IUP	IUP	IUP	50	ECP	IUP	IUP	83	IUP	IUP	IUP
17	IUP	IUP	IUP	51	IUP	IUP	IUP	84	IUP	IUP	IUP
18	IUP	IUP	IUP	52	IUP	IUP	IUP	85	IUP	IUP	IUP
19	IUP	IUP	IUP	53	IUP	IUP	IUP	86	IUP	IUP	IUP
20	IUP	IUP	IUP	54	IUP	IUP	IUP	87	IUP	IUP	IUP
21	ECP	IUP	ECP	55	IUP	IUP	IUP	88	IUP	ECP	IUP
22	IUP	IUP	ECP	56	ECP	ECP	ECP	89	IUP	IUP	IUP
23	IUP	IUP	IUP	57	ECP	ECP	ECP	90	IUP	IUP	IUP
24	ECP	ECP	ECP	58	IUP	IUP	IUP	91	IUP	IUP	IUP
25	IUP	IUP	IUP	59	IUP	IUP	IUP	92	IUP	IUP	IUP
26	IUP	IUP	IUP	60	IUP	IUP	IUP	93	ECP	ECP	ECP
27	IUP	IUP	IUP	61	IUP	IUP	IUP	94	IUP	IUP	IUP
28	IUP	IUP	IUP	62	IUP	IUP	IUP	95	IUP	IUP	IUP
29	ECP	ECP	ECP	63	IUP	IUP	IUP	96	IUP	IUP	IUP
30	IUP	IUP	IUP	64	IUP	IUP	IUP	97	IUP	IUP	IUP
31	IUP	IUP	IUP	65	IUP	IUP	IUP	98	ECP	ECP	ECP
32	IUP	IUP	IUP	66	ECP	IUP	IUP	99	ECP	IUP	ECP
33	IUP	IUP	IUP	67	IUP	IUP	IUP	100	ECP	IUP	IUP
34	IUP	IUP	IUP								

(*) TC represents the Patient's "True" Category

Appendix B

Software Solutions

This appendix provides a brief discussion of the software solutions available to researchers for computing inter-rater reliability coefficients. The list of software packages presented here is far from being exhaustive. It merely represents my short list of products that I recommend the readers of this book to consider. Many packages offer several options for computing agreement coefficients, although the number of built-in procedures is quite limited. Specialized add-in packages, functions, or macros written by independent researcher-programmers compensate this deficiency to some extent. Among the statistical packages considered here are R, SAS, SPSS, and STATA, with a particular emphasis on R and SAS. I will also mention some freely-available online calculators, which generally have limited capability. For MS Excel, AgreeStat developed by the author of this book, is a user-friendly Excel-based software that is commercially available in Windows and Mac versions. The Mac version of AgreeStat requires Mac Office 2011 or a more recent version.

B.1 The R Software

The R package has become an immensely popular statistical package across the world. If you are going to do statistical analysis on a regular basis for many years, and you do not know which statistical software to learn, this is one you will want to give a very serious consideration to. No doubt. You will enjoy the assistance of an extended online support group where you will be able to ask questions. Moreover, the product is entirely free, and can be downloaded at http://www.r-project.com . Numerous quality books have been published to help practitioners and scientists learn how to use it.

R is an interactive computing environment that makes a large collection of statistical functions available to you. Using R is about finding the right function and learning how to use it. R gives you the opportunity to develop your own functions for performing routine tasks as well as develop completely new packages for advanced users. Those who are new to R might be interested in the PDF file entitled "Using R for Introductory Statistics" prepared by John Verzani. It provides a short and friendly introduction to the R package as well as a good overview of its capabilities.

It can be downloaded at,

http://cran.r-project.org/doc/contrib/Verzani-SimpleR.pdf

As a courtesy service to the readers of this book, I decided to write a series of R functions that compute all chance-corrected agreement coefficients presented in this book. Standard errors, confidence intervals, as well as p-values associated with these coefficients are calculated by these functions. These R functions can all be downloaded from the webpage www.agreestat.com/book4/ . They are organized in three R script files, corresponding to the three ways your ratings must be organized:

- **agree.coeff2.r**

  The functions contained in this script file compute various agreement coefficients and their standard errors when dealing with two raters, and ratings that are organized in a contingency table (or a square matrix) showing counts of subjects by rater and category. You may use this format if each rater rated all subjects. Otherwise subjects rated by one rater and not by the other may not be properly classified. In this case, you should have two columns of raw scores, and use one of the functions in the script file agree.coeff3.raw.r.

- **agree.coeff3.dist.r**

  The functions contained in this script file compute various agreement coefficients and their standard errors when dealing with multiple raters, and ratings that are organized in the form of an $n \times q$ table showing counts of raters by subject and category. Here n represents the number of subjects and q the number of categories.

- **agree.coeff3.raw.r**

  The functions contained in this script file compute various agreement coefficients and their standard errors when dealing with multiple raters, and rating data organized in the form of an $n \times r$ table showing the (alphanumeric) raw ratings that the raters assigned to the subjects. Here n represents the number of subjects and r the number of raters. The data is presented in the form of n rows containing r ratings each.

- **weights.gen.r**

  The functions in this script file generate various weights to be used when computing weighted agreement coefficients.

In order to use any of the functions contained in these script files, you need to read the appropriate script into R. If you want to use the functions contained in "agree.coeff2.r" for example, then you will read this file into R as follows:

```
>source("C:\\AdvancedAnalytics\\R Scripts\\agree.coeff2.r")
```

R FUNCTIONS IN SCRIPT FILE agree.coeff2.r

If your analysis is limited to two raters, then you may organize your data in a contingency table that shows the count of subjects by rater and by category. Table B.1 is an example of such data where two neurologists classified 65 patients who suffer from Multiple Sclerosis into 4 diagnostic categories.

Table B.1: Diagnostic Classification of Multiple Sclerosis Patients by Two Neurologists[a]

New Orleans Neurologist	Winnipeg Neurologist			
	1	2	3	4
1	5	3	0	0
2	3	11	4	0
3	2	13	3	4
4	1	2	4	14

[a]From Landis & Koch (1977)

Here is the list of functions in the script file `agree.coeff2.r`:

(1) `kappa2.table` (for Cohen's unweighted and weighted kappa coefficients)

(2) `scott2.table` (for Scott's unweighted and weighted Pi coefficients)

(3) `gwet.ac1.table` (for Gwet's unweighted and weighted AC_1 coefficients)

(4) `bp2.table` (for Brennan-Prediger unweighted and weighted coefficients)

(5) `krippen2.table` (for Krippendorff alpha coefficients)

All these functions operate the same way. Therefore, only the first of these functions named `kappa2.table` is discussed here in details. The same discussion applies to the other functions as well.

`kappa2.table`:   *Cohen's kappa coefficient for 2 raters*

Description

This function calculates the unweighted as well as the weighted Cohen's kappa coefficients for 2 raters whose ratings are summarized in a square contingency table such as Table B.1. Some cells may have 0 values. However, the number of rows and columns must be equal.

Usage

```
kappa2.table(ratings,weights=diag(ncol(ratings)),conflev=0.95,
        N=Inf,print=TRUE)
```

Arguments

Of all arguments that this function takes, only the first one is required. The remaining arguments are all optional.

- `ratings`: A $q \times q$ matrix, where q is the number of categories. This is the only argument you must specify if you want the unweighted analysis,

- `weights`: A $q \times q$ matrix of weights. The default argument is the diagonal matrix where all diagonal numbers equal to 1, and all off-diagonal numbers equal to 0. This special weight matrix leads to the unweighted analysis. You may specify your own $q \times q$ weight matrix here as `weights=own.weights`. If you want to use quadratic weights with Table B.1 data for example, then the weights parameter would be `weights=quadratic.weights(1:4)`. You may want to look at the `weights.gen.r` script for a complete reference of all weight functions.

- `conflev`: The confidence level associated with the agreement coefficient's confidence interval.

- `N`: An optional parameter representing the total number of subjects in the target subject population. Its default value is infinity, which for all practical purposes assumes the target subject population to be very large and will not require any finite-population correction when computing the standard error.

- `print`: An optional logical parameter which takes the default value of TRUE if you also want the function to output the results on the screen. Set this parameter to FALSE if you do not want the results to be displayed on the screen. Setting this parameter to FALSE is recommended if this function is used as part of another routine.

Details

`kappa2.table` can accept data in the form of a matrix or in the form of a data frame as long as the input data supplied can be interpreted as a square matrix. To do the weighted analysis, you may create your own weight matrix, or use one of the many existing weight-generating functions in the `weights.ge.r` script file. Each weight function takes a single mandatory parameter, which is a vector containing all categories used in the study. *The weight functions always sort all numeric-type category vectors in ascending order. Consequently, the weighted coefficients are computed properly only if the positions of the columns and rows in the input dataset are in the same order as the corresponding categories in the sorted category vector. For alphanumeric-type category vectors, they are assumed to be already ranked following an order that is meaningful to the researcher. That is adjacent columns and adjacent rows are associated with categories that can be considered as partial agreement.*

Value

Calling the function `kappa2.table` returns the following 5 values:

- `pa`: the percent agreement.
- `pe`: the percent chance agreement.
- `kappa`: Cohen's kappa coefficient.
- `stderr`: the standard error of Cohen's kappa.
- `p.value`: the p-value of the kappa coefficient.

Examples

```
>ratings<-matrix(c(5, 3, 0, 0, # creates a matrix with Table B.1 data
+                   3, 11, 4, 0,
+                   2, 13, 3, 4,
+                   1, 2, 4, 14),ncol=4,byrow=T)
```

```
# to compute unweighted kappa, its standard error and more
>kappa2.table(ratings)
```

The results displayed on the screen will look like this:
```
Cohen's Kappa Coefficient
=========================
Percent agreement: 0.4782609 Percent chance agreement: 0.2583491
Kappa coefficient: 0.2965166 Standard error: 0.07850387
95% Confidence Interval: ( 0.1398645, 0.4531686)
P-value: 0.0003361083
```

```
# to compute weighted kappa with quadratic weights
>kappa2.table(ratings,quadratic.weights(1:4))
# the above call assumes the script file weights.gen.r was read into R, and
```
the results obtained are the following:
```
Cohen's Kappa Coefficient
=========================
Percent agreement: 0.9098229 Percent chance agreement: 0.7591542
Kappa coefficient: 0.6255814 Standard error: 0.07873187
95% Confidence Interval: ( 0.4684744, 0.7826884)
P-value: 2.749756e-11
```

R FUNCTIONS IN SCRIPT FILE **agree.coeff3.dist.r**

If your experiment involves three raters or more you can no longer summarize the ratings in a contingency table as previously done for the case of two raters. One option is to present that data in the form of a table where each row represents one subject, each column represents one category, and each table cell represents the number of raters who classified the specified subject into the specified category. Such a table shows the distribution of raters by subject and by category. Table B.2 is an example of such data where six raters classified 4 patients into 5 diagnostic categories.

Table B.2: Distribution of 6 Raters by Subject and Category[a]

Subject	Category				
	Depression	Personality Disorder	Schizophrenia	Neurosis	Other
A	0	0	0	6	0
B	0	1	4	0	1
C	2	0	4	0	0
D	0	3	3	0	0

[a]An extract of Table 1 of Fleiss (1971)

The following functions contained in the script file **agree.coeff3.dist.r** are what you will need to analyze rating data such as described in Table B.2:

(1) **fleiss.kappa.dist** (for Fleiss's unweighted and weighted kappa coefficients)

(3) **gwet.ac1.dist** (for Gwet's unweighted and weighted AC_1 coefficients)

(4) **bp.coeff.dist** (for Brennan-Prediger unweighted and weighted coefficients)

(5) **krippen.alpha.dist** (for Krippendorff unweighted and weighted alpha coefficients)

All these functions operate the same way. Therefore, only the first of these functions named **fleiss.kappa.dist** is discussed here in details. The same discussion applies to the other functions as well.

---

fleiss.kappa.dist: *Fleiss' kappa coefficient for multiple raters*

Description

This function calculates the unweighted as well as the weighted Fleiss' generalized kappa coefficients for multiple raters whose ratings are presented in the form of a distribution of raters by subject and category such as in Table B.2. A table cell may have a 0 value if none of the raters classified the subject into the category associated with that cell. The number of raters may vary by subject leading to a table with different row totals. That will be the case when the experiment generated missing ratings, with subjects being rated by a different number of raters.

Usage

```
fleiss.kappa.dist(ratings,weights="unweighted",conflev=0.95,
        N=Inf,print=TRUE)
```

Arguments

Of all arguments used by this function, only the first one is required, the remaining arguments being all optional. If your goal is limited to unweighted statistics, then the simple function call `fleiss.kappa.dist(ratings)` *is sufficient to produce Fleiss' generalized kappa along with it standard error, confidence interval, and p-value.*

- `ratings`: This is an $n \times q$ matrix or data frame (or matrix), where n is the number of subjects, and q the number of categories. This is the only argument that must be specified if you want an unweighted analysis,

- `weights`: This is a $q \times q$ matrix of weights. The default argument is "unweighted". With this option, the function will create a diagonal weight matrix with all diagonal numbers equal to 1, and all off-diagonal numbers equal to 0. This special weight matrix leads to the unweighted analysis. You may create your own $q \times q$ weight matrix (e.g. `own.weights`) and assign it to the weights parameter as `weights=own.weights`. If you want to use quadratic weights with Table B.2 data for example, then the weights parameter would be `weights=quadratic.weights(1:5)`. You may want to look at the `weights.gen.r` script for a complete reference of all weight functions available.

- `conflev`: The confidence level associated with the agreement coefficient's confidence interval.

- `N`: An optional parameter representing the total number of subjects in the target subject population. Its default value is infinity, which for all practical purposes assumes the target subject population to be very large and will not require any finite-population correction when computing the standard error.

- `print`: An optional logical parameter which takes the default value of TRUE if you also want the function to output the results on the screen. Set this parameter to FALSE if you do not want the results to be displayed on the screen.

Details

fleiss.kappa.dist can accept input data in the form of a matrix or in the form of a data frame as long as the input data supplied can be interpreted as a matrix. To do the weighted analysis, you may create your own weight matrix, or use one of the many existing weight-generating functions in the weights.ge.r script. Each weight function takes a single mandatory parameter, which is a vector containing all categories used in the study. *The weight functions always sort all numeric-type category vectors in ascending order. Consequently, the weighted coefficients are computed properly only if column positions in the input dataset match those of the corresponding categories in the sorted category vector. For alphanumeric-type category vectors, they are assumed to already be ranked following an order that is meaningful to the researcher.*

Value

Calling function fleiss.kappa.dist returns the following 5 values:

- pa: the percent agreement.
- pe: the percent chance agreement.
- fleiss.kappa: Fleiss' generalized kappa coefficient.
- stderr: the standard error of Fleiss' kappa.
- p.value: the p-value of Fleiss' kappa coefficient.

Examples

```
# creates a matrix with Table B.2 data
>ratings<-matrix(c(0, 0, 0, 6, 0,
+                  0, 1, 4, 0, 1,
+                  2, 0, 4, 0, 0,
+                  0, 3, 3, 0, 0),ncol=5,byrow=T)
```

```
# to compute unweighted Fleiss' kappa, its standard error and more
>fleiss.kappa.dist(ratings)
```

The results displayed on the screen will look like this:
```
Fleiss' Kappa Coefficient
=========================
Percent agreement: 0.5666667 Percent chance agreement: 0.3090278
Fleiss kappa coefficient: 0.3728643 Standard error: 0.2457742
95% Confidence Interval: ( -0.409299 , 1 )
P-value: 0.2265189
```

```
# to compute weighted kappa with quadratic weights
>fleiss.kappa.dist(ratings,quadratic.weights(1:5))
# the call above assumes the script file weights.gen.r was read into R, and
```

generates the following results:
```
Fleiss' Kappa Coefficient
==========================
Percent agreement: 0.9270833 Percent chance agreement: 0.8854167
Fleiss kappa coefficient: 0.3636364 Standard error: 0.2525845
Weights:
1 0.9375 0.75 0.4375 0
0.9375 1 0.9375 0.75 0.4375
0.75 0.9375 1 0.9375 0.75
0.4375 0.75 0.9375 1 0.9375
0 0.4375 0.75 0.9375 1

95% Confidence Interval: ( -0.4402002 , 1)
P-value: 0.2455769
```

R FUNCTIONS IN SCRIPT FILE agree.coeff3.raw.r

If your analysis is based on three raters or more we previously saw that one option is to organize your data as a distribution of raters by subject and by category. Alternatively, you may report the raw ratings in a table where each row represents a subject, each column a rater, and each table cell the actual rating assigned by the rater to the subject. Table B.3 is an example of such data where 5 raters classified 4 subjects into 3 categories labeled as {1, 2, 3}.

Table B.3: Rating of Four Subjects by Five Raters[a]

	Raters				
Subject	I	II	III	IV	V
A	2	2	3	2	2
B	2	2	2	2	2
C	2	2	2	2	1
D	1	2	2	2	2

[a]This is Table 2 of Finn (1970)

The following functions contained in the script file agree.coeff3.raw.r are what you will need to analyze rating data such as described in Table B.3:

(1) fleiss.kappa.raw (for Fleiss's unweighted and weighted kappa coefficients)

(3) gwet.ac1.raw (for Gwet's unweighted and weighted AC_1 coefficients)

(4) bp.coeff.raw (for Brennan-Prediger unweighted and weighted coefficients)

(5) `krippen.alpha.raw` (for Krippendorff unweighted and weighted alpha coefficients)

(5) `conger.kappa.raw` (for Conger's unweighted and weighted kappa coefficients)

All these functions operate the same way. Therefore, only the first of these functions named `fleiss.kappa.raw` is discussed here in details. The same discussion applies to the other functions as well.

`fleiss.kappa.raw`: *Fleiss' kappa coefficient for multiple raters & raw ratings*

Description

This function calculates the unweighted as well as the weighted Fleiss' generalized kappa coefficients for multiple raters whose raw ratings are listed horizontally for each subject such as in Table B.3. A table cell may be missing if a rater did not rate a particular subject. When the ratings are alphanumeric then the blank character is treated as a missing value.

Usage

```
fleiss.kappa.raw(ratings,weights="unweighted",conflev=0.95,
        N=Inf,print=TRUE)
```

Arguments

*Of all arguments used by this function, only the first one is required. The remaining arguments being all optional. If your goal is limited to unweighted statistics, then the simple function call **fleiss.kappa.raw(ratings)** is sufficient to produce Fleiss' generalized kappa along with its standard error, confidence interval, and p-value.*

- `ratings`: This is an $n \times r$ matrix or data frame (or matrix), where n is the number of subjects, and r the number of raters. This is the only argument that is required if you want an unweighted analysis.

- `weights`: This is a $q \times q$ matrix of weights. The default argument is "unweighted", and there is no need to specify it explicitly when the unweighted analysis is what you want. The `weights` parameter can take any of the following values "quadratic", "linear", "ordinal", "radical", "ratio", "circular", or "bipolar". You may refer to the previous chapters for an explicit definition of these different weights. You will need to read the `weights.gen.r` script into R before this function can perform a weighted analysis.

When the input data is in the form of raw ratings, you may not have a direct way of obtaining a list of all categories involved in the experiment, especially if the dataset is large. This makes it more difficult although not impossible to define your own weight matrix.

- `conflev`: The confidence level associated with the agreement coefficient's confidence interval.

- `N`: An optional parameter representing the total number of subjects in the target subject population. Its default value is infinity, which for all practical purposes assumes the target subject population to be very large and will not require any finite-population correction when computing the standard error.

- `print`: An optional logical parameter which takes the default value of TRUE if you also want the function to output the results on the screen. Set this parameter to FALSE if you do not want the results to be displayed on the screen.

Details

`fleiss.kappa.raw` can accept data in the form of a matrix or in the form of a data frame as long as the input data supplied can be interpreted as a matrix. The ratings may be of numeric or alphanumeric types. To perform the weighted analysis, you need to assign one the values mentioned above to the weights parameter. If you have the list of categories in your dataset, you may even create your own weight matrix, or use one of the many existing weight-generating functions in the `weights.ge.r` script. Each weight function takes a single mandatory parameter, which is a vector containing all categories used in the study. *The weight functions always sort all numeric-type category vectors in ascending order. I assume here that adjacent categories on the sorted list represent a higher degree of agreement than two categories that are farther apart.*

Value

Calling function `fleiss.kappa.raw` returns the following 5 values:

- `pa`: the percent agreement.

- `pe`: the percent chance agreement.

- `fleiss.kappa`: Fleiss' generalized kappa coefficient.

- `stderr`: the standard error of Fleiss' kappa.

- `p.value`: the p-value of Fleiss' kappa coefficient.

Examples

```
# creates a matrix with Table B.3 data
>table.b.3<-matrix(c(
+                    2, 2, 3, 2, 2,
+                    2, 2, 2, 2, 2,
```

```
+                    2, 2, 2, 2, 1,
+                    1, 2, 2, 2, 2),ncol=5,byrow=TRUE)
```

to compute unweighted Fleiss' kappa, its standard error and more
```
>fleiss.kappa.raw(ratings)
```

The results displayed on the screen will look like this:
```
Fleiss' Kappa Coefficient
==========================
Percent agreement: 0.7 Percent chance agreement: 0.735
Fleiss kappa coefficient: -0.1320755 Standard error : 0.05375461
95% Confidence Interval: ( -0.3031466 , 0.03899568 )
P-value: 1.908890
```

to compute weighted kappa with quadratic weights
```
>fleiss.kappa.dist(ratings,weights="quadratic")
```
the above call assumes that the script file `weights.gen.r` was previously read into R, and generates the following results:
```
Fleiss' Kappa Coefficient
============================
Percent agreement: 0.925 Percent chance agreement: 0.92625
Fleiss kappa coefficient: -0.01694915 Standard error: 0.06525606
Weights: quadratic
95% Confidence Interval: ( -0.2246230 , 0.1907247 )
P-value: 1.188125
```

B.2   AgreeStat for Excel

AgreeStat is a commercial Excel-based software developed by the author of this book. This software is menu-driven and user-friendly. It can compute various chance-corrected agreement coefficients, and many versions of intraclass correlation coefficients. The current version can be tested by downloading a trial copy from AgreeStat's webpage http://www.agreestat.com/agreestat.html, and is available for both Windows and Mac operating systems. For the Mac edition, the user will need to have Excel 2011 or a later version of Microsoft Office. AgreeStat's webpage contains a wealth of information about the different features of this software.

B.3   Online Calculators

Several websites have implemented the kappa coefficient. Although most of them are limited to the original two-rater version of Cohen (1960), a few have implemented Fleiss' extension to multiple raters as well. These online calculators are rarely maintained and do not always implement the latest techniques. Only a few online calculators are mentioned here. Interested readers could find many more minor and very limited calculators with a simple Google search.

- http://www.statstodo.com/CohenKappa_Pgm.php

  This online program is simple and very intuitive. It only implements two coefficients, which are the original kappa coefficient of Cohen (1960) for two raters, and its multiple-rater extension proposed by Fleiss (1971) . This program gives the user the opportunity to input the data in the form of a raw list of ratings for each subject, or in the form of a summary table of counts. However, this program always uses the summary table of counts to perform all calculations. Even if raw ratings are supplied by the user, the program will convert them to a summary table of counts.

  There are a few issues that users of this program must be aware of:

  ⇒ This program does not appear to use the correct standard error expressions for Cohen's kappa that were published by Fleiss et al. (1969) . Therefore the standard errors associated with kappa that this program produces are incorrect.

  ⇒ For FLeiss' generalized kappa, the program uses the standard error expression of Fleiss (1971). This expression too is incorrect. The correct expression is provided in chapter 5 of this book.

  ⇒ This program assumes that each rater rated all subjects. Therefore, you may need to eliminate from your dataset all subjects that were not rated by all raters. The program will not do it for you.

  ⇒ This program automatically creates the 95% confidence interval with no possibility of specifying another confidence level.

- ReCal ("Reliability Calculator"): http://dfreelon.org/utils/recalfront/
  This is an online utility that essentially computes the percent agreement, Fleiss' extension of kappa for multiple raters, Cohen's kappa (for 2 raters), the average of all Cohen's pairwise kappa, and Krippendorff's alpha. This online calculator seems to be used primarily by researchers and students in the field of communication and is very intuitive.

  ReCal does not appear to be flexible regarding the way input ratings must be organized. You must supply a matrix of raw ratings where each row represents the subject and each column the rater. No standard error, confidence interval or *p*-value are computed, which could be a problem for more sophisticated users.

B.4 SAS Software

SAS is one of the major statistical software packages on the market today. It is a massive software system that has been around for many decades, and which is very expensive. It would be unwise to consider acquiring this product for the sole purpose of computing inter-rater reliability coefficients. Those who already have access to it, will certainly want to know about its capability as far as computing inter-rater reliability coefficients is concerned. SAS does not offer many built-in procedures for calculating inter-rater reliability coefficients. Actually the FREQ Procedure is the only option available and is limited to the original two-rater version of kappa suggested by Cohen (1960). A SAS macro program is necessary if you need to go beyond the basics.

The use of SAS for the purpose of calculating inter-rater reliability coefficients has been discussed extensively in Gwet (2010*c*). The reader would find in this manuscript a wealth of information regarding the advantages and disadvantages of using SAS to compute inter-rater reliability coefficients, as well as some options for calculating many of the coefficients discussed in this book.

B.5 SPSS & STATA

SPSS is also among the major statistical software packages on the market today. Just like SAS, it has been around for a while, and specializes in the social sciences. SPSS offers more built-in procedures for computing inter-rater reliability coefficients than SAS, although not many alternatives to the two-rater kappa of Cohen (1960) can be found. Not many SPSS macro programs were developed by independent programmers to implement some of well-known agreement coefficients.

STATA is another major statistical software packages, which is more recent than SAS and SPSS, and which specializes in the medical field. The document http://www.stata.com/manuals13/rkappa.pdf summarizes well what STATA has to offer in the area inter-rater reliability. Unlike SAS and SPSS, STATA has a built-in procedure for computing the multiple-rater version of kappa proposed by Fleiss (1971). Once again, unless you are already a STATA user, it would be unwise to acquire this major software for the sole purpose of computing inter-rater reliability coefficients.

B.6   Concluding Remarks

In this appendix I reviewed some of what I consider to be among the most interesting software options for researchers involved in inter-rater reliability assessment. Numerous researchers have made it known to me over the years that they wanted to have R functions that implement the different coefficients and associated standard errors that I proposed in the earlier editions of this book. It is the main reason why I developed the R functions presented in this appendix. Additional R functions will eventually be developed for the calculation of intraclass correlation coefficients. AgreeStat was developed for Excel users and those who are primarily interested in user-friendly menu-driven software packages. It implements almost all techniques discussed in this book, and additional information can be found about it at `www.agreestat.com/agreestat.html`.

Before using a particular software package for calculating inter-rater reliability coefficients, researchers need to find out how that package handles missing ratings. Many programs made available to the general public do not have a well-defined strategy for dealing with missing ratings, which are known to be an important problem in many inter-rater reliability experiments. Even some existing R functions proposed in some publicly-available R packages such as `irr` or `concord` tend to exclude from analysis any subject that was not rated by all raters. This crude strategy may eliminate a substantial amount of data collected by the researcher. A better strategy consists of using every single data point that was gathered as recommended throughout this book.

Bibliography

[1] Aickin, M. (1990), "Maximum Likelihood Estimation of Agreement in the Constant Predictive Probability Model, and Its Relation to Cohen's Kappa." *Biometrics*, **46**, 293-302.

[2] Agresti, A. (1988), "A Model Agreement Between Ratings on an Ordinal Scale." *Biometrics*, **44**, 539-548.

[3] Agresti, A. (1992), "Modeling patterns of agreement and disagreement." *Statistical Methods in Medical Research*,**1**, 201-218.

[4] Altman, D. G. (1991). *Practical Statistics for Medical Research*. Chapman and Hall.

[5] Benini, R. (1901). *Principii di Demongraphia: Manuali Barbera Di Scienze Giuridiche Sociali e Politiche* (No. 29). Firenze, Italy : G. Barbera.

[6] Bennett, E. M., Alpert, R., and Goldstein, A. C. (1954), "Communications through limited response questioning." *Public Opinion Quarterly*, **18**, 303-308.

[7] Berry, K. J., and Mielke, Jr., P. W. (1988), "A Generalization of Cohen's Kappa Agreement Measure To Interval Measurement and Multiple Raters," *Educational and Psychological Measurement*, **48**, 921-933.

[8] Bland, M. J., Altman, D. G. (1986), "Statistical Methods for Assessing Agreement between two Methods of Clinical Measurement." *Lancet*, **1**, 307-310.

[9] Bland, M. J., Altman, D. G. (1996), "Statistics Notes: Measurement error." *British Medical Journal*, **312**, p. 1654.

[10] Brennan, R. L., and Prediger, D. J. (1981). "Coefficient Kappa : some uses, misuses, and alternatives." *Educational and Psychological Measurement*, **41**, 687-699.

[11] Byrt, T., Bishop, J., and Carlin, J. B. (1993). "Bias, prevalence and Kappa." *Journal of Clinical Epidemiology*,46, 423-429.

[12] Cantor, A. B. (1996). "Sample-Size Calculations for Cohen's Kappa.", *Psychological Methods*, **1**, 150-153.

[13] Carletta, J. (1996). "Assessing Agreement on Classification Tasks: the Kappa Statistic." *Computational Linguistics*,**22**, 1-6.

[14] Carmines, E. G., and Zeller, R. A. (1979), *Reliability and Validity Assessment*, Sage Publications.

[15] Cicchetti, D. V., and Feinstein, A. R. (1990). "High Agreement but low Kappa : II. Resolving the paradoxes." *Journal of Clinical Epidemiology*, 43, 551-558.

[16] Cochran, W. G. (1977). *Sampling Techniques*, John Wiley & Sons, Inc. : New York.

[17] Cohen, J. (1960). "A coefficient of agreement for nominal scales." *Educational and Psychological Measurement*, 20, 37-46.

[18] Cohen, J. (1968). "Weighted kappa : Nominal scale agreement with provision for scaled disagreement or partial credit." *Psychological Bulletin*, 70, 213-220.

[19] Conger, A. J. (1980), "Integration and Generalization of Kappas for Multiple Raters," *Psychological Bulletin*, **88**, 322-328.

[20] Cronbach, L. J. (1951), "Coefficient Alpha, and the Internal Structure," *Psychometrika*, **16**(3), 297-334.

[21] Doros, G. and Lew, R. (2010), "Design Based on Intr-Class Correlation Coefficients." *American Journal of Biostatistics*, **1**(1), 1-8.

[22] Eckes, T. (2011). *Introduction to Many-Facet Rasch Measurement*. Peter Lang, Internationaler Verlag der Wissenschaften.

[23] Efron, B. (1979). "Bootstrap methods : another look at the jackknife." *Annals of statistics*, **7**, 1-26.

[24] Everitt, B. S. (1992). *The Analysis of Contingency Tables (2nd Ed.)* Chapman and Hall, London.

[25] Feinstein, A. R., and Cicchetti, D. V. (1990), "High agreement but low kappa : I. The problems of two paradoxes," *Journal of Clinical Epidemiology*, **43**, 543-549.

[26] Fenning, S., Craig, T. J., Tanenberg-Karant, M., & Bromet, E. J. (1994). "Comparison of facility and research diagnoses in first-admission psychotic patients," *American Journal of Psychiatry*, **151**, 1423-1429.

[27] Finn, R. H. (1970), "A Note on Estimating the Reliability of Categorical Data," *Educational and Psychological Measurement*, **30**, 71-76.

[28] Flack, V. F. (1987), "Confidence intervals for the interrater agreement measure kappa," *Communications in Statistics - Theory and Methods*, **16**, 953-968.

[29] Flack, V. F., Afifi, A. A., Lachenbruch, P. A., and Schouten, H. J. A. (1988), "Sample Size Determinations for the Two Rater Kappa Statistic," *Psychometrika*, **53**, 321-325.

[30] Fleiss, J. L. (1971). "Measuring nominal scale agreement among many raters", *Psychological Bulletin*, **76**, 378-382.

[31] Fleiss, J. L. (1981). *Statistical Methods for Rates and Proportions*. John Wiley & Sons.

[32] Fleiss, J. L., Cohen, J., and Everitt, B. S. (1969). "Large sample standard errors of kappa and weighted kappa," *Psychological Bulletin*, **72**, 323-327.

[33] Fleiss, J. L., and Davies, M. (1982). "Jackknifing Functions of Multinomial Frequencies, with an Application to a Measure of Concordance," *American Journal of Epidemiology*, **115**, 841-845.

[34] Fleiss, J. L., Levin, B., and Paik, M. C. (2003). *Statistical Methods for Rates and Proportions* (3rd ed.). Wiley Series in Probability and Statistics.

[35] Fleiss, J. L., Nee, J. C. M., and Landis, J. R. (1979). "The large sample variance of kappa in the case of different sets of raters." *Psychological Bulletin*, **86**, 974-977.

[36] Friedman, M. (1937). "The use of ranks to avoid the assumption of normality implicit in the analysis of variance." *Journal of the American Statistical Association*, **32 (200)**, 675-701.

[37] Gartner, J. B. (1991). "The standard error of Cohen's kappa." *Statistics in Medicine*, **10**, 767-775.

[38] Giraudeau, B., and Mary, J. Y. (2001). "Planning a reproducibility study: how many subjects and how many replicates per subject for an expected width of the 95 per cent confidence interval of the intraclass correlation coefficient." *Statistics in Medicine*, **20**, 3205-3214.

[39] Goodman, L. A., and Kruskal, W. H. (1954). "Measures of Association in Cross Classifications." *Journal of the American Statistical Association*, **49**, 1732-1769.

[40] Grove, W. M., Andreasen, N. C., McDonald-Scott, P., Keller, M. B., and Shapiro, R. W. (1981). "Reliability Studies of Psychiatric Diagnosis." *Archives of General Psychiatry*, **38**, 408-413.

[41] Guttman, L. (1945). "The test-retest reliability of qualitative data." *Psychometrika*, **11**, 81-95.

[42] Gwet, K. L. (2008a). "Computing inter-rater reliability and its variance in the presence of high agreement." *British Journal of Mathematical and Statistical Psychology*, **61**, 29-48.

[43] Gwet, K. L. (2008b). "Variance estimation of nominal-scale inter-rater reliability with random selection of raters." *Psychometrika*, **73**, 407-430.

[44] Gwet, K. L. (2008c). Intrarater Reliability. In R. B. D'Agostino, L. Sullivan, and J. Massaro (Eds.), *Wiley Encyclopedia of Clinical Trials* (pp. 473-485). Wiley-Interscience

[45] Gwet, K. L. (2010*a*). *How to Compute Intraclass Correlation Using Excel: A Practical Guide to Inter-Rater Reliability Assessment for Quantitative Data*, Advanced Analytics, LLC.

[46] Gwet, K. L. (2010*b*). *The Practical Guide to Statistics: Basic Concepts, Methods, and Meaning*, Advanced Analytics, LLC.

[47] Gwet, K. L. (2010*c*). *Inter-Rater Reliability Using SAS: A Practical Guide for Nominal, Ordinal, and Interval Data*, Advanced Analytics, LLC.

[48] Hale, C. A., and Fleiss, J. L. (1993). "Interval estimation under two study designs for kappa with binary classifications," *Biometrics*, **49**, 523-533.

[49] Holley, J.W., and Guilford, J. P. (1964), "A note on the G index of agreement." *Educational and Psychological Measurement*, **24**, 749-753.

[50] Holsti, O.R. (1969). *Content Analysis for the Social Sciences and Humanities*, Reading, MA: Addison-Wesley.

[51] Hubert, L., "Kappa revisited." *Psychological Bulletin*, **84**, 289-297.

[52] Janson, S., and Vegelius, J. (1979). "On generalizations of the G index and the PHI coefficient to nominal scales." *Multivariate Behavioral Research*, **14**, 255-269.

[53] Janson, H., and Olsson, U. (2001). "A Measure of Agreement for Interval or Nominal Multivariate Observations," *Educational and Psychological Measurement*, **61**, 277-289.

[54] Janson, H., and Olsson, U. (2004). "A Measure of Agreement for Interval or Nominal Multivariate Observations by Different Sets of Judges," *Educational and Psychological Measurement*, **64**, 62-70.

[55] Jung, H. W. (2003). "Evaluating interrater agreement in SPICE-based assessments," *Computer Standards & Interfaces*, **25**, 477-499.

[56] Kendall, M. G. (1938). "A New Measure of Rank Correlation," *Biometrika*, **30**, 81-93.

[57] Kendall, M. G., and Babington-Smith, B. (1939). "The Problem of *m* Rankings," *Annals of Mathematical Statistics*, **10**, 275-287.

[58] Kolmogorov, A. N. (1999). The Theory of Probability. In A. D. Aleksandrov, A. N. Kolmogorov, and M. A. Lavrent'ev (Eds.), *Mathematics - Its Contents, Methods and Meaning* (Chapter XI, pp. 229-264). Dover Publications - Dover Books on Mathematics.

[59] Kraemer, H. C. (1979). "Ramifications of a population model for κ as a coefficient of reliability," *Psychometrika*, **44**, 461-472.

[60] Kraemer, H. C., Peryakoil, V. S., and Noda, A. (2002). "Kappa Coefficients in Medical Research," *Statistics in Medicine*, **21**, 2109-2129.

[61] Krippendorff, K. (1970). "Estimating the reliability, systematic error, and random error of interval data," *Educational and Psychological Measurement*, **30**, 61-70.

[62] Krippendorff, K. (1978). "Reliability of binary attribute data," *Biometrics*, **34**, 142-144.

[63] Krippendorff, K. (2004). *Content Analysis: An Introduction to Its Methodology*, Thousand Oaks, Calif, USA.

[64] Krippendorff, K. (2011). "Computing Krippendorff's alpha reliability." http://www.asc.upenn.edu/usr/krippendorff/mwebreliability5.pdf

[65] Krippendorff, K. (2011). "Agreement and Information in the Reliability of Coding," *Communication Methods and Measures*, **5.2**, 1-20.

[66] Krippendorff, K. (2012). *Content Analysis: An Introduction to Its Methodology, 3rd. Edition*, Thousand Oaks, CA: SAGE Publications, Inc.

[67] Kruskal, W. H. (1952). "A nonparametric test for the several sample problem," *Annals of Mathematical Statistics*, **23**, 525-540.

[68] Kruskal, W. H., and Wallis, W. A. (1952). "Use of ranks in one-criterion variance analysis," *Journal of the American Statistical Association*, **47**, 583-621.

[69] Kuder, G. F., and Richardson, M. W. (1937). "The Theory of the Estimation of Test Reliability," *Psychometrika*, **2**, 151-160.

[70] Landis, J. R, and Koch G. (1977). "The measurement of observer agreement for categorical data," *Biometrics*, **33**, 159-174.

[71] Lee, J. J., and Tu, Z. N. (1994). "A better confidence interval for kappa (κ) on measuring agreement between two raters with binary outcomes." *Journal of Computational and Graphical Statistics*, **3**, 301-321.

[72] Leone, M.A., Gaviani, P., and Ciccone, G. (2006). "Inter-coder agreement for ICD-9-CM coding of stroke," *Neurological Sciences*, **27**, 445-448.

[73] Lindeman, R. H., Meranda, P. F., and Gold, R. Z. (1980). *Introduction to Bivariate and Multivariate Analysis*, Glenview, IL: Scott, Foresman and Company.

[74] Likert, R. (1932). "A Technique for the Measurement of Attitudes." *Archives of Psychology*, **140**, 1-55.

[75] Lindsay,B. G., Markatou, M., Ray, S., Yang, K., Chen, S. (2008). "Quadratic Distances on Probabilities: A Unified Foundation." *The Annals of Statistics*, **36**, 983-1006.

[76] Lipsitz, S. R., Laird, N. M., and Brennan, T. A. (1994). "Simple moment estimates of the κ-coefficient and its variance," *Applied Statistics*, **43**, 309-323.

[77] Light, R. J. (1971). "Measures of response agreement for qualitative data : some generalizations and alternatives," *Psychological Bulletin*, **76**, 365-377.

[78] Likert, R. (1931). "A Technique for the Measurement of Attitudes," *Archives of Psychology*, New York: Columbia University Press.

[79] Mann, H., and Whitney, D. (1947). "On a test of whether one of two random variables is stochastically larger than the other." *Annals of Mathematical Statistics*, **18**, 50-60.

[80] Marascuilo, L. A., and McSweeney, L. (1977). *Nonparametric and Distribution-free Methods for the Social Sciences*. Monterey, CA: Brooks/Cole Publishing Company.

[81] Maxwell, A. E. (1977). "Coefficient of agreement between observers and their interpretation." *British Journal of Psychiatry*, **130**, 79-83.

[82] McCarthy, P. J. (1966). "Replication : An approach to the analysis of data from complex surveys." National Center for Health Statistics, Washington, D.C., Series, 2, 14.

[83] McGraw, K. O., and Wong, S. P. (1996). "Forming Inferences About Some Intraclass Correlation Coefficients." *Psychological Methods*, **1**, 30-46.

[84] McIver, J. P., and Carmines, E. G. (1981). *Unidimensional Scaling*, Thousand Oaks, CA: Sage.

[85] Metropolis, N., and Ulam, S. (1949). "The Monte-Carlo Method." *Journal of the American Statistical Association*, **44**, 335-341.

[86] Miller, R. G. (1974). "The jackknife - a review." *Biometrika*, **61**, 1-15.

[87] Neyman, J. (1934). "On the Two Different Aspects of the Representative Method : the Method of Stratified Sampling and the Method of Purposive Selection." *Journal of the Royal Statistical Society*, **97**, 558-606.

[88] Nunnally, J. C. (1978). *Psychometric Theory (2nd ed.)*. New York: McGraw-Hill.

[89] Osgood, C.E. (1959). The Representational Model and Relevant Research Methods. In I. de Sola Pool (Ed.), *Trends in Content Analysis* (pp. 33-88). Urbana: University of Illinois Press.

[90] Park, H. M., and Jung, H. W. (2003). "Evaluating Interrater Agreement with Intraclass Correlation Coefficient in SPICE-based Software Process Assessment," *Proceedings of the Third International Conference On Quality Software*, 308-314.

[91] Pearson, K. (1896). "Mathematical contributions to the theory of evolution - III. Regression, heredity and panmixia," *Philosophical Transactions of the Royal Society of London*, Series A 187, 253-318.

[92] Pearson, K. (1900). "On the Criterion that a given System of Deviations from the Probable in the Case of a Correlated System of Variables is such that it can

Reasonably be Supposed to have arisen in a Random Sampling," *Philosophical Magazine*, 5, 157-175.

[93] Perreault, W.D., and Leigh, L.E. (1989). "Reliability of nominal data based on qualitative judgments," *Journal of Marketing Research*, **26**, 135-148.

[94] Quenouille, M. H. (1949). Approximate tests of correlation in time series. *Journal of The Royal Statistical Society*, Series B, 11, 68-84.

[95] Quenouille, M. H. (1956). "Notes on bias in estimation." *Biometrika*, **61**, 353-360.

[96] Rowland, W. J. (1984), "The relationships among nuptial coloration, aggression, and courtship in male Threespine Sticklebacks," *Canadian Journal of Zoology*, **51**, 453-466.

[97] Särndal, C. E., Swensson, B., and Wretman, J. (2003). *Model Assisted Survey Sampling*, Springer-Verlag New York, Inc.

[98] Satterthwaite, F. E. (1946), "An Approximate Distribution of Estimates of Variance Components," *Biometrics*, **2**, 110-114.

[99] Schouten, H. J. A. (1986), "Nominal scale agreement among observers," *Psychometrika*, **51**, 453-466.

[100] Schuster, C. and von Eye, A. (2001). "Models for ordinal agreement data," *Biometrical Journal*, **43**(7), 795-808.

[101] Scott, W. A. (1955). "Reliability of content analysis : the case of nominal scale coding." *Public Opinion Quarterly*, **XIX**, 321-325.

[102] Searle, S. R. (1997). *Linear Models (Wiley Classics Library)*. Wiley-Interscience: John Wiley & Sons, Inc.

[103] Shoukri, M. M (2010). *Measures of Interobserver Agreement and Reliability, Second Edition (Chapman & Hall/CRC Biostatistics Series)*. CRC Press.

[104] Shrout, P. E., and Fleiss, J. L. (1979), "Intraclass Correlations: Uses in Assessing Rater Reliability." *Psychological Bulletin*, **86**(2), 420-428.

[105] Siegel, S., and Castellan, N. J., Jr. (1988). *Nonparametric Statistics for the Behavioral Sciences* (2nd ed.). New York: McGraw-Hill Book Company.

[106] Sim J., and Wright C. C. (2005), "The kappa statistic in reliability studies : use, interpretation, and sample size requirements." *Physical Therapy* **85**(3), 257-268.

[107] Spearman, C. (1904), "The Proof and Measurement of Association between two Things." *American Journal of Psychology*, **15**, 72-101.

[108] Stein, C.R., Devore, R.B., and Wojcik, B.E. (2005). Calculation of the Kappa Statistic for Inter-Rater Reliability: The Case Where Raters Can Select Multiple Responses from a Large Number of Categories. In *SAS Institute Inc.*

2005. Proceedings of the Thirtieth Annual SAS® Users Group International Conference. Cary, NC : SAS Institute Inc .

[109] Tanner, M.A. and Young, M.A. (1985). "Modeling agreement among raters," *Journal of American Statistical Association*, **80**, 175-180.

[110] Traub, R. E. (1994). *Reliability for the Social Sciences: Theory and Applications*, Sage Publications, Beverly Hills.

[111] Tukey, J. W. (1958). "Bias and confidence in not quite large samples (Abstract)." *Annals of Mathematical Statistics*, **29**, 614.

[112] von Eye, A., and Mun, E. Y. (2006). *Analyzing Rater Agreement: Manifest Variable Methods*, Lawrence Erlbaum Associates; Pap/Cdr edition.

[113] Wallis, W. A. (1939). "The Correlation Ratio for Ranked Data," *Journal of the American Statistical Association*, **34**, 533-538.

[114] Wilcoxon, F. (1949). *Some Rapid Approximate Statistical Procedures.* Stamford, CT: Stamford Research Laboratories, American Cyanamid Corporation.

[115] Zhao, X., Liu, J.S., and Deng, K. (2013). Assumptions behind Intercoder Reliability Indices. In C.T. Salmon (Ed.), *Communication Yearbook*, **36** (pp. 419-480). Routledge

List of Notations

Author Index

Subject Index

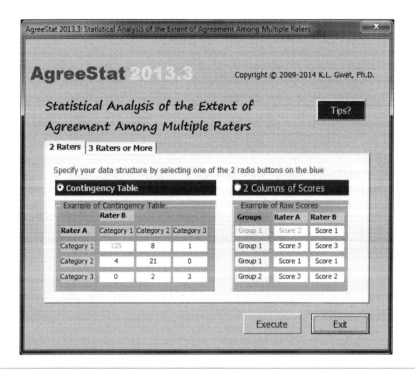

- Download **AgreeStat**, the Point-And-Click Excel VBA program for the statistical analysis of inter-rater reliability data. It can be downloaded by visiting the web page **www.agreestat.com**. **AgreeStat** is available in both Windows and Mac platforms, and is compatible with Windows Excel 2007 or later, and with Mac Excel 2011 or later.

- **AgreeStat** is integrated in a stand-alone Excel workbook, and does not require any installation.

- At **www.agreestat.com** you may also download some of the author's research papers on inter-rater reliability.

- Users of the statistical package r, may download useful r function by visiting the web page **http://www.agreestat.com/r_functions.html**.

- For updates on recent ideas and techniques, you may also want to visit the author's blog **http://inter-rater-reliability.blogspot.com/**.

- Corrections to this book, and other book-related materials can be found at **www.agreestat.com/book4/**

Made in the USA
Middletown, DE
27 October 2017